ABBREVIATIONS USED IN CONTROL OF COMMUNICABLE DISEASES IN MAN

BSL	=	Biosafety level (i.e., BSL 1, 2, 3, 4)
CA	=	cold hemagglutinins
CAT scan	=	computerized axial tomography
CDC	=	Centers for Disease Control
CNS	=	central nervous system
ca.	=	circa
cm	=	centimeter
CF	=	complement fixation
CIOMS	=	Council for International Organizations of Medical Sciences
co-trimoxazole	=	TMP-SMX (trimethoprim-sulfamethoxazole)
CSF	=	cerebrospinal fluid
CIE	=	counterimmunoelectrophoresis
CT scan	=	computerized tomography
cu mm	=	cubic millimeter
DTP	=	Diphtheria and Tetanus Toxoids and Pertussis Vaccine Adsorbed USP
EIA	=	enzyme immunoassay
EM	=	electron microscopy
EPI	=	Expanded Programme Immunizations, WHO
ESR	=	erythrocyte sedimentation rate
ELISA	=	enzyme-linked immunosorbent assay
FA	=	direct fluorescent or immunofluorescent antibody test
FAO	=	Food and Agriculture Organization of the United Nations
g	=	gram
GI	=	gastrointestinal
HA	=	hemagglutination
HAI/HI	=	hemagglutination inhibition
HIV	=	human immunodeficiency virus
IEM	=	immune electron microscopy
IF	=	immunofluorescent testing
IFA	=	indirect immunofluorescent antibody test
IgA	=	immunoglobulin class A
IgG	=	immunoglobulin class G
IgM	=	immunoglobulin class M
IG	=	immune globulin (serum)
IHA	=	indirect hemagglutination

i

IM	=	intramuscular
IU	=	international unit
IV	=	intravenous
kb	=	kilobase
kg	=	kilogram
LA	=	latex agglutination
lbs	=	pounds
m	=	meter
meq	=	milliequivalents
mg	=	milligram
μg	=	microgram
ml	=	milliliter
mm	=	millimeter
μm	=	micrometer
nm	=	nanometer
ppm	=	parts per million
RBC	=	red blood cell
RIA	=	radioimmunoassay
sp. or spp.	=	species
UNDP	=	United Nations Development Programme
USA	=	United States of America
USDA	=	US Department of Agriculture
UK	=	United Kingdom
URI	=	upper respiratory infection
USPHS	=	US Public Health Service
USSR	=	Union of Soviet Socialist Republic
UV	=	ultraviolet
v.	=	versus
WHO	=	World Health Organization
WBC	=	white blood cell

Control of Communicable Diseases in Man

Abram S. Benenson, editor

Fifteenth Edition   1990

An official report of the American Public Health Association

American Public Health Association
1015 Fifteenth Street, NW
Washington, DC 20005

American Public Health Association
1015 Fifteenth Street, NW
Washington, DC 20005

William H. McBeath, MD, MPH
Executive Director

Printed and bound in the United States of America.

Design: Donya Melanson Associates, Boston, MA
Typesetting: Byrd PrePress, Springfield, VA
Set in: Garamond
Printing and Binding; Crest Litho, Inc., Watervliet, NY
Cover Note: The cover illustrates four basic aspects of
communicable disease control—grain: proper nutrition;
flask: research; syringe: prevention and treatment; hand
and soap: sanitation.
ISBN 0-87553-170-9

100M 9/90

v

WALTER R. DOWDLE, Ph.D.
    Deputy Director
    Centers for Disease Control
    Atlanta GA 30333
ALFRED S. EVANS, M.D., M.P.H., FACE
    John Rodman Paul Professor of Epidemiology, Emeritus
    Yale University School of Medicine
    60 College Street
    New Haven CT 06510
JAMES L. HADLER, M.D., M.P.H.
    Chief, Epidemiology Section
    State Department of Health Services
    150 Washington Street
    Hartford CT 06106
SCOTT B. HALSTEAD, M.D.
    Acting Director, Health Sciences Division
    The Rockefeller Foundation
    1133 Avenue of the Americas
    New York NY 10036
RICHARD B. HORNICK, M.D.
    Vice President, Medical Education Administration
    Orlando Regional Medical Center
    1414 South Kuhl Avenue
    Orlando FL 32806-2093
WILLIAM S. JORDAN, Jr., M.D.
    Emeritus Director, Microbiology and Infectious Diseases Program
    National Institute of Allergy and Infectious Disease
    National Institutes of Health
    Bethesda MD 20892
MYRON M. LEVINE, M.D., D.T.P.H.
    Professor and Director
    Center for Vaccine Development
    University of Maryland School of Medicine
    10 South Pine Street
    Baltimore MD 21201

EDWARD A. MORTIMER, Jr., M.D.
    Professor and Vice Chairman, Department of Epidemiology and
    Biostatistics
    Professor, Department of Pediatrics
    Case Western Reserve University School of Medicine
    2119 Abington Road
    Cleveland OH 44106-2333
ROBERT E. SHOPE, M.D.
    Professor of Epidemiology
    Department of Epidemiology and Public Health
    Yale University School of Medicine
    Box 3333
    New Haven CT 06510
JAMES H. STEELE, D.V.M., M.P.H.
    Professor, Environmental Sciences
    Center for Infectious Diseases
    School of Public Health
    University of Texas
    Houston TX 77030
WILLIAM D. TIGERTT, M.D.
    Editor, American Journal of Tropical Medicine and Hygiene
    15 Charles Plaza - Suite 2202
    Baltimore MD 21201

LIAISON REPRESENTATIVES

George W. Beran, D.V.M., Ph.D., L.H.D.
    Conference of Public Health Veterinarians
Walter R. Dowdle, Ph.D.
    US Public Health Service
Robert Hall, BSc (Med), MB, BS, DipRACOG, MPII, FRACMA
    Department of Community Services and Health, Australia
F. J. López-Antuñano, M.D., M.P.H.
    Pan American Health Organization
Joseph Losos, M.D., D.E.CH., FCRP(C) FACPM
    Department of National Health and Welfare, Canada
Donald O. Lyman, M.D., D.T.P.H.
    Association of State and Territorial Health Officials
Arvind C. Patel, M.B., Ch.B, M.R.N.Z.C.G.P., M.C.C.M.(N.Z.)
    Department of Health, New Zealand

R. G. Penn, M.B., Ch.B.
   Department of Health and Social Security, England
LT COL Michael R. Peterson, D.V.M., M.P.H., Dr.P.H.
   US Department of Defense
Stanley A. Plotkin, M.D.
   American Academy of Pediatrics
Daniel Reid, M.B., Ch.B., FFCM, FRCP, DPH
   Scottish Home and Health Department, Scotland
G. Torrigiani, M.D., Ph.D.
   World Health Organization

TABLE OF CONTENTS

FOREWORD TO THE FIFTEENTH EDITION

The current fifteenth edition of *CCDM* marks the 75th anniversary of this renowned public health standard. Public health workers across the nation and around the world have long found practical utility and reference value in repeated use of this classic work.

Control of Communicable Diseases in Man has its origin in a pamphlet prepared early in this century by Francis Curtis, then health officer of Newton, Massachusetts. Copies of the popular pamphlet circulated among local health officers in New England. In 1916, Robert N. Hoyt, then health officer of Manchester, New Hampshire, persuaded the APHA annual meeting in Cincinnati to undertake preparation of a national version with the potentially broader utility and added authority to be had through sponsorship by the American Public Health Association.

A resulting 1917 report of the APHA Committee on Standard Regulations became the first edition of today's *CCDM*. It was approved by the USPHS, and published in *Public Health Reports* of October 21, 1917 (32:41:1706–1733). Reprints were available from the Government Printing Office for five cents. A modest publication of 30 pages, it listed control measures for the 38 communicable diseases then officially reportable in the United States.

Since then, APHA has undertaken periodic revision and expansion of *CCDM* as community needs and scientific knowledge have increased. Editions of this popular handbook have been published in English, Spanish, French, Portuguese, Japanese, Arabic, and Italian. It has been officially adopted for authorized use by many state and provincial health departments, national ministries of health, military medical services, and academic institutions. The present revision covers more than 200 diseases in well over 500 pages.

All who use this manual owe a great professional debt to the hundreds of scientists who through the years have contributed generously of their time and expertise to its substance. Without their voluntary service, there would be no *CCDM*. For this edition, their names are listed and their roles described hereinafter. Such recognition is small compensation for their effort, but it represents a sincere expression of appreciation from grateful colleagues for a job well done.

Highest commendation is reserved for the Editor. Historically, only three individuals have been chosen to serve in that capacity, each an internationally distinguished statesperson of epidemiology:

Haven Emerson	editions 1 through 7	(35 years)
John Gordon	editions 8 through 10	(15 years)
Abram S. Benenson	editions 11 through 15	(20 years)

Recent editions are clear testimony to Dr. Benenson's selfless commitment to professional service in the public interest. On behalf of all who use or benefit from this book, we acclaim with sincerest gratitude his exceptional contributions to the Association, to the profession, and to the public.

William H. McBeath, MD, MPH
Executive Director
American Public Health Association

PREFACE TO THE FIFTEENTH EDITION

The *Control of Communicable Diseases in Man* was first published by the American Public Health Association in 1917 to present the essential facts needed to control communicable diseases of man. Quinquennial revisions (this the fifteenth) assure that the information and recommended practices remain abreast of the advances in our scientific knowledge and of the changes in social and socioeconomic conditions. The book is intended to provide health workers a ready source of information on how to recognize a specific disease, then how to manage the patients so that they do not become sources for new cases, and to provide guidance for their treatment to preserve lives. It is not intended to replace more inclusive textbooks but to be a source of basic information on which initial action can be taken.

The primary aim of the editors is to provide an accurate, informative text for public health workers in official and voluntary health agencies, including physicians, dentists, veterinarians, sanitary engineers, public health nurses, social workers, health educators and sanitarians; and for physicians, dentists and veterinarians in private practice who are concerned with the control of communicable diseases. The book is also designed for those serving with the armed forces at home and abroad, and for health workers stationed in foreign countries. School administrators and students of medicine and public health will also find the material useful.

A second function of this book is to furnish public health administrators a guide and a source of materials for preparing regulations and legal requirements for the control and management of communicable disease and for developing programs for health education of the public. In some jurisdictions, the control measures recommended in this book constitute a component of the health regulations. At the other end of the scale, the need of field workers for a handy reference determines the format of the manual and a size to fit in the pocket.

The events in the five years since the last edition was published have proven that communicable diseases are far from extinct and are presently causing more disease and deaths. The spread of the acquired immunodeficiency syndrome or, more properly, HIV infection, continues unabated; Lyme disease is affecting more and more people and is recognized over more and more of the earth's surface; measles, instead of being eradicated from the USA, has become epidemic. Streptococcal disease had seemed to have lost its threat as the cause of potentially serious complications, but now we are seeing a resurgence of acute rheumatic fever and increasing reports of fatal toxic septicemias.

On the positive side, molecular biology studies are providing an understanding of the events of infection and immunity. New effective drugs are being designed, based on specific identified targets in the pathogenetic sequence. However, continuing surveillance of the pathogens is needed to detect changes by which the organisms become resistant to a previously effective drug.

The disease coverage of this manual is intended to be global, including rare and exotic diseases. The jet plane and increasing international travel have created the situation where all travelers can return home within the incubation period of every infectious disease. Smallpox, even though it has been eradicated globally, is still included in this edition lest the disease appear again through some mischance; it is essential that there be a readily available source of information for rapid recognition and appropriate immediate action. Sources of information on exotic diseases may not be readily available to the practitioner; this book attempts to fill some of the gap until more extensive information can be acquired.

This manual is published by the American Public Health Association, but the presentation aims to be international. The production of this volume involves active participation by the WHO, the Pan American Health Organization (PAHO) and the health authorities of the major English-speaking countries. It is officially translated into French, Spanish and Portuguese; it has also been translated into many other languages. Toward this end, to avoid confusions based on disease nosology in different languages, each disease is identified by the numbers assigned by the World Health Organization *International Classification of Disease*, 9th Revision, Clinical Modification (ICD-9 CM). However, during the life of this edition, ICD-10 will come into effect in 1993, but is not available now. The English names used for the diseases are those recommended by the Council for International Organizations of Medical Sciences (CIOMS) and the World Health Organization (WHO) in *International Nomenclature of Diseases;* Volume II (Part 2, Mycoses, 1st edition, 1982, and Part 3, Viral Diseases, 1st edition, 1983) has been used as much as possible, unless the recommended name is too different from that in current use. In that case, the recommended name is shown as the first synonym.

The development of the text is a group effort by a large number of outstanding scientists who receive no remuneration for their efforts other than knowing the impact on public health and the lives saved. The members of the editorial board, selected for their expertise (and that of their associates) on specific diseases, were each assigned chapters for review and updating. After review and some editing by the editor and associate editor, these chapters were sent to all members of the editorial board and to the liaison representatives who had been designated by the various health agencies in the USA (governmental and nongovernmental), WHO, PAHO, and the health departments of Australia, Canada, New Zealand, Scotland and the United Kingdom. Many chapters were sent by the recipient to those most experienced in a given disease within their group or country; these colleagues have given freely of their time and effort. The many comments and criticisms were then considered in preparing the penultimate versions; those which raised problem issues were again distributed to the 28 people involved. After resolution of disagreement, the final drafts were reviewed by the original reviewer and submitted to the printer. While this edition presents the composite efforts of many individuals, named and not named, in many countries, the task of adjudicating among conflicting suggestions fell to the editor, who accepts the responsibility for having possibly rejected suggestions which consequently will be proven to have been correct.

While the perspective of the book is concerned with the problems in the United States, diseases do not respect international borders. An increasing number of diseases, such as influenza, must be considered on a global basis; toward this end, WHO has established a network of *International Collaborating Centres* which can provide national authorities with the services of consultation, collection and analysis of information, assistance in the establishment of standards, production and distribution of standard and reference material, exchange of information, training and organization of collaborative research, and information dissemination regarding the incidence of specific diseases. The diseases covered by these centers are indicated in section 9E of the appropriate chapters; WHO should be approached for further details about the available services.

While this manual is not intended to be a therapeutic guide, the currently best clinical management, especially of the exotic diseases, is indicated in section 9B7 of each disease presentation. Since the drugs needed for treatment of some rare or exotic diseases may not be available commercially within the United States, the Director of the Centers for Disease Control (CDC) of the U.S. Public Health Service (USPHS) has established the CDC Drug Service to provide access to rarely used drugs on an Investigational New Drug (IND) basis. These can be obtained by calling (404) 639-3670 or 3356, or at night, for emergency requests only, (404) 639-2888. The items available from this source are specified under the appropriate disease discussion. Some immunoprophylactic or immunotherapeutic agents are also available from CDC. Since several of the drugs and immunobiologics are considered "Emergency Life Saving" products, they are also dispensed from the US Quarantine Stations, located in international air terminals in seven major cities throughout the USA. (Requests are made through CDC.)

While the format of earlier editions (and sometimes the original words written by the previous editors, Haven Emerson and John E. Gordon) is retained, every chapter has been carefully updated. New sections have been added; these include TWAR pneumonia, campylobacteriosis, ehrlichiosis, and erythema infectiosum. The naming of several diseases has been changed to seek conformity with CIOMS-WHO nomenclature recommendations.

Scope and Contents - The presentation is standardized. Each disease is briefly identified with regard to clinical features, differentiation from allied or related conditions and laboratory diagnostic procedures. These laboratory procedures are snowballing as newer procedures for identifying the pathogen (such as the polymerase chain reaction and antigen capture techniques) and for detecting specific antibodies (such as the use of synthetic antigens) come into common use; this edition lists those procedures most frequently in use in diagnostic laboratories at the present time. Subsequent standard sections identify the *infectious agent, occurrence, reservoir, mode of transmission, incubation period, period of communicability* of the disease, and *susceptibility and resistance* of the host. *Methods of control* are described under the following five headings:

A. *Preventive measures:* Applicable generally to individuals and groups when and where the particular disease may occur in sporadic, endemic or epidemic form, and whether or not the disease is an active threat at the moment; e.g., chlorination of water supplies, pasteurization of milk, control of rodents and arthropods, animal management, immunization procedures, and health education of the public.

B. *Control of patient, contacts and the immediate environment:* Those measures designed to prevent spread of the disease to other persons, arthropods or animals from infected individuals; recommendations on the appropriate management of contacts to assure earliest possible preventive measures or management to prevent disease dissemination during the incubation period; and to detect any carriers and their management to minimize disease spread. Specific or best current treatment is outlined to minimize the period of communicability and to reduce morbidity and mortality. Recommendations for isolation have been based largely on the *CDC Guideline for Isolation Precautions in Hospitals* by Julia S. Garner and Bryan P. Simmons and *CDC Guideline for Infection Control in Hospital Personnel* by Walter W. Williams (in one volume). While the category-specific isolation precautions are epitomized in the section on definitions (after Zygomycosis, this volume), review of the original publications, available from the Superintendent of Documents, U.S. Government Printing Office, Washington DC 20402, may be desirable.

C. **Epidemic measures:** Those procedures of emergency character designed to limit the spread of a communicable disease which has developed widely in a group or community, or within an area, state or nation. These measures are not applicable when the disease occurs sporadically among widely separated individuals or separated by considerable intervals of time.

D. **Disaster implications:** The likelihood that the disease might constitute a major problem in a disaster or catastrophic situation and whether there would be need for specific preventive actions.

E. **International measures:** Such controls of international travelers, immigrants, goods, animals and animal products and their means of transport based on provisions of international health regulations, conventions, intergovernmental agreements or national laws; also any controls that may protect populations of one country against the known risk of infection from another country where a disease may be present in endemic or epidemic form. This section indicates any special programs, such as WHO Collaborating Centres, which might be operational.

Reporting of Communicable Diseases - The first step in the control of a communicable disease is its rapid identification, followed by notification to the local health authority that the disease exists within the particular jurisdiction. Administrative practices on the diseases to be reported and how they should be reported may vary greatly from one region to another because of different conditions and different disease frequencies. This manual presents a basic scheme of reporting, directed toward a practical working procedure rather than ideal practice. The purpose is to provide necessary and timely information to permit the institution of appropriate control measures by responsible health authorities, as well as to encourage uniformity in morbidity reporting so that data between different health jurisdictions within a country and between nations can be validly compared.

A reporting system functions at four levels. The first is the collection of the basic data in the local community where the disease occurs. The data are next assembled at district, state or provincial level. The third stage is the aggregation of the information under national auspices. Finally, for certain prescribed diseases, report is made by the national health authority to the World Health Organization.

Consideration here is limited to the first level of the reporting system - the collection of the basic data at the local level, which is the fundamental part of any reporting scheme and because this manual is primarily for local health workers. The basic data sought at the local level are of two kinds (also see Definitions, Report of a disease):

1. *Report of Cases:* Each local health authority, in conformity with regulations of higher authority, will determine what diseases are to be reported as a routine and regular procedure, who is responsible for reporting, the nature of the report required and the manner in which reports are forwarded to the next superior jurisdiction.

Physicians are required to report all notifiable illnesses which come to their attention; in addition, the statutes or regulations of many localities require reporting by hospital, householder, or other persons having knowledge of a case of a reportable disease. Within hospitals, a specific officer should be charged with the responsibility for submitting required reports. These may be case reports or collective reports.

Case reports of a communicable disease provide minimal identifying data of name, address, diagnosis, age, sex and date of report for each patient and, in some instances, suspects; dates of onset and basis for diagnosis are useful. The right of privacy of the individual must be respected.

Collective reports are the assembled number of cases, by diagnosis, occurring within a prescribed time and without individual identifying data, e.g., "20 cases of malaria, week ending October 6."

2. *Report of Epidemics:* In addition to the requirement for individual case reports, any unusual or group expression of illness which may be of public concern (see Definitions, Epidemic) should be reported to the local health authority by the most expeditious means, whether it is included or not in the list of diseases officially reportable in the particular locality; and whether it is a well-known identified disease or an indefinite or unknown clinical entity (see Class 4, below).

For reporting purposes, the diseases listed in this manual are distributed among the following five classes, according to the practical benefit which can be derived from reporting. These classes are referred to by number throughout the text, under section 9B1 of each disease. The purpose is to provide a scheme on the basis of which each health jurisdiction may determine its list of regularly reportable diseases.

Class 1: Case Report Universally Required by International Health Regulations or as a Disease under Surveillance by WHO.

This class can be divided into:

1.   Those diseases subject to the International Health Regulations (1969), Third Annotated Edition, 1983, WHO, Geneva; i.e, the internationally quarantinable diseases - plague, cholera,

yellow fever and smallpox; and

1A. Diseases under Surveillance by WHO, established by the 22d World Health Assembly - louse-borne typhus fever and relapsing fever, paralytic poliomyelitis, malaria and viral influenza.

An obligatory case report is made to the health authority by telephone, telegraph, or other rapid means; in an epidemic situation, collective reports of subsequent cases in a local area on a daily or weekly basis may be requested by the next superior jurisdiction, as, for example, in a cholera epidemic. The local health authority forwards the initial report to the next superior jurisdiction by the most expeditious means if it is the first recognized case in the local area or is the first case outside the limits of a local area already reported; otherwise, weekly by mail or telegraphically in unusual situations.

Class 2: Case Report Regularly Required Wherever the Disease Occurs

Two subclasses are recognized, based on the relative urgency for investigation of contacts and source of infection, or for starting control measures.

2A. Case report to local health authority by telephone, telegraph, or other rapid means. These are forwarded to next superior jurisdiction weekly by mail, except that the first recognized case in an area or the first case outside the limits of known affected local area is reported by telephone or telegraph; examples - typhoid fever, diphtheria.

2B. Case report by most practicable means; forwarded to next superior jurisdiction as a collective report, weekly by mail; examples - brucellosis, leprosy.

Class 3: Selectively Reportable in Recognized Endemic Areas

In many states and countries, diseases of this class are not reportable. Reporting may be prescribed in particular regions, states or countries by reason of undue frequency or severity. Three subclasses are recognized; 3A and 3B are primarily useful under conditions of established endemicity as a means leading toward prompt control measures and to judge the effectiveness of control programs. The main purpose of 3C is to stimulate control measures or to acquire essential epidemiologic data.

3A. Case report by telephone, telegraph, or other rapid means in specified areas where the disease ranks in importance with

Class 2A; not reportable in many countries; examples - scrub typhus, Argentine and Bolivian hemorrhagic fever.

3B. Case report by most practicable means; forwarded to next superior jurisdiction as a collective report by mail weekly or monthly; not reportable in many countries; examples - bartonellosis, coccidioidomycosis.

3C. Collective report weekly by mail to local health authority; forwarded to next superior jurisdiction by mail weekly, monthly, quarterly, or sometimes annually; examples - schistosomiasis, fasciolopsiasis.

Class 4: Obligatory Report of Epidemics - No Case Report Required

Prompt report of outbreaks of particular public health importance by telephone, telegraph, or other rapid means; forwarded to next superior jurisdiction by telephone or telegraph. Pertinent data include number of cases, time frame, approximate population involved and apparent mode of spread; examples - staphylococcal food poisoning, adenoviral keratoconjunctivitis, unidentified syndrome.

Class 5: Official Report Not Ordinarily Justifiable

Diseases of this class are of two general kinds: those typically sporadic and uncommon, often not directly transmissible from person to person (chromoblastomycosis); or those of such epidemiologic nature as to offer no special practical measures for control (common cold).

Diseases are often made reportable but the information gathered is put to no practical use, and with no feed-back to those who provided the data. This leads to deterioration in the general level of reporting, even for diseases of much importance. Better case reporting results when official reporting is restricted to those diseases for which control services are provided or potential control procedures are under evaluation, or epidemiologic information is needed for a definite purpose.

ACKNOWLEDGEMENTS

Grateful acknowledgement is hereby made to all the experts, both within and without the American Public Health Associaton, and within and without the USA, who have prepared and critically reviewed sections in their area of expertise. The conscientious efforts of the Editorial Committee and of the national and international Liaison Representatives (who contributed not only their own effort but called on the experts in their various countries) provided information to make the final product of greatest value. Special recognition must be made to the participation of Dr. Lew Legters, my associate editor, and especially to my research associate, Charlotte Shindledecker Seidman, who again managed the nuts and bolts of digging out needed information as well as assuring that everything fit together in the end, as she had for the 14th edition. My sincere appreciation must also be expressed to the staff of the San Diego State University Foundation for their administrative support.

Special recognition is due my wife, Regina v.A. Benenson (whose van Aalten family crest appears as the chapter dividers), for the many solitary nights she spent while this and the four previous editions were taking shape!

ACQUIRED IMMUNODEFICIENCY SYNDROME

ICD-9 042-044

(HIV infection, AIDS)

1. **Identification**—AIDS is a severe, life-threatening clinical condition, first recognized as a distinct syndrome in 1981. This syndrome represents the late clinical stage of infection with the human immunodeficiency virus (HIV), which most often results in progressive damage to the immune and other organ systems, especially the CNS.

Within several weeks to several months after infection with HIV, many persons develop an acute self-limited mononucleosis-like illness lasting for a week or two. Infected persons may then be free of clinical signs or symptoms for many months to years before other clinical manifestations, including opportunistic infections and constitutional and neurologic symptoms appear. The severity of HIV-related illnesses is, in general, directly correlated with the degree of immune system dysfunction. Onset of clinical illness is usually insidious with non-specific symptoms such as lymphadenopathy, anorexia, chronic diarrhea, weight loss, fever and fatigue. However, this constellation of non-specific symptoms is usually not sufficient by itself for a diagnosis of AIDS. These latter signs and symptoms in an HIV-infected person have been referred to as AIDS-related complex (ARC), or "symptomatic HIV infection."

More than a dozen opportunistic infections and several cancers are considered to be sufficiently specific indicators of the underlying immunodeficiency to be included in the case definition of AIDS. These opportunistic infections include: *Pneumocystis carinii* pneumonia, chronic cryptosporidiosis, toxoplasmosis of the CNS, esophageal or lower respiratory tract candidiasis, disseminated or CNS cryptococcosis, disseminated atypical mycobacteriosis, pulmonary or GI or CNS or ocular cytomegalovirus (CMV) infection, chronic ulcerative mucocutaneous or disseminated herpes simplex infection and progressive multifocal leukoencephalopathy; cancers include Kaposi's sarcoma, primary B-cell lymphoma limited to the brain and non-Hodgkin's lymphoma. These diseases, if diagnosed by standard histologic and/or culture techniques, were accepted as meeting the surveillance definition of AIDS developed by CDC, if other known causes of immunodeficiency were ruled out.

In 1987, this definition was revised to include additional indicator diseases (such as wasting syndrome, extrapulmonary tuberculosis and neurologic disease such as HIV dementia or sensory neuropathy) and to accept as a presumptive diagnosis some of the indicator diseases if laboratory tests such as HIV antibody assays showed evidence of HIV infection. The case definition may be revised again as more clinical information becomes available. For example, recurrent bacterial septicemia or pneumonia (already AIDS-indicator diagnoses in pediatric AIDS) and pulmonary tuberculosis are being investigated as major manifestations of HIV-related immunodeficiency.

The proportion of human immunodeficiency virus (HIV)-infected persons who will ultimately develop AIDS is not precisely known. Cohort studies of HIV-infected adults carried out before specific antiviral therapy was available indicated that about 15-20% developed AIDS within 5 years, and about 50% within 7-10 years. Beyond 10 years, it was projected that the vast majority of infected persons may develop AIDS within another 5 to 10 years. With modern therapy, these incubation periods are almost certain to be longer by several years. Without specific therapy, the case fatality rate of AIDS has been very high and most patients (80-90%) have died within 3-5 years after the diagnosis of AIDS is made.

This description and case definition apply to adult AIDS cases primarily in industrialized countries. In developing countries, which often lack adequate laboratory facilities for the histologic or culture diagnosis of the specified surrogate indicator diseases, WHO has developed a clinical case definition of AIDS for public health reporting that relies on specific combinations of major and minor signs/symptoms and diseases for a diagnosis of AIDS. The clinical manifestations of AIDS in infants and young children overlap with failure to thrive, inherited immunodeficiencies and other childhood health problems. CDC has published pediatric case definitions.

Serologic tests for antibodies to HIV have been commercially available since 1985. The most commonly used screening test (EIA or ELISA) is highly sensitive and specific. However, when this test is reactive, it must be supplemented by a more specific test such as the Western blot or indirect immunofluorescence assay. A nonreactive supplemental test negates the reactive EIA test; a positive reaction supports it, and an indeterminate result in the Western blot test calls for further evaluation.

Most persons infected with HIV develop detectable antibodies within 1 to 3 months; occasionally, there may be a more prolonged interval. Other tests to detect HIV infections during the period after infection but prior to seroconversion are being developed, such as serologic tests for circulating HIV antigen (p24) and the polymerase chain reaction (PCR) for viral nucleic acid sequences. These tests show promise, but questions regarding sensitivity, specificity and interpretation remain.

The absolute T-helper cell count is used most often to evaluate the severity of HIV infection and to help clinicians make decisions regarding therapy. Other laboratory findings, such as lymphopenia, hypergammaglobulinemia, p24 antigenemia, anergy to mitogens and antigens, and an inversion of the helper/suppressor T-lymphocyte ratio due to an absolute decrease in T-helper lymphocytes, usually precede clinical findings. Other non-specific tests that may have some prognostic value include assays for serum β-2-microglobulin and IgA, and urine neopterin.

2. **Infectious agent**—Human immunodeficiency virus (HIV), a retrovirus. Two types have been identified: type 1 (HIV-1) and type 2 (HIV-2). These viruses are serologically and geographically relatively distinct, but have similar epidemiologic and pathologic characteristics.

3. **Occurrence**—The syndrome was first reported in 1981, but isolated cases occurred in the USA and in several other areas of the world (Haiti, Africa and Europe) during the 1970s; by mid-1990, over 130,000 cases had been reported in the USA. Although the USA has recorded the largest number of cases, AIDS has been recorded in virtually all countries, among all races, ages and social classes. Worldwide, WHO estimated that close to 600,000 cases (with about half in sub-Saharan Africa) had occurred by 1990.

In the USA, as of 1990, nearly all patients with AIDS fall into the following categories: homosexual or bisexual men (about 70%), intravenous drug users (20%), heterosexual contacts of infected partners (4%), children born to infected mothers (1%) and patients with hemophilia (1%). Other individuals at risk include pre-1985 transfusion recipients. Nearly 90% of all persons with AIDS are 20-49 years of age; 93% of the cases of Kaposi's sarcoma (the most commonly diagnosed cancer in AIDS patients) have occurred among homosexual or bisexual men. It is estimated that, by 1990, about 1 million people were HIV-infected in the USA, and 6 to 8 million worldwide.

HIV-1 infection is found in the Americas, Europe, sub-Saharan Africa and most other countries; HIV-2 has been found primarily in West Africa, with some cases in Western and other African countries that are linked epidemiologically to West Africa.

4. **Reservoir**—Humans.

5. **Mode of transmission**—Routine social or community contact with an HIV-infected person carries no risk of transmission; only sexual exposure and exposure to blood or tissues carries a risk. The routes of transmission of HIV are analogous to those of hepatitis B virus (HBV). Epidemiologic evidence indicates that HIV can be transmitted from person to person through sexual contact, sharing HIV-contaminated intravenous needles and syringes, and through transfusion of infected blood or its components. Clotting factor concentrates manufactured from unscreened plasma were a significant source of HIV infection for persons with hemophilia; donor screening, effective heat treatment and other processing of concentrates have virtually eliminated this risk since 1985. While virus has on occasion been found in saliva, tears, urine and bronchial secretions, transmission after contact with these secretions has not been reported. There are a number of co-factors that may contribute to the transmission and for clinical outcomes of HIV infection; these include other sexually transmitted agents. There is no laboratory or

epidemiologic evidence to indicate that biting insects have transmitted HIV infection.

From 25% to 35% of infants born to HIV-infected mothers are infected before, during, or shortly after birth. After direct exposure of health care workers to HIV-infected blood through injury with needles and other sharp objects, the rate of seroconversion is <0.5%, much lower than the risk of HBV infection (about 25%) after a similar exposure.

6. **Incubation period**—Variable. Although the time from infection to the development of detectable antibodies is generally 1-3 months, the time from HIV infection to diagnosis of AIDS has an observed range of about 2 months to 10 years or longer. About half of infected persons will have developed AIDS 10 years after infection in the absence of specific antiviral treatment. The median incubation period in infected infants is shorter than in adults. Treatment lengthens the incubation period.

7. **Period of communicability**—Unknown; presumed to begin early after onset of HIV infection and extend throughout life. Epidemiologic evidence suggests that communicability increases with increasing immune deficiency, clinical symptoms and perhaps genital ulcer disease.

8. **Susceptibility and resistance**—Unknown, but susceptibility presumed to be general. Race does not appear to affect susceptibility to HIV infection or AIDS. Presence of other sexually transmitted diseases, especially those with ulcerations, may increase susceptibility, as may the presence of the penile foreskin. No recovered cases have been conclusively documented; degree of immunity is unknown.

9. **Methods of control**—

A. *Preventive measures:*

1) Public and school health education must stress the facts that having multiple sexual partners and sharing drug paraphernalia increase the risk of infection with HIV, and must provide students with the skills needed to avoid or reduce risky behaviors.

2) Avoid sexual intercourse (anal, vaginal or oral) with persons known or suspected to be infected with HIV. Use latex condoms with nonpetroleum-based lubricants and a spermicide to reduce the risk of sexual transmission. The risk from oral sex is not easily quantifiable, but is presumed to be low. There is no risk of HIV transmission in a long-term mutually monogamous relationship between two persons known not to be infected with HIV.

3) Expansion of treatment facilities for drug users may reduce HIV transmission. Such measures as instructing

needle users in decontamination methods and "needle exchange" programs should be considered and evaluated.

4) Anonymous and/or confidential HIV counseling and testing sites are in operation in all states of the USA. Counseling, HIV testing and medical referrals should be offered routinely in sexually transmitted disease (STD), tuberculosis and drug treatment clinics; those offering prenatal care or family planning services; facilities that offer services to gay men; and in communities where HIV seroprevalence is high.

5) Regulations have been established by the US Food and Drug Administration (FDA) to prevent HIV contamination of plasma and blood. All donated units must be tested for HIV antibody; only donations testing negative can be used. Persons who have engaged in behaviors that place them at increased risk of HIV infection must not donate plasma, blood, organs for transplantation, tissue or cells (including semen for artificial insemination). Organizations collecting plasma, blood or organs (including sperm banks, milk banks, bone banks, etc.) should inform potential donors of this recommendation and must test all donors. When possible, donations of sperm, milk or bone should be frozen and stored for at least 3 months. Donors testing negative after that interval can be considered not to have been infected at the time of donation.

6) Physicians should adhere strictly to medical indications for transfusions. The use of autologous transfusions should be considered.

7) Only clotting factor products that have been screened and treated to inactivate HIV should be used.

8) Care should be taken in handling, using and disposing of needles or other sharp instruments. Health care workers should wear latex gloves if there is contact with blood or fluids that are visibly bloody. Any patient's blood on the worker's skin should be washed off with soap and water without delay.

9) WHO recommends immunization of asymptomatic HIV-infected children with the EPI vaccines; those who are symptomatic should not receive BCG vaccine. In the USA, BCG and oral polio vaccines are not recommended for HIV-infected children regardless of symptoms; live MMR vaccines are recommended for all HIV-infected children.

B. *Control of patient, contacts and the immediate environment:*

1) Report to local health authority: Official report of cases of

AIDS is obligatory in all health jurisdictions in the USA and in most countries. Most states in the USA have also implemented or are considering requiring reporting of HIV infections. Official report may be required in some countries or provinces, Class 2B (see Preface).

2) Isolation: Universal precautions apply to all patients. Observe additional precautions appropriate for specific infections that occur in AIDS patients.

3) Concurrent disinfection: Of equipment contaminated with blood, and excretions and secretions visibly contaminated with blood.

4) Quarantine: None. Tissue donation: Patients and their sexual partners should not donate blood, plasma, organs for transplantation, tissues, cells, semen for artificial insemination or breast milk for human milk banks.

5) Immunization of contacts: None.

6) Investigation of contacts and source of infection: In the USA, notification of sexual and needle-sharing partners should be conducted either by the HIV-infected individual (partner referral), or by health care providers and health departments (provider referral).

7) Specific treatment: Rapid progress is being reported in drug treatment for asymptomatic and symptomatic HIV infection. Early diagnosis of infection and referral for medical evaluation are indicated. Consult more current sources of information for appropriate drugs, schedules and doses. There is no known treatment for the underlying immune deficiency. Selected antiviral agents, such as zidovudine (azidothymidine, AZT), prolong life, reduce the risk of opportunistic infections and may prolong the incubation period. Otherwise, treatment consists of specific measures for the opportunistic diseases that result from HIV infection. Prophylactic use of oral cotrimoxazole or aerosolized pentamidine have been recommended for the prevention of *Pneumocystis carinii* pneumonia. All HIV-infected persons should receive tuberculin skin tests and be evaluated for active disease if the skin test is positive and be placed on anti-tuberculous therapy, or evaluated for preventive therapy if the skin test is negative.

C. *Epidemic measures:* HIV is currently pandemic, with large numbers of infections reported in the Americas, Europe, Africa and SE Asia. See 9A, above, for recommendations.

D. *Disaster implications:* Emergency personnel should follow the same universal precautions as health workers; if latex gloves are not available and skin surfaces contact blood, this should be washed off as soon as possible. Masks, visors, etc., are indicated when performing procedures that may involve spurting or splashing of blood or bloody fluids. Emergency transfusion services should use blood donations that are screened for HIV antibody; when it is not possible to test donated blood for HIV antibody, donations should be accepted only from donors who have engaged in no HIV risk behaviors and preferably from donors who have previously tested negative for HIV antibodies.

E. **International measures:** A global prevention and control program coordinated by WHO was initiated in 1987. As of 1990, virtually all countries throughout the world have developed an AIDS prevention and control program. Several nations have instituted requirements for AIDS or HIV examinations for entry by foreign travelers (mainly those applying for resident or longer-term visas, such as for work or study); WHO has not endorsed these measures.

ACTINOMYCOSIS   ICD-9 039

1. **Identification**—A chronic bacterial disease most frequently localized in jaw, thorax or abdomen (liver); bloodborne spread with generalized disease may occur. The lesions are firmly indurated areas of purulence and fibrosis that spread slowly to contiguous tissues; eventually, draining sinuses may be formed which penetrate to the surface. Discharges from sinus tracts may contain "sulfur granules," i.e., colonies of the infectious agent.

Diagnosis is made by demonstrating slim, non-spore-forming Gram-positive bacilli, with or without branching, or "sulfur granules" in tissue or pus, and by isolating the micro-organisms from samples of appropriate clinical materials not contaminated with normal flora during collection. The clinical findings and culture allow distinction between actinomycosis and actinomycetoma, very different diseases. (See Mycetoma.)

2. **Infectious agents**—*Actinomyces israelii* is the usual human pathogen; *A. naeslundii, A. meyeri* and *Arachnia propionica (Actinomyces propionicus)* also have been reported to cause human actinomycosis. All species are Gram-positive, non-acid-fast, anaerobic to micro-aerophilic, higher bacteria which may be part of the normal oral flora.

3. **Occurrence**—An infrequent human disease, occurring sporadically

throughout the world. All races, both sexes, and all age groups may be affected; greatest frequency is from 15 to 35 years of age; the ratio of males to females is approximately 2/1. Cases in cattle, horses and other animals are caused by other *Actinomyces* species.

4 **Reservoir**—The natural reservoir of *A. israelii* and other agents is man. In the normal oral cavity, the organisms grow as saprophytes in and around carious teeth, in dental plaque, and in tonsillar crypts, without apparent penetration or cellular response in adjacent tissues. Sample surveys in the USA, Sweden and other countries have demonstrated *A. israelii* microscopically in granules from crypts of 40% of extirpated tonsils, and, by anaerobic culture, from as many as 30–48% of specimens of saliva or material from carious teeth. *A. israelii* has been found in the vaginal secretions of approximately 10% of women using intrauterine devices. No external environmental reservoir such as straw or soil has been demonstrated.

5. **Mode of transmission**—Presumably the agent passes by contact from person to person as a part of the normal oral flora. From the oral cavity, the organism may be swallowed, inhaled, or introduced into jaw tissues by injury or at the site of neglected or irritating dental defects. The source of clinical disease is endogenous.

6. **Incubation period**—Irregular; probably many years after colonization in the oral tissues, and days or months after precipitating trauma and actual penetration of tissues.

7. **Period of communicability**—Time and manner in which *Actinomyces* and *Arachnia* species become a part of the normal oral flora are unknown; except for rare instances of human bite, not related to specific exposure to an infected person.

8. **Susceptibility and resistance**—Natural susceptibility is low. Immunity following attack has not been demonstrated.

9. **Methods of control**—

   A. *Preventive measures:* None, except that maintenance of good dental hygiene, particularly removal of accumulating dental plaque, will reduce risk of infection around teeth.

   B. *Control of patient, contacts and the immediate environment:*

   1) Report to local health authority: Official report not ordinarily justifiable, Class 5 (see Preface).
   2) Isolation: None.
   3) Concurrent disinfection: None.
   4) Quarantine: None.
   5) Immunization of contacts: None.

    6) Investigation of contacts and source of infection: Not profitable.

    7) Specific treatment: No spontaneous recovery. Prolonged administration of penicillin in high doses is usually effective; tetracycline, erythromycin and cephalosporin antibiotics are alternatives. Surgical drainage of abscesses is often necessary.

C. **Epidemic measures:** Not applicable, a sporadic disease.

D. **Disaster implications:** None.

E. **International measures:** None.

AMEBIASIS ICD-9 006

1. **Identification**—An infection with a protozoan parasite that exists in two forms: the hardy, infective cyst and the more fragile, potentially pathogenic trophozoite. The parasite may act as a commensal or invade the tissues, giving rise to intestinal or extra-intestinal disease. Most infections are asymptomatic, but may become clinically important under certain circumstances. Intestinal disease varies from acute or fulminating dysentery with fever, chills and bloody or mucoid diarrhea (amebic dysentery), to mild abdominal discomfort with diarrhea containing blood or mucus alternating with periods of constipation or remission. Amebic granulomata (ameboma), sometimes mistaken for carcinoma, may occur in the wall of the large intestine in patients with intermittent dysentery or colitis of long duration. Ulceration of the skin, usually in the perianal region, occurs rarely by direct extension from intestinal lesions. Dissemination via the bloodstream may occur, producing abscess of the liver or, less commonly, of the lung or brain.

Amebic colitis is often confused with various forms of inflammatory bowel disease such as ulcerative colitis; special care should be taken to distinguish the two diseases since corticosteroids may exacerbate the amebic colitis. Amebiasis can also mimic numerous other noninfectious and infectious diseases. Conversely, the presence of amebae may be misinterpreted as the cause of diarrhea in a person whose primary enteric illness is the result of another condition.

Diagnosis is made by microscopic demonstration of trophozoites or cysts in fresh or suitably preserved fecal specimens, smears of aspirates or scrapings obtained by proctoscopy, aspirates of abscesses or sections of tissue; the presence of trophozoites containing RBCs is indicative of invasive amebiasis. Examination should be done on fresh specimens by a trained microscopist since the organism must be differentiated from nonpathogenic amebae and macrophages. Cultures on special media are not routinely used. Use of reference laboratory services may be required. Many serologic tests are available as adjuncts in diagnosing extraintestinal amebiasis such as liver abscess where stool examination is often negative. Scintillography, ultrasonography and CAT scanning, in addition to conventional x-ray techniques, are helpful in revealing the presence and location of an amebic liver abscess, and can be considered diagnostic when associated with a high titer of specific antibodies.

2. **Infectious agent**—*Entamoeba histolytica*, a parasitic organism not to be confused with *E. hartmanni*, *E. coli*, or other intestinal protozoa. Virulence of amebic strains tends to correlate with the isozyme phenotype of the parasite. Eight potentially pathogenic and 11 non-pathogenic zymodemes have been identified from stool samples from four continents. Most asymptomatic cyst-passers carry non-pathogenic strains.

3. **Occurrence**—Amebiasis is ubiquitous. Invasive amebiasis is mostly a disease of young adults, especially males. It is rare below age 5 years and especially below 2 years, when dystentery is due mostly to *Shigellae*. Published prevalence rates of cyst passage vary widely from place to place. In general, rates are higher in areas with poor sanitation, such as parts of the tropics; in mental institutions; and among sexually promiscuous male homosexuals. In areas with good sanitation, amebic infections tend to cluster in households and institutions. The proportion of cyst passers who have clinical disease is usually low.

4. **Reservoir**—Man; usually a chronically ill or asymptomatic cyst passer.

5. **Mode of transmission**—Outbreaks result mainly from ingestion of fecally contaminated water containing amebic cysts. Endemic spread is by hand-to-mouth transfer of feces, by contaminated raw vegetables, possibly by soiled hands of foodhandlers, and perhaps occasionally by water. Transmission may occur sexually by oral-anal contact. Patients with acute amebic dysentery pose only limited danger to others because of the absence of cysts in dysenteric stools and the fragility of trophozoites.

6. **Incubation period**—Variable; from a few days to several months or years; commonly 2-4 weeks.

7. **Period of communicability**—During the period of cyst passing, which may continue for years; however, this may apply only to nonpathogenic strains.

8. **Susceptibility and resistance**—Although susceptibility to infection is general, most persons harboring the organism do not develop disease, probably related to the zymodeme of the organism carried. Susceptibility to reinfection has been demonstrated.

9. **Methods of control—**

   A. *Preventive measures:*

   1) Educate the general public in personal hygiene, particularly in sanitary disposal of feces, and in handwashing after defecation and before preparing or eating food. Disseminate information regarding the risks involved in eating uncleaned or uncooked fruits and vegetables and in drinking water of questionable purity.

   2) Teach known carriers the need for thorough handwashing after defecation; treat if symptoms develop.

   3) Educate high-risk groups to avoid sexual practices that may permit fecal-oral transmission.

   4) Dispose of human feces in a sanitary manner.

   5) Protect public water supplies from fecal contamination. Sand filtration of water removes nearly all cysts, and diatomaceous earth filters remove them completely. Chlorination of water as generally practiced in municipal water treatment does not always kill cysts; small quantities of water as in canteens or Lyster bags are best treated with prescribed concentrations of iodine, either liquid (8 drops of 2% tincture of iodine/quart of water or 12.5 ml/liter of a saturated aqueous solution of iodine crystals), or as water purification tablets (a tablet of tetraglycine hydroperiodide, Globaline®, per quart of water). A contact period of at least 10 minutes (30 minutes if cold) should be allowed to elapse before drinking the water. Portable filters with <1.0 μm pore sizes are effective. Water of undetermined quality can be made safe by boiling.

   6) Health agencies should supervise the sanitary practices of persons preparing and serving food in public eating places and the general cleanliness of the premises involved. Routine examination of foodhandlers as a control measure is impractical.

   7) Disinfectant dips for fruits and vegetables are of unproved value in preventing transmission of *E. histolytica*. Thorough washing with potable water and keeping them dry may help; cysts are killed by desiccation and temperatures above 50°C (122°F).

   8) Use of chemoprophylactic agents is not advised.

   B. *Control of patient, contacts and the immediate environment:*

   1) Report to local health authority: In selected endemic areas; in many states (USA) and countries not reportable, Class 3C (see Preface).

2) Isolation: For hospitalized patients, enteric precautions in the handling of feces and contaminated clothing and bed linen. Exclusion of infected individuals from foodhandling and from direct care of hospitalized and institutionalized patients. Release to return to work in a sensitive occupation when chemotherapy is completed.

3) Concurrent disinfection: Sanitary disposal of feces.

4) Quarantine: None.

5) Immunization of contacts: Not applicable.

6) Investigation of contacts and source of infection: Household members and other suspected contacts should have adequate microscopic examination of feces.

7) Specific treatment: Acute amebic dysentery is best treated with metronidazole (Flagyl®) followed by iodoquinol (Diodoquin®) if cyst passage persists. Dehydroemetine (Mebadin®) followed by iodoquinol is a suitable alternative treatment. Extra-intestinal amebiasis should be treated with metronidazole, or a combination of dehydroemetine plus chloroquine (Aralen®). Occasionally, abscesses may require surgical aspiration. Asymptomatic carriers may be treated with iodoquinol or diloxanide furoate (Furamide®).

   Metronidazole is best not used during the first trimester of pregnancy; however, there has been no proof of teratogenicity in humans. Dehydroemetine is contraindicated during pregnancy. Diloxanide furoate and dehydroemetine are available from the CDC Drug Service, CDC, Atlanta (see Preface).

C. *Epidemic measures:* Any group of cases requires prompt laboratory confirmation to exclude other etiologic agents (as has frequently occurred) and epidemiologic investigation to determine source of infection and mode of transmission. If a common vehicle is indicated, such as water or food, appropriate measures should be taken to correct the situation.

D. *Disaster implications:* Disruption of normal sanitary facilities and food controls will favor an outbreak of amebiasis, especially in population groups with large numbers of cyst passers.

E. *International measures:* None.

ANGIOSTRONGYLIASIS   ICD-9 128.8
(Eosinophilic meningoencephalitis, Eosinophilic meningitis)

1. **Identification**—A disease of the CNS due to a nematode; meninges are predominantly involved. Invasion may be asymptomatic or mildly symptomatic; it is more commonly characterized by severe headache, stiffness of neck and back and various paresthesias. Temporary facial paralysis occurs in 5% of patients. Low-grade fever may be present. The worm has been found in the CSF and the eye. CSF usually exhibits pleocytosis with 25-100% eosinophils; blood eosinophilia is not always present, but has reached 82%. Illness may last a few days to several months. Deaths have rarely been reported.

Differential diagnosis includes tuberculous meningitis, cerebral toxoplasmosis, coccidioidal meningitis, aseptic meningitis, syphilis, cerebral cysticercosis, paragonimiasis, echinococcosis and gnathostomiasis.

Diagnosis, especially in endemic areas, is suggested by eosinophils in the CSF and a history of eating raw molluscs; immunodiagnostic tests are presumptive; demonstration of the worms in the CSF or at autopsy is confirmatory.

2. **Infectious agent**—*Angiostrongylus cantonensis,* a nematode (lungworm of rats). The third-stage larvae are infective to man.

3. **Occurrence**—The disease is endemic in Hawaii, Tahiti, many other Pacific islands, Vietnam, Thailand, Malaysia, China, Indonesia, Taiwan, the Philippines and Cuba. The nematode is found as far north as Japan, as far south as Brisbane, Australia, and in Africa as far west as the Ivory Coast. Also reported in Madagascar, Egypt, Puerto Rico, Brazil and New Orleans.

4. **Reservoir**—The rat (*Rattus* and *Bandicota* spp.).

5. **Mode of transmission**—Ingestion of raw or insufficiently cooked snails, slugs or land planarians, which are intermediate or transport hosts harboring infective larvae. Prawns, fish and land crabs that have ingested snails or slugs may also transport the infective larvae. Lettuce and other leafy vegetables contaminated by small molluscs may serve as a source of infection. The molluscs are infected by first-stage larvae excreted by an infected rodent; when third-stage larvae have developed, rodents (and people) are infected when they ingest infected molluscs. In the rat, the larvae migrate to the brain and mature to the adult stage; the young adults migrate to the surface of the brain and through the venous system to reach their final site in the pulmonary arteries.

After mating, eggs deposited by female worms hatch in terminal branches of the pulmonary arteries, the first-stage larvae enter the bronchial system and pass up the trachea, are swallowed and passed in the feces. In people, the cycle rarely goes beyond the CNS stage.

6. **Incubation period**—Usually 1-3 weeks; it may be longer or shorter.

7. **Period of communicability**—Not transmitted from person to person.

8. **Susceptibility and resistance**—Susceptibility to infection is general. Malnutrition and debilitating diseases may contribute to an increase in severity, even to a fatal outcome.

9. **Methods of control**—

   A. *Preventive measures:*

      1) Educate the general public in preparation of seafoods and both aquatic and terrestrial snails.
      2) Control rats.
      3) Boil snails, prawns, fish and crabs for 3-5 minutes, or freeze at -15°C (5°F) for 24 hours; this is effective in killing the larvae.
      4) Avoid eating raw foods which have been contaminated by snails or slugs; thorough cleansing of lettuce and other greens to eliminate molluscs and their products does not always eliminate infective larvae.

   B. *Control of patient, contacts and the immediate environment:*

      1) Report to local health authority: Official report not ordinarily justifiable, Class 5 (see Preface).
      2) Isolation: None.
      3) Concurrent disinfection: Not necessary.
      4) Quarantine: None.
      5) Immunization of contacts: Not applicable.
      6) Investigation of contacts and source of infection: The source of food involved and its preparation should be investigated.
      7) Specific treatment: Albendazole may be effective.

   C. *Epidemic measures:* Any grouping of several cases in a particular geographic area or institution warrants prompt epidemiologic investigation.

   D. *Disaster implications:* None.

   E. *International measures:* None.

ABDOMINAL ANGIOSTRONGYLIASIS   ICD-9 128.8

Since 1967, a syndrome similar to appendicitis has been recognized in Costa Rica, predominantly among children under the age of 13, with abdominal pain and tenderness in the right iliac fossa and flank, fever, anorexia, vomiting, abdominal rigidity, a tumor-like mass in the right lower quadrant, and pain on rectal examination. Leukocytosis is generally between 20,000 to 30,000/cu mm, with eosinophils ranging from 11% to 61%. On surgery, yellow granulations are found in the subserosa of the intestinal wall, and eggs and larvae of *Angiostrongylus costaricensis* are found in lymph nodes, intestinal wall, omentum, etc.; adult worms are in the small arteries, generally in the ileocecal area. The infection has been recognized in people in Central and S America.

The reservoir of this parasite is a rodent (the cotton rat, *Sigmodon hispidus,* among which the worm is present in southern USA); slugs are the usual intermediate hosts. The adults live in the mesenteric arteries in the cecal area, and the eggs are carried into the intestinal wall. On embryonation, the first-stage larvae migrate to the lumen, are excreted in the feces and ingested by a slug. Within the slug, the larvae develop to the third-stage which is infective to rats and people. The infective larvae are found in the slug's slime (mucus) left on soil or other surfaces; when ingested by people, the infective larvae penetrate the gut wall, maturing in the lymphatic nodes and vessels. The adult worms migrate to the mesenteric arterioles of the ileocecal region where oviposition occurs. In people, most of the eggs and larvae degenerate and cause a granulomatous reaction. There is no specific treatment; surgical intervention is sometimes necessary.

ANISAKIASIS   ICD-9 127.1

1. **Identification**—A parasitic disease of the human GI tract usually manifested by cramping abdominal pain and vomiting, resulting from the ingestion of uncooked marine fish containing larval ascaridoid nematodes. The motile larvae burrow into the stomach wall producing acute ulceration with nausea, vomiting and epigastric pain, sometimes with hematemesis. They may migrate upward and attach in the oropharynx causing cough. In the small intestine, they cause eosinophilic abscesses, and the symptoms may mimic appendicitis or regional enteritis. At times they perforate into the peritoneal cavity; rarely they involve the large bowel.

Diagnosis is made by recognition of the 2 cm-long larva invading the oropharynx, or by visualizing the larva through gastroscopic examination or in surgically removed tissue.

2. **Infectious agents**—Larval nematodes of the subfamily Anisakidinae, genera *Anisakis, Contracaecum, Pseudoterranova,* and *Hysterothylacium.*

3. **Occurrence**—The disease occurs in individuals who eat uncooked

and inadequately treated (frozen, salted, marinated, smoked) saltwater fish, squid, or octopus. This is common in Japan (sushi and sashimi), the Netherlands (herring), Scandinavia (gravlax), and on the Pacific coast of Latin America (ceviche). Several hundred cases have been described in Japan. Formerly, the disease was frequently seen in the Netherlands. Cases are now seen with increasing frequency throughout western Europe and the USA, with the growing consumption of raw fish.

4. **Reservoir**—Anisakidinae are widely distributed in nature, but only certain of those which are parasitic in sea mammals constitute a major threat to man. The natural life cycle involves transmission of larvae by predation through small crustaceans to squid, octopus or fish, then to sea mammals, with people as incidental hosts.

5. **Mode of transmission**—The infective larvae live in the abdominal mesenteries of fish; often after death of their host, they invade the body muscles of the fish. When ingested by people and liberated by digestion in the stomach, they may penetrate the gastric or intestinal mucosa.

6. **Incubation period**—Gastric symptoms may develop within a few hours after ingestion. Symptoms referable to the small and large bowel occur within a few days or weeks, depending on the size and location of the larva.

7. **Period of communicability**—Direct transmission from person to person does not occur.

8. **Susceptibility and resistance**—Apparently universal susceptibility.

9. **Methods of control**—

   A. *Preventive measures:*

   1) Avoid ingestion of inadequately cooked marine fish. Heating to 60°C (140°F) for 10 minutes or freezing at -20°C (-4°F) for at least 5 days kills the larvae. The latter control method is used with success in the Netherlands.
   2) Candling is recommended for fishery products in which parasites can be found.
   3) Cleaning (evisceration) of fish as soon as possible after they are caught reduces the number of larvae penetrating into the muscles from the mesenteries.

   B. *Control of patient, contacts and the immediate environment:*

   1) Report to local health authority: Not ordinarily justifiable, Class 5 (see Preface). However, a case or cases recognized in an area not previously known to be involved, or any in an area where control measures are in effect, should be reported.

2) Isolation: None.
3) Concurrent disinfection: None.
4) Quarantine: None.
5) Immunization of contacts: None.
6) Investigation of contacts and source of infection: None. Examination of others possibly exposed at the same time may be productive.
7) Specific treatment: Gastroscopic removal of larvae; excision of lesions.

C. *Epidemic measures:* None.

D. *Disaster implications:* None.

E. *International measures:* None.

ANTHRAX　　　　　　　　　　　　　ICD-9 022
(Malignant pustule, Malignant edema, Woolsorters' disease, Ragpickers' disease, Charbon)

1. Identification—An acute bacterial disease usually affecting the skin, but may rarely involve the mediastinum or intestinal tract. In cutaneous anthrax, itching of an exposed skin surface occurs first, followed by a lesion which becomes papular, then vesiculated, and in 2-6 days develops into a depressed black eschar. The eschar is usually surrounded by mild to moderate edema, sometimes with small secondary vesicles. Pain is unusual and, if present, is due to edema or secondary infection. The lesion has been confused with human orf (see Orf virus disease). Untreated infections may spread to regional lymph nodes and to the bloodstream with an overwhelming septicemia. Involvement of the meninges can occur. Untreated cutaneous anthrax has a case fatality rate between 5 and 20%, but with effective antibiotic therapy, few deaths occur. The lesion evolves through typical local changes even after the initiation of antibiotic therapy.

Initial symptoms of inhalation anthrax are mild and nonspecific, resembling a common URI; acute symptoms of respiratory distress, x-ray evidence of mediastinal widening, fever and shock follow in 3-5 days, with death shortly thereafter. Intestinal anthrax is rare and more difficult to recognize, except that it tends to occur in explosive outbreaks; abdominal distress is followed by fever, signs of septicemia and death in the typical case. An oropharyngeal form of primary disease has been described.

Laboratory confirmation is made by demonstration of the causative organism in blood, lesions or discharges by direct Gram-stained smears or by culture or inoculation of mice, guinea pigs or rabbits. The bacillus can be identified by FA techniques. Fourfold or greater titer rise in paired sera by electrophoretic immunotrans blots or ELISA may be helpful.

2. **Infectious agent**—*Bacillus anthracis,* a Gram-positive, encapsulated, spore-forming, nonmotile rod.

3. **Occurrence**—An infrequent and sporadic human infection in most industrial countries. Primarily an occupational hazard of workers who process hides, hair (especially from goats), bone and bone products and wool; and of veterinarians and agriculture and wildlife workers who handle infected animals. Human anthrax is endemic in those agricultural regions of the world where anthrax in animals is common, including countries in Europe, Asia and Africa. New areas of infection in livestock may develop through introduction of animal feed containing contaminated bone meal. Environmental events such as floods may provoke epizootics.

4. **Reservoir**—Animals, including wildlife such as elephants, hippopotami and impalas; cattle, sheep, goats and other animals with septicemic infection shed postmortem. The spores of *B. anthracis,* which are very resistant to adverse environmental conditions and disinfection, may remain viable in contaminated soil areas for many years after the source-animal infection has terminated. There is evidence of environmental multiplication of *B. anthracis* under favorable soil pH, nutrient and temperature conditions. Dried or otherwise processed skins and hides of infected animals may harbor the spores for years.

5. **Mode of transmission**—The infection of the skin is by contact with (1) tissues of animals (cattle, sheep, goats, horses, pigs and others) dying of the disease and possibly by biting flies which had partially fed on such animals; (2) contaminated hair, wool, hides, or products made from them such as drums, brushes, etc.; or (3) soil associated with infected animals, or contaminated bone meal used in gardening. Inhalation anthrax results from inhalation of spores. Intestinal and oropharyngeal anthrax arise from ingestion of contaminated meat; there is no evidence that milk from infected animals transmits anthrax. The disease spreads among grazing animals through contaminated soil and feed, and among omnivorous and carnivorous animals through contaminated meat, bone meal or other feeds. Vultures have been reported to spread the organism from one area to another. Accidental infections may occur among laboratory workers.

6. **Incubation period**—Two to 7 days; most cases occur within 48 hours after exposure.

7. **Period of communicability**—No evidence of transmission from

person to person. Articles and soil contaminated with spores may remain infective for years.

8. Susceptibility and resistance—Uncertain; there is some evidence of inapparent infection among persons in frequent contact with the infectious agent; second attacks have not been documented.

9. Methods of control—

A. *Preventive measures:*

1) Immunize high-risk persons with a cell-free vaccine prepared from a culture filtrate containing the protective antigen (available in the USA from the Michigan Department of Public Health, Division of Bio Products, 3500 N. Logan—Box 30035, Lansing MI 48909). This is effective in preventing cutaneous and possibly inhalation anthrax; it is recommended for veterinarians and those handling potentially contaminated industrial raw materials.

2) Educate employees handling potentially contaminated articles about personal cleanliness, modes of anthrax transmission and care of skin abrasions.

3) Control dust and properly ventilate in hazardous industries, especially those which handle raw animal fibers. Maintain continuing medical supervision of employees, with prompt medical care of all suspicious skin lesions. Use protective clothing and adequate facilities for washing and changing clothes after work. Locate eating facilities away from places of work. Vaporized formaldehyde has been employed for terminal disinfection of textile mills contaminated with *B. anthracis.*

4) Thoroughly wash, disinfect or sterilize hair, wool or hides, and bone meal or other feed of animal origin prior to processing.

5) Do not sell the hides of animals exposed to anthrax nor use their carcasses as food or feed supplements (i.e., as bone or blood meal).

6) If anthrax is suspected, do not necropsy the animal but aseptically collect a jugular blood sample for culture. Avoid contamination of the area. If a necropsy is inadvertently performed, autoclave or incinerate all instruments or materials. Deeply bury carcasses at the site of death if possible; do not burn on open field. Decontaminate soil seeded by carcasses or discharges with 5% lye, anhydrous calcium oxide (quicklime), or bury deeply with the carcass. In burial, cover carcass with quicklime.

7) Promptly vaccinate and annually revaccinate all animals at risk. Treat symptomatic animals with penicillin or tetra-

cyclines; vaccinate these animals after cessation of therapy. Treatment in lieu of vaccination may be used for animals exposed to a discrete source of infection such as a contaminated commercial feed.

8) Control effluents and trade wastes of rendering plants handling potentially infected animals and those from factories that manufacture products from hair, wool or hides likely to be contaminated.

B. *Control of patient, contacts and the immediate environment:*

1) Report to local health authority: Case report obligatory in most states and countries, Class 2A (see Preface). Also report to appropriate livestock or agriculture authority.

2) Isolation: Drainage/secretion precautions for duration of illness for cutaneous and inhalation anthrax.

3) Concurrent disinfection: Of discharges from lesions and articles soiled therewith. Spores require steam sterilization or burning to assure destruction. Terminal cleaning.

4) Quarantine: None.

5) Immunization of contacts: None.

6) Investigation of contacts and source of infection: Search for history of exposure to infected animals or animal products and trace to place of origin. In a manufacturing plant, inspect for adequacy of preventive measures as outlined in 9A, above.

7) Specific treatment: Penicillin is the drug of choice and is given for 5 to 7 days. Tetracyclines, erythromycin and chloramphenicol are also effective.

C. *Epidemic measures:* Outbreaks may be an occupational hazard of animal husbandry: The occasional epidemics in the USA are local industrial outbreaks among employees who work with animal products, especially goat hair. Outbreaks related to the handling and consumption of meat from infected cattle have occurred in Asia, Africa and the USSR.

D. *Disaster implications:* None, except in case of floods in previously infected areas.

E. *International measures:* Sterilize imported bone meal before use as animal feed. Disinfect wool, hair, hides and other products when indicated and practical; formaldehyde, ethylene oxide and cobalt irradiation have been used.

ARTHROPOD-BORNE VIRAL DISEASES
(Arboviral Diseases)

Introduction

A large number of arboviruses are known to produce clinical and subclinical infection in man, and the number is growing rapidly. There are four main clinical syndromes:

(1) An acute CNS disease ranging in severity from mild aseptic meningitis to encephalitis with coma, paralysis and death;

(2) acute benign fevers of short duration, many resembling dengue fever with and without an exanthem, although on occasion some may give rise to a more serious illness with CNS involvement or hemorrhages;

(3) hemorrhagic fevers, which include acute febrile diseases with extensive hemorrhagic involvement, external or internal, frequently serious, and associated with capillary leakage, shock and significantly high case fatality rates (all of them may cause liver damage, but in yellow fever, hepatic damage is most severe and is accompanied by frank jaundice); and

(4) polyarthritis and rash, with or without fever and of variable duration, benign or with arthralgic sequelae lasting several weeks to months. These clinical features form the basis of presentation in these chapters.

Most of these viruses cause zoonoses, and infections of people are accidentally acquired through an arthropod vector, with man an unimportant host in the cycle. In the presence of viremia and a suitable vector, a few may become epidemic. Sometimes man can serve as the principal source of virus amplification and vector infection. Most of the viruses are mosquito-borne, several are tick-borne and others are sandfly-borne. A few are transmitted by *Culicoides* species (midges, gnats). Laboratory infections occur, some by aerosols.

Although the agents differ, these diseases share common epidemiologic factors (related chiefly to the vector) in their transmission cycles which are important in control. Consequently, the selected diseases under each clinical syndrome are arranged in four groups: mosquito- and midge-borne, tick-borne, sandfly-borne and unknown. Diseases of major importance are described individually, or in groups with similar clinical and epidemiologic features.

Viruses believed to be associated with human disease are listed in the accompanying table with type of vector, the predominant character of recognized disease and the geographic distribution. In some instances, observed cases are too few to be certain of the usual clinical reaction. Some have been recognized only through laboratory-acquired exposure. None is included where evidence of human infection is based solely on serologic survey; otherwise, the number would be much greater. Those which cause diseases covered in subsequent chapters are marked on the table by an asterisk; some of the less important or less well-studied are not discussed in the text.

Over 100 viruses presently classified as arboviruses produce disease in man. Most of these are further classified by antigenic relationships, morphology and replicative mechanisms into families and genera, of which Togaviridae *(Alphavirus)* and Flaviviridae *(Flavivirus)* are the best known. These two genera contain some agents causing predominantly encephalitis and others causing predominantly other febrile illnesses. Alphaviruses are mosquito-borne; flaviviruses include both mosquito-borne and tick-borne agents and some agents without recognized vectors. Viruses of the family Bunyaviridae and of several other groups produce principally febrile diseases or hemorrhagic fevers.

DISEASES IN MAN CAUSED BY ARTHROPOD-BORNE VIRUSES

Virus Group	Name of Virus	Vector	Disease in Man	Where Found
TOGAVIRIDAE *Alphavirus*				
	*Chikungunya	Mosquito	Fever, arthritis, hemorrhagic fever	Africa, SE Asia, Philippines
	*Eastern equine encephalomyelitis	Mosquito	Encephalitis	Americas
	Everglades	Mosquito	Encephalitis	Florida (USA)
	*Mayaro (Uruma)	Mosquito	Fever, arthritis, rash	S America
	Mucambo	Mosquito	Fever	S America
	*O'nyong-nyong	Mosquito	Fever, arthralgia	Africa
	*Ross River	Mosquito	Arthritis, rash	Australia, S Pacific
	Semliki Forest	Mosquito	Encephalitis	Africa
	*Sindbis (Ockelbo)	Mosquito	Fever, arthritis, rash	Africa, India, SE Asia, Philippines, Australia, USSR, Europe
	Tonate	Mosquito	Fever	S America
	*Venezuelan equine encephalomyelitis	Mosquito	Fever, encephalitis	Americas
	*Western equine encephalomyelitis	Mosquito	Encephalitis	Americas

*Asterisked groups and viruses are discussed in the text. See index for page numbers.

DISEASES IN MAN CAUSED BY ARTHROPOD-BORNE VIRUSES

Virus Group	Name of Virus	Vector	Disease in Man	Where Found
FLAVIVIRIDAE *Flavivirus*				
	Apoi	Unknown	Encephalitis	Japan
	*Banzi	Mosquito	Fever	Africa
	Rio Bravo (Bat salivary gland)	Unknown	Encephalitis, aseptic meningitis	USA, Trinidad
	Bussuquara	Mosquito	Fever	S America
	Dakar bat	Unknown	Fever	Africa
	*Dengue 1,2,3 and 4	Mosquito	Fever, hemorrhagic fever, rash	Throughout tropics
	Ilheus	Mosquito	Fever, encephalitis	S & Central America
	*Japanese encephalitis	Mosquito	Encephalitis	Asia, Pacific Is.
	Koutango	Mosquito	Fever, rash	Africa
	*Kunjin	Mosquito	Fever, encephalitis	Australia, Sarawak
	*Kyasanur Forest disease	Tick	Hemorrhagic fever, meningoencephalitis	India
	*Louping ill	Tick	Encephalitis	UK
	*Murray Valley encephalitis	Mosquito	Encephalitis	Australia, New Guinea
	Negishi	Unknown	Encephalitis	Japan
	*Omsk hemorrhagic fever	Tick	Hemorrhagic fever	USSR
	*Powassan	Tick	Encephalitis	Canada, USA, USSR

FLAVIVIRIDAE
Flavivirus (cont.)

*Rocio	Mosquito	Encephalitis	Brazil
Sepik	Mosquito	Fever	New Guinea
*Spondweni	Mosquito	Fever	Africa
*St. Louis encephalitis	Mosquito	Encephalitis, hepatitis	Americas
*Tick-borne encephalitis			
*European subtype	Tick	Encephalitis	Europe
*Far Eastern subtype	Tick	Encephalitis	Europe, Asia
Usutu	Mosquito	Fever	Africa
Wesselsbron	Mosquito	Fever	Africa, Asia
*West Nile	Mosquito	Fever, encephalitis, rash, hepatitis	Africa, Indian subcontinent, Middle East, Europe
*Yellow Fever	Mosquito	Hemorrhagic fever	Africa, S & Central America
*Zika	Mosquito	Fever	Africa, SE Asia

BUNYAVIRIDAE
Bunyavirus

*Anopheles A group			
*Group C			
Tacaiuma	Mosquito	Fever	S America
Apeu	Mosquito	Fever	S America
Caraparu	Mosquito	Fever	S America
Itaqui	Mosquito	Fever	S America
Madrid	Mosquito	Fever	Panamá

*Asterisked groups and viruses are discussed in the text. See index for page numbers.

DISEASES IN MAN CAUSED BY ARTHROPOD-BORNE VIRUSES

Virus Group	Name of Virus	Vector	Disease in Man	Where Found
BUNYAVIRIDAE				
Bunyavirus				
*Group C (*cont.*)	Marituba	Mosquito	Fever	S America
	Murutucu	Mosquito	Fever	S America
	Nepuyo	Mosquito	Fever	S and Central America
	Oriboca	Mosquito	Fever	S America
	Ossa	Mosquito	Fever	Panamá
	Restan	Mosquito	Fever	Trinidad
Bunyamwera group	*Bunyamwera	Mosquito	Fever	Africa
	Germiston	Mosquito	Fever	Africa
	Ilesha	Unknown	Fever, rash	Africa
	Shokwe	Mosquito	Fever	Africa
	Tensaw	Mosquito	Encephalitis	N America
	Wyeomyia	Mosquito	Fever	S America, Panamá
Bwamba Group	*Bwamba	Mosquito	Fever, rash	Africa
	Pongola	Mosquito	Fever	Africa
California Group	*California encephalitis	Mosquito	Encephalitis	USA
	Guaroa	Mosquito	Fever	S America, Panamá
	Inkoo	Mosquito	Fever	Scandinavia
	*Jamestown Canyon	Mosquito	Encephalitis	USA, Canada

BUNYAVIRIDAE

	Virus	Disease	Vector	Distribution
California Group (*cont.*)	*LaCrosse	Encephalitis	Mosquito	USA
	*Snowshoe hare	Encephalitis	Mosquito	USA, Canada, China, USSR Europe, Africa
	Tahyna	Fever	Mosquito	
Guama group	Catu	Fever	Mosquito	S America
	Guama	Fever	Mosquito	S America
Simbu group	*Oropouche	Fever, meningitis	*Culicoides*	S America, Panamá Africa, Asia
	Shuni	Fever	Mosquito, *Culicoides*	
Phlebovirus (*Sandfly fever group)	Alenquer	Fever	Unknown	S America
	Candiru	Fever	Unknown	S America
	Chagres	Fever	Phlebotomine	Central America
	SF-Naples type	Fever	Phlebotomine	Europe, Africa, Asia
	Punta Toro	Fever	Phlebotomine	Panamá
	Rift Valley fever	Fever, hemorrhage, encephalitis, retinitis	Mosquito	Africa
	SF-Sicilian type	Fever	Phlebotomine	Europe, Africa, Asia
	Toscana	Aseptic meningitis	Phlebotomine	Italy

*Asterisked groups and viruses are discussed in the text. See index for page numbers.

DISEASES IN MAN CAUSED BY ARTHROPOD-BORNE VIRUSES

Virus Group	Name of Virus	Vector	Disease in Man	Where Found
BUNYAVIRIDAE				
Nairovirus	*Nairobi sheep disease	Tick	Fever	Africa, India
	*Dugbe	Tick	Fever	Africa
	*Crimean-Congo hemorrhagic fever	Tick	Hemorrhagic fever	Europe, Africa Central Asia, Middle East
Unclassified	Bangui	Unknown	Fever, rash	Africa
	*Bhanja	Tick	Fever, encephalitis	Africa, Europe, Asia
	Issk-Kul (Keterah)	Tick	Fever	Asia
	Kasokero	Unknown	Fever	Africa
	Nyando	Mosquito	Fever	Africa
	Tamdy	Tick	Fever	USSR
	Tataguine	Mosquito	Fever, rash	Africa
	Wanowrie	Tick	Fever, hemorrhage	Middle East, Asia
REOVIRIDAE (*Orbivirus*)				
Bluetongue Group	Bluetongue	*Culicoides*	Fever	Worldwide
*Changuinola group	Changuinola	Phlebotomine	Fever	Central America

REOVIRIDAE (*Orbivirus*) (*cont.*)

*Kemerovo group			
	Kemerovo	Tick	Fever	USSR
	Lipovnik	Tick	Fever, meningitis	Europe
*Colorado Tick fever			
	Colorado tick fever	Tick	Fever	USA, Canada
Ungrouped			
	Orungo	Mosquito	Fever	Africa
RHABDOVIRIDAE			
Vesicular stomatitis group			
	*Vesicular stomatitis, Indiana & New Jersey	Phlebotomine	Fever, encephalitis	Americas
	Vesicular stomatitis, Alagoas	Phlebotomine	Fever	S America
	*Chandipura	Mosquito	Fever	India, Africa
	Piry	Mosquito	Fever	S America
LeDantec group			
	LeDantec	Unknown	Encephalitis	Senegal
ORTHOMYXOVIRIDAE			
	Dhori	Tick	Fever	Africa, Europe, Asia
	*Thogoto	Tick	Meningitis	Africa, Europe
NOT CLASSIFIED			
	*Quaranfil	Tick	Fever	Africa

*Asterisked groups and viruses are discussed in the text. See index for page numbers.

ARTHROPOD-BORNE VIRAL ARTHRITIS AND RASH

ICD-9 066.3

(Ross River disease, Epidemic polyarthritis and rash, Ross River fever)

1. **Identification**—A self-limited viral disease characterized by arthritis, primarily in the wrist, knee, ankle and small joints of the extremities, which lasts from days to months. In many patients, the onset of arthritis is followed in 1-10 days by a maculopapular rash, usually non-pruritic, affecting mainly the trunk and limbs. Buccal and palatal enanthema may occur. The rash resolves within 7 to 10 days, followed by a fine desquamation. Fever is sometimes absent. Cervical lymphadenopathy occurs frequently. Paresthesias and tenderness of palms and soles are present in a small percentage of cases.

Serologic tests show a rise in titer to alphaviruses; the virus may be isolated from the blood of acutely ill patients in mosquitoes or mosquito cell culture.

2. **Infectious agent**—Ross River virus; Sindbis, chikungunya and o'nyong-nyong viruses cause a similar illness and are described in the section on Arthropod-borne viral fevers.

3. **Occurrence**—Major outbreaks have occurred in Australia in the Murray Valley, coastal New South Wales, Northern Territory and Queensland, chiefly from January to May. Sporadic cases occur in other coastal regions of Australia and New Guinea. In 1979, a major outbreak occurred in Fiji and spread to other Pacific islands, including Tonga and the Cook Islands, with 15,000 cases in American Samoa in 1979-80.

4. **Reservoir**—Probably macropods (e.g., kangaroos); possibly other marsupials and wild rodents. Transovarian transmission in *Aedes vigilax* has been demonstrated in the laboratory, making an insect reservoir a possibility.

5. **Mode of transmission**—Transmitted by *Culex annulirostris, Ae.vigilax, Ae. polynesiensis* and other *Aedes* spp. of mosquitoes.

6. **Incubation period**—Three to 11 days.

7. **Period of communicability**—No evidence of transmission from person to person.

8. **Susceptibility and resistance**—Recovery is universal and followed by lasting immunity; second attacks are unknown. Inapparent infections are common, especially in children, among whom the disease is rare. Arthritis occurs more frequently among adult females and in persons with HLA DR7 Gm $a^+x^+b^+$ phenotypes.

9. **Methods of control—**

A. *Preventive measures:* The general measures applicable to mosquito-borne viral encephalitides (see I9A 1-5 and 8).

B. *Control of patient, contacts and the immediate environment:*

1) Report to local health authority: In selected endemic areas; in many countries not a reportable disease, Class 3B (see Preface).
2) Isolation: Protect patients from mosquitoes to avoid further transmission.
3) Concurrent disinfection: None.
4) Quarantine: None.
5) Immunization of contacts: None.
6) Investigation of contacts and source of infection: Search for unreported or undiagnosed cases where the patient had lived during the 2 weeks prior to onset; check all family members serologically.
7) Specific treatment: None.

C. *Epidemic measures:* Same as for arthropod-borne viral fevers (see Dengue, 9C).

D. *Disaster implications:* None.

E. *International measures:* WHO Collaborating Centres (see Preface).

ARTHROPOD-BORNE VIRAL ENCEPHALITIDES
I. MOSQUITO-BORNE ARBOVIRAL ENCEPHALITIDES   ICD-9 062

EASTERN EQUINE ENCEPHALITIS, WESTERN EQUINE ENCEPHALITIS LACROSSE ENCEPHALITIS, JAMESTOWN CANYON ENCEPHALITIS, CALIFORNIA ENCEPHALITIS, JAPANESE ENCEPHALITIS, MURRAY VALLEY ENCEPHALITIS (AUSTRALIAN ENCEPHALITIS), ST. LOUIS ENCEPHALITIS AND ROCIO ENCEPHALITIS

1. **Identification—**A group of acute inflammatory viral diseases of short duration involving parts of the brain, spinal cord and meninges. Signs and symptoms are similar, but vary in severity and rate of progression. Most infections are asymptomatic; mild cases often occur as febrile headache or aseptic meningitis. Severe infections are usually

marked by acute onset, headache, high fever, meningeal signs, stupor, disorientation, coma, spasticity, tremors, occasionally convulsions (especially in infants) and spastic, but rarely flaccid, paralysis. Case fatality rates range from 0.3 to 60%; those with Japanese (JE), Murray Valley (MV) and eastern equine (EEE) encephalitis viral infections are highest. Neurologic sequelae occur with variable frequency depending on age and infecting agent; they tend to be most severe in infants infected with JE, WEE and EEE viruses; the elderly are at greatest risk of encephalitis after St. Louis encephalitis (SLE) or EEE virus infection. LaCrosse virus infections generally occur in children <15 years of age; seizure disorder may follow. Mild leukocytosis is usual in these diseases; leukocytes in the CSF range from 50 to 500/cu mm, occasionally ≥1,000/cu mm in infants infected with EEE virus.

These diseases require differentiation from the tick-borne encephalitides (see below); encephalitic and nonparalytic poliomyelitis; rabies; mumps meningoencephalitis; lymphocytic choriomeningitis; aseptic meningitis due to enteroviruses; herpes encephalitis; postvaccinal or postinfection encephalitides; and bacterial, mycoplasmal, protozoal, leptospiral and mycotic meningitides or encephalitides. Venezuelan equine encephalomyelitis, Rift Valley fever and West Nile viruses, producing primarily arthropod-borne viral fever (see Arthropod-borne viral fevers), are sometimes responsible for encephalitis.

Specific identification is made by demonstrating specific IgM in acute phase serum or CSF, or antibody rises between early and late specimens of serum by neutralization, CF, HI, FA, ELISA or other serologic tests. Cross-reactions may occur within a virus group. Virus may sometimes be isolated by inoculation of suckling mice or cell culture with the brain tissue of fatal cases, rarely with blood or CSF after symptoms have appeared; histopathologic changes are not specific for individual viruses.

2. **Infectious agents**—Each disease is caused by a specific virus in one of three groups: EEE and western equine encephalomyelitis (WEE) in the alphaviruses; JE, Kunjin, MV encephalitis, St. Louis (SLE) and Rocio in the flaviviruses; and LaCrosse, California encephalitis, Jamestown Canyon and snowshoe hare viruses in the California group of bunyaviruses.

3. **Occurrence**—EEE is recognized in eastern and north central USA and adjacent Canada, in scattered areas of Central and S America and in the Caribbean Islands; WEE in western and central USA, Canada and Argentina; JE in western Pacific Islands from Japan to the Philippines and in many areas of eastern Asia from Korea to Indonesia, China and India with the vectors often breeding in rice paddies; Kunjin and MV encephalitis in parts of Australia and New Guinea; SLE in most of the USA, Ontario (Canada) and also in Trinidad, Jamaica, Panamá and Brazil; Rocio encephalitis in Brazil. LaCrosse encephalitis is acquired from forest- and tire-breeding mosquitoes in the USA. Cases occur in temperate latitudes in summer and early fall, and are commonly limited to areas and years of

high temperature and many mosquitoes.

4. **Reservoir**—LaCrosse virus overwinters in *Aedes* eggs; the true reservoir or means of winter carry-over for other viruses is unknown, possibly in birds, rodents, bats, reptiles, amphibians or surviving mosquito eggs or adults, probably differing for each virus.

5. **Mode of transmission**—By the bite of infective mosquitoes. Most important vectors are: for EEE in the USA and Canada—probably *Culiseta melanura* from bird to bird, and one or more *Aedes* and *Coquillettidia* spp. from birds or animals to man; for WEE in western USA and Canada—*Culex tarsalis;* for JE—*C. tritaeniorhynchus, C. vishnui* complex, and also *C. gelidus* in the tropics; for MV—probably *C. annulirostris;* for SLE in the USA—*C. tarsalis,* the *C. pipiens-quinquefasciatus* complex, and *C. nigripalpus;* for LaCrosse—*Ae. triseriatus.* Mosquitoes acquire the infection from wild birds or small mammals (LaCrosse virus), but pigs are important for JE. LaCrosse virus is transovarially and venereally transmitted in *Ae. triseriatus.*

6. **Incubation period**—Usually 5-15 days.

7. **Period of communicability**—Not directly transmitted from person to person. Virus is not usually demonstrable in the blood of man after onset of disease. Mosquitoes remain infective for life. Viremia in birds usually lasts 2-5 days, but may be prolonged in bats, reptiles and amphibia, particularly if interrupted by hibernation. Horses develop active disease with the two equine viruses and with JE, but viremia is rarely present in high titer or for long periods; therefore, man and horses are uncommon sources of mosquito infection.

8. **Susceptibility and resistance**—Susceptibility to clinical disease is usually highest in infancy and old age; inapparent or undiagnosed infection is more common at other ages. Susceptibility varies with virus; e.g, LaCrosse encephalitis is usually a disease of children, while severity of SLE increases with age. Infection results in homologous immunity. In highly endemic areas, adults are largely immune to local strains by reason of mild and inapparent infection; susceptibles are mainly children.

9. **Methods of control**—

   A. *Preventive measures:*

      1) Educate the public as to mode of spread and control.
      2) Destroy larvae and eliminate breeding places of known and suspected vector mosquitoes.
      3) Kill mosquitoes by space and residual spraying of human habitations (see Malaria, 9A1).
      4) Screen sleeping and living quarters; use mosquito bednets.

5) Avoid exposure to mosquitoes during hours of biting, or use repellents (see Malaria, 9A4).

6) In endemic areas, immunize domestic animals or house them away from living quarters; e.g., pigs in JE-endemic areas.

7) Mouse-brain inactivated vaccine against JE encephalitis for children is used in Japan, Korea, Thailand, India and Taiwan; cell culture vaccines are used in Taiwan and China. A vaccine against JE is expected to become available in the USA in spring 1990, for travelers to endemic areas.

   For those under continued intensive exposure, EEE and WEE vaccines (inactivated, dried) are available from the U.S. Army Medical Research Institute for Infectious Disease, Fort Detrick, Frederick MD.

8) Passively protect accidentally exposed laboratory workers by human or animal immune serum.

B. *Control of patient, contacts and the immediate environment:*

1) Report to local health authority: Case report obligatory in most states (USA) and in some countries, Class 2A (see Preface). Report under the appropriate disease; or as encephalitis, other forms; or as aseptic meningitis, with etiology or clinical type specified when known.

2) Isolation: None; virus is not usually found in blood, secretions or discharges during clinical disease. Enteric precautions are appropriate until enterovirus meningoencephalitis (q.v.) is ruled out.

3) Concurrent disinfection: None.

4) Quarantine: None.

5) Immunization of contacts: None.

6) Investigation of contacts and source of infection: Search for missed cases and the presence of vector mosquitoes; test for viremia in both febrile and asymptomatic family members. Primarily a community problem (see 9C, below).

7) Specific treatment: None.

C. *Epidemic measures:*

1) Identification of infection among horses or birds and recognition of human cases in the community have epidemiologic value by indicating frequency of infection and areas involved. Immunization of horses probably does not limit spread of the virus in the community.

2) Fogging or spraying from aircraft with suitable insecticides has shown promise for aborting urban epidemics of SLE.

D. **Disaster implications:** None.

E. **International measures:** Spray with insecticide those airplanes arriving from recognized areas of prevalence. WHO Collaborating Centres (see Preface).

II. TICK-BORNE ARBOVIRAL ENCEPHALITIDES   ICD-9 063
FAR EASTERN TICK-BORNE ENCEPHALITIS (RUSSIAN SPRING-SUMMER ENCEPHALITIS), CENTRAL EUROPEAN TICK-BORNE ENCEPHALITIS, LOUPING ILL, POWASSAN VIRUS ENCEPHALITIS

1. **Identification**—A group of viral diseases clinically resembling the mosquito-borne encephalitides, except that the Far Eastern tick-borne subtype is often associated with focal epilepsy, flaccid paralysis (particularly of the shoulder girdle) and other residua. Central European tick-borne encephalitis (diphasic milk fever or diphasic meningoencephalitis) has a longer course, averaging 3 weeks. The initial febrile stage is not associated with symptoms referable to the CNS, and a second phase of fever and meningoencephalitis follows 4-10 days after apparent recovery; fatality and severe residua are less frequent than for the Far Eastern tick-borne disease. Louping ill in man also has a diphasic pattern and is relatively mild.

Specific identification is made by demonstration of specific IgM in acute phase serum or CSF, by serologic tests of paired sera, or by isolation of virus from blood during acute illness by inoculation of suckling mice or tissue culture. Common serologic tests do not differentiate members of this group but do distinguish the group from most other similar diseases.

2. **Infectious agents**—A complex within the flaviviruses; minor antigenic differences exist, more with Powassan than others, but viruses causing these diseases are closely related.

3. **Occurrence**—Disease of the CNS caused by this virus complex is distributed spottily over much of the USSR, other parts of eastern and central Europe, Scandinavia and the UK. In general, the Far Eastern subtype has a more eastern or Asian distribution, diphasic meningoencephalitis predominates in Europe, while louping ill occurs chiefly in the British Isles, but recently has been recognized in Western Europe. Powassan virus is present in Canada, the USA and the USSR. Seasonal incidence depends on activity of the tick vectors. *Ixodes persulcatus* is usually active in spring and early summer, while infections from *I. ricinus* bites occur in both early summer and early autumn, and infections from *I. cookei* bites peak from June to September.

Areas of highest incidence are those where man has intimate association with large numbers of infected ticks, generally in rural or forested areas, but also in some urban populations. Local epidemics of central European tick-borne encephalitis have occurred among persons consuming unpasteurized milk and dairy products from goats and sheep, thus the name diphasic milk fever. The age pattern varies widely in different regions and is influenced by opportunity for exposure to ticks, consumption of milk from infected animals, or by previously acquired immunity. Laboratory infections are common, some with serious sequelae, others fatal.

4. **Reservoir**—The tick or a combination of tick and mammal appears to be the true reservoir; transovarian tick passage of some viruses in the USSR has been demonstrated. Sheep and deer are the hosts most involved in louping ill. Rodents and sometimes other mammals and birds give rise to tick infections in Europe and Asia.

5. **Mode of transmission**—By the bite of infective ticks, or by consumption of milk from certain infected animals. *Ixodes persulcatus* is the principal vector in eastern USSR, and *I. ricinus* in western USSR and other parts of Europe; the latter is also the vector of louping ill of sheep in Scotland. *I. cookei* is the principal vector in eastern Canada and the USA. Larval ticks usually ingest virus by feeding on rodents, sometimes other mammals and birds. Adult ticks may acquire infection from man. Raw milk may be a vehicle for diphasic meningoencephalitis.

6. **Incubation period**—Usually 7-14 days.

7. **Period of communicability**—Not directly transmitted from person to person. A tick infected at any stage remains infective for life. Viremia in a variety of vertebrates may last for several days; in man, up to 7-10 days.

8. **Susceptibility and resistance**—Both sexes and all ages are susceptible. Infection, whether inapparent or overt, leads to immunity.

9. **Methods of control**—

    A. *Preventive measures:*

       1) See Lyme disease, 9A1-2, for measures against ticks.
       2) Inactivated virus vaccines have been used extensively in central Europe and the USSR with reported safety and effectiveness.
       3) Boil or pasteurize milk of susceptible animals in areas where diphasic meningoencephalitis occurs.

    B. *Control of patient, contacts and the immediate environment:*

       1) Report to local health authority: In selected endemic areas; in most countries not a reportable disease, Class 3B (see Preface).
       2) Isolation: None, after tick removal.

3) Concurrent disinfection: None.
4) Quarantine: None.
5) Immunization of contacts: None.
6) Investigation of contacts and source of infection: Search for missed cases, presence of tick vectors and animals excreting virus in milk.
7) Specific treatment: None.

C. **Epidemic measures:** See Lyme disease, 9C.

D. **Disaster implications:** None.

E. **International measures:** WHO Collaborating Centres (see Preface).

ARTHROPOD-BORNE VIRAL FEVERS

I. MOSQUITO-BORNE AND CULICOIDES-BORNE ARBOVIRAL FEVERS:

Yellow fever, dengue and chikungunya are presented separately.

I A. VENEZUELAN EQUINE   ICD-9 066.2 ENCEPHALOMYELITIS VIRUS DISEASE

(Venezuelan equine encephalitis, Venezuelan equine fever)

1. **Identification**—Clinical manifestations of this viral infection are influenza-like, with an abrupt onset of severe headache, chills, fever, myalgia, retro-orbital pain, nausea and vomiting. Conjunctival and pharyngeal injection are the only physical signs. Most infections are relatively mild, with symptoms lasting 3-5 days. Some cases may have a diphasic fever course; after a few days of fever, particularly in children, CNS involvement may appear, ranging from somnolence to frank encephalitis with disorientation, convulsions, paralysis, coma and death. During the 1971 Texas outbreak, 3 of 40 patients studied had severe CNS involvement, with sequelae of personality change and/or paralysis.

Diagnosis is suspected on clinical and epidemiologic grounds (exposure in an area where an equine epizootic occurred), and confirmed by virus isolation, rise in antibody titer, or detection of specific IgM. Virus can be isolated in cell culture from blood and nasopharyngeal washings during the first 72 hours of symptoms; acute and convalescent sera 10 days apart reveal a rising antibody titer. Laboratory infections occur unless proper containment facilities are used.

2. **Infectious agent**—Venezuelan equine encephalomyelitis virus, an alphavirus, with epizootic and enzootic serotypes.

3. **Occurrence**—Endemic in northern S America, Trinidad, Central America and Panamá, Mexico and Florida. The disease appears as epizootics, principally in northern and western S America; the epizootic in 1970-71 spread through Central America into the USA.

4. **Reservoir**—A rodent-mosquito cycle maintains the enzootic serotypes. Epizootic serotypes are transmitted in a cycle involving horses, which serve as the major source of virus to provide large-scale infection of mosquitoes, which in turn infect man.

5. **Mode of transmission**—By the bite of an infected mosquito. Viruses of the complex have been isolated from a number of genera, including *Culex (Melanoconion), Aedes, Mansonia, Psorophora, Haemagogus, Sabethes* and *Anopheles*. Laboratory infections by aerosols are common; there is no evidence of aerosol transmission from horses to man.

6. **Incubation period**—Usually 2-6 days; can be as short as one day.

7. **Period of communicability**—Human cases are infectious for mosquitoes for at least 72 hours; the mosquitoes probably transmit virus throughout life. Person-to-person transmission may occur but has not been proven. Virus is present in the pharyngeal secretions.

8. **Susceptibility and resistance**—Susceptibility is general. Mild infections and subsequent immunity occur frequently in endemic areas. Children are at greatest risk for developing CNS infection.

9. **Methods of control**—

A. *Preventive measures:*

1) Use general mosquito-control procedures.
2) Avoid forested endemic areas, especially at dusk and dawn.
3) An investigational attenuated virus vaccine (TC-83) for Venezuelan equine encephalomyelitis has been used effectively to protect laboratory workers and other adults at high risk. (Available in the USA from the U.S. Army Medical Research Institute for Infectious Disease, Fort Detrick, Frederick MD.) This vaccine proved to be effective in protecting horses during the 1970-71 epizootic; control of infection in horses effectively prevented additional human cases.

B. *Control of patient, contacts and the immediate environment:*

1) Report to local health authority: In selected endemic areas; in most countries not a reportable disease, Class 3B (see Preface).
2) Isolation: Blood/body fluid precautions. Patients should be treated in a screened room or in quarters treated with a residual insecticide for at least 5 days after onset, or until afebrile.
3) Concurrent disinfection: None.
4) Quarantine: None.
5) Immunization of contacts: None.
6) Investigation of contacts and source of infection: Search for unreported or undiagnosed cases.
7) Specific treatment: None.

C. *Epidemic measures:*

1) Determine extent of the infected areas; immunize horses and/or restrict their movement from the affected area.
2) Conduct a community survey to determine density of vector mosquitoes, their breeding places and effective control measures.
3) Establish an intensive, appropriate mosquito-control program.
4) Use repellents for those exposed to mosquitoes.
5) Identify the disease among horses and prevent mosquito feeding.

D. *Disaster implications:* None.

E. *International measures:* Vaccinate animals and restrict their movement from epizootic areas to areas free of the disease.

I B. OTHER MOSQUITO-BORNE AND *CULICOIDES*-BORNE FEVERS ICD-9 066.3

BUNYAMWERA VIRAL FEVER, BWAMBA VIRUS DISEASE, CHIKUNGUNYA VIRUS DISEASE, MAYARO VIRUS DISEASE (MAYARO FEVER, URUMA FEVER), O'NYONG-NYONG, RIFT VALLEY FEVER, WEST NILE FEVER, GROUP C VIRUS DISEASE, OROPOUCHE VIRUS DISEASE, SINDBIS (OCKELBO) VIRUS DISEASE AND OTHERS.

1. **Identification**—A group of febrile viral illnesses usually lasting a week or less, many of which are dengue-like (see table in the arbovirus introduction for mosquito-borne viruses). Usual onset is with headache, malaise, arthralgia or myalgia, and occasionally, nausea and vomiting; generally some conjunctivitis and photophobia. Fever may or may not be

diphasic (saddleback). Rashes are common in infections with West Nile, Mayaro, Sindbis, chikungunya and o'nyong-nyong viruses. Polyarthritis is a characteristic feature of infections with chikungunya, Sindbis and Mayaro viruses.

Minor hemorrhages have been attributed to chikungunya virus disease in SE Asia and India (see under Dengue hemorrhagic fever). In chikungunya virus disease, leukopenia is common; convalescence is frequently prolonged. Meningoencephalitis occasionally complicates West Nile and Oropouche virus infections. Rift Valley fever (RVF) cases may develop encephalitis, hemorrhage, or retinitis. Several group C viruses are reported to produce weakness in the lower limbs; they are rarely fatal, except in cases with encephalitis or hemorrhage especially from RVF. Epidemics of chikungunya, o'nyong-nyong, RVF and Oropouche fever may involve thousands of patients.

Serologic tests differentiate other fevers of viral or unknown origin, but chikungunya, o'nyong-nyong, and other alphaviruses are difficult to distinguish from one another. In some infections, a specific diagnosis is possible during the febrile period by virus isolation from blood by inoculation of suckling mice or cell culture. Laboratory infections occur with many of these viruses.

2. **Infectious agents**—Each disease is caused by a distinct virus of the same name as the disease. West Nile, Banzi, Kunjin, Spondweni and Zika viruses are flaviviruses; the closely related chikungunya and o'nyong-nyong, along with Mayaro and Sindbis, are alphaviruses. Group C bunyaviruses are Apeu, Caraparu, Itaqui, Madrid, Marituba, Murutucu, Nepuyo, Oriboca, Ossa and Restan. Oropouche is a Simbu group bunyavirus; RVF is in the sandfly fever group. Others in smaller groups are listed in the introductory table.

3. **Occurrence**—West Nile virus is present in Egypt, Israel, India, France and is probably widespread in parts of Africa, the northern Mediterranean area and Asia. Chikungunya virus is found in Africa, India, SE Asia and the Philippine Islands; Sindbis occurs throughout the Old World and in Australia; Rift Valley, o'nyong-nyong, Bwamba and Bunyamwera fevers thus far have been identified only in Africa. Mayaro and group C virus fevers occur in tropical S America, Panamá and Trinidad. Oropouche fever is found in Trinidad, Panamá and Brazil; Kunjin virus in Australia. Seasonal incidence depends on vector prevalence. Occurrence is primarily rural and forest, although occasionally RVF, Oropouche and chikungunya occur in explosive urban and suburban outbreaks.

4. **Reservoir**—Unknown for some viruses. Most are maintained in a continuous vertebrate-mosquito cycle in tropical environments. Oropouche virus may be transmitted by *Culicoides*. Birds are a source of mosquito infection for West Nile and Sindbis viruses, and rodents for group C viruses.

5. **Mode of transmission**—In most instances, by bite of an infective mosquito; for chikungunya—*Aedes aegypti* and possibly others; West Nile—*Culex univittatus* in Egypt and *C. pipiens molestus* in Israel; o'nyong-nyong—*Anopheles* spp. ; Mayaro—*Mansonia* and *Haemagogus* spp.; Sindbis virus—various *Culex* spp., especially *C. univittatus,* also *C. morsitans* and *Ae. communis;* Bunyamwera—*Aedes* spp.; group C viruses—species of *Aedes* and *Culex (Melanoconion).* For Rift Valley (in sheep and other animals)—a large number of potential vectors including various *Aedes* mosquitoes; *Ae. mcintoshi* may be infected transovarially and account for maintenance of RVF virus in enzootic foci. Many human infections of RVF are associated with handling infective material of animal origin during necropsy and butchering. *Culex pipiens* was implicated in a 1977 epidemic of RVF in Egypt with at least 600 deaths; mechanical transmission by hematophagous flies and transmission by aerosols or contact with highly infective blood may contribute to the explosive nature of RVF outbreaks.

6. **Incubation period**—Usually 3-12 days.

7. **Period of communicability**—Not directly transmitted from person to person. Infected mosquitoes probably transmit virus throughout life. Viremia, essential for vector infection, is present for many of these viruses during early clinical illness in man.

8. **Susceptibility and resistance**—Susceptibility appears to be general, in both sexes and throughout life. Inapparent infections and mild but undiagnosed disease are common. Infection leads to immunity; susceptibles in highly endemic areas are mainly young children.

9. **Methods of control**—

   A. *Preventive measures:*

      1) Follow the general measures applicable to mosquito-borne viral encephalitides (9A1-6 and 9A8). For RVF, precautions in care and handling of infected animals and their products, as well as human acute-phase blood, are important.

      2) An experimental inactivated cell culture vaccine is used in humans for RVF; live and inactivated vaccines are used for sheep, goats and cattle.

   B. *Control of patient, contacts and the immediate environment:*

      1) Report to local health authority: In selected endemic areas; in most countries not a reportable disease, Class 3B (see Preface). For RVF, notify WHO, FAO and the International Office of Epizootics (OIE) in Paris.

      2) Isolation: Blood and body fluid precautions. Keep patient in screened room or in quarters treated with an insecti-

cide for at least 5 days after onset or until afebrile. Blood of hemorrhagic RVF patients may be infectious.

3) Concurrent disinfection: None.
4) Quarantine: None.
5) Immunization of contacts: None.
6) Investigation of contacts and source of infection: Determine place of residence of patient during fortnight before onset. Search for unreported or undiagnosed cases.
7) Specific treatment: None.

C. *Epidemic measures:*

1) Conduct a community survey to determine density of vector mosquitoes, identify their breeding places and promote their elimination.
2) Use mosquito repellents for persons exposed because of occupation or otherwise to bites of vectors.
3) Identification of the disease among sheep and other animals (Rift Valley), and serologic surveys of birds (West Nile) or rodents (group C viruses) have epidemiologic value by indicating prevalence of infection and areas involved.
4) Immunize sheep, goats and cattle against RVF.

D. *Disaster implications:* None.

E. *International measures:* For RVF, vaccinate animals and restrict their movement from enzootic areas to those free from disease, and do not butcher sick animals; for others, none except enforcement of international agreements designed to prevent transfer of mosquitoes by ships, airplanes and land transport. WHO Collaborating Centres (see Preface).

II. TICK-BORNE ARBOVIRAL FEVERS   ICD-9 066.1
COLORADO TICK FEVER AND OTHER TICK-BORNE FEVERS

1. Identification—Colorado tick fever is an acute febrile, often diphasic, dengue-like viral disease with infrequent rash. A brief remission is usual, followed by a second bout of fever lasting 2-3 days; neutropenia and thrombocytopenia almost always occur on the fourth to fifth day of fever. Characteristically, it is a moderately severe disease, but rarely severe in children, with occasional encephalitis, myocarditis or tendency to bleed. Deaths are rare. Bhanja virus can cause severe neurologic disease and death; CNS infections also occur with Kemerovo and Thogoto viruses (the latter may cause hepatitis).

Laboratory confirmation of Colorado tick fever is made by isolation of virus from blood by inoculation of suckling mice or cell cultures or demonstration of antigen in erythrocytes by IF; CF and neutralizing antibodies do not appear for ≥2 weeks. Clinical manifestations of other types and diagnostic methods vary only slightly, except that serum is used for virus isolation.

2. **Infectious agents**—The viruses of Colorado tick fever and Nairobi sheep disease (Ganjam), and the Kemerovo, Lipovnik, Quaranfil, Bhanja, Thogoto and Dugbe viruses.

3. **Occurrence**—For Colorado tick fever, areas above 5000 feet elevation in western Canada and in Washington, Oregon, Idaho, Montana, California, Nevada, Utah, Wyoming, Colorado, New Mexico and S Dakota in the USA; it is endemic in occurrence and common in much of the affected area. Virus has been isolated from *Dermacentor andersoni* ticks in Alberta and British Columbia. Most frequent in adult males, but also affects women and children; seasonal incidence parallels the period of greatest tick activity. (Geographic distribution of other viruses is shown in the introductory table.)

4. **Reservoir**—For Colorado tick fever, small mammals, ground squirrels, porcupine, chipmunk and *Peromyscus* spp.; also ticks, principally *D. andersoni*.

5. **Mode of transmission**—To man by bite of an infective vector tick. In Colorado tick fever, immature ticks *(D. andersoni)* acquire infection by feeding on infected viremic animals; they remain infected transstadially and transmit virus to man by feeding as adult ticks.

6. **Incubation period**—Usually 4-5 days.

7. **Period of communicability**—Not directly transmitted from person to person, except by transfusion. The wildlife cycle is maintained by ticks, which remain infective throughout life. Virus is present in blood during the course of the fever and, in Colorado tick fever, in erythrocytes from 2-16 weeks or more after onset.

8. **Susceptibility and resistance**—Susceptibility apparently is universal. Second attacks are rare. Experimental reinfection is unsuccessful.

9. **Methods of control**—

   A. *Preventive measures:* Control of ticks and rodent hosts (see Lyme disease, 9A1-2).

   B. *Control of patient, contacts and the immediate environment:*

   1) Report to local health authority: In endemic areas (USA);

in most states and countries not a reportable disease, Class 3B (see Preface).

2) Isolation: Blood and body fluid precautions. No blood donations for 4 months.

3) Concurrent disinfection: None; remove ticks from patients.

4) Quarantine: None.

5) Immunization of contacts: None.

6) Investigation of contacts and source of infection: Identification of tick-infested areas.

7) Specific treatment: None.

C. **Epidemic measures:** Not applicable.

D. **Disaster implications:** None.

E. **International measures:** WHO Collaborating Centres (see Preface).

III. PHLEBOTOMINE-BORNE ARBOVIRAL FEVERS

SANDFLY FEVER   ICD-9 066.0
(Phlebotomus fever, Pappataci fever)

CHANGUINOLA VIRUS DISEASE   ICD-9 066.0
(Changuinola fever)

VESICULAR STOMATITIS VIRUS   ICD-9 066.8
DISEASE
(Vesicular stomatitis fever, VSV)

1. **Identification**—A group of arboviral diseases with a 3-4 day fever "grippe." Headache, with fever of 38.3°-39.5°C (101°-103°F), sometimes higher, retrobulbar pain on motion of the eyes, injected sclerae, malaise, nausea, and pain in the limbs and back are characteristic. Pharyngitis, oral mucosal vesicular lesions and cervical adenopathy are characteristic of VSV infections. Leukopenia is usual on the fourth to fifth day after onset of fever. Symptoms may be alarming, but death is unknown. Complete recovery may be preceded by prolonged mental depression. Encephalitis may occur following Toscana and Chandipura virus infections.

Diagnosis is suspected by the clinical picture and the occurrence of multiple similar cases. Diagnosis may be confirmed by detection of specific IgM, by titer rise in serologic tests or by isolation of virus from blood in newborn mice or in cell culture; for VSV infections, from throat swabs and vesicular fluid.

2. **Infectious agents**—The sandfly fever group of viruses; at least seven related immunologic types (Naples, Sicilian, Candiru, Chagres, Alenquer, Toscana and Punta Toro) have been isolated from man and differentiated. In addition, Changuinola virus (orbivirus) and vesicular

stomatitis virus of the Indiana type (rhabdovirus), both of which produce febrile disease in man, have been isolated from *Lutzomyia* species. Chandipura virus is a rhabdovirus.

3. **Occurrence**—In those parts of Europe, Africa and Asia where the vector exists; also in Central and S America, where closely related viral agents are present. A disease of subtropical and tropical areas with long periods of hot, dry weather in Europe and Africa, and rainforest in the New World tropics; distributed in a belt extending around the Mediterranean and eastward into Myanmar (Burma) and China. The disease is seasonal, between April and October, and is prone to appear as a disease of troops and travelers from nonendemic areas.

4. **Reservoir**—Principal reservoir is the man-sandfly complex; an animal reservoir is suspected, but not yet demonstrated, except that arboreal rodents and nonhuman primates may harbor New World sandfly fever viruses, and possibly vesicular stomatitis virus. Rodents (gerbils) have been implicated as a reservoir for Old World sandfly viruses. Transovarian transmission of some viruses has been demonstrated in phlebotomines.

5. **Mode of transmission**—By bite of an infective sandfly. The vector of the classic viruses is a small, hairy, blood-sucking midge (*Phlebotomus papatasi*, the common sandfly), which bites at night and has a limited flight range. Sandflies of the genus *Sergentomyia* also have been found to be infected and may be vectors. Members of the genus *Lutzomyia* are involved in Central and S America.

6. **Incubation period**—Up to 6 days, usually 3-4 days, rarely less.

7. **Period of communicability**—Virus is present in the blood of an infected person at least 24 hours before and 24 hours after onset of fever. Phlebotomines become infective about 7 days after biting an infected person and remain so for their normal life span of about one month.

8. **Susceptibility and resistance**—Susceptibility is essentially universal; homologous acquired immunity is possibly lasting. Relative resistance of native populations in sandfly areas is probably attributable to infection early in life.

9. **Methods of control**—

   A.   ***Preventive measures:*** Control of sandflies is the important consideration (see Leishmaniasis, Cutaneous, 9A1).

   B.   ***Control of patient, contacts and the immediate environment:***

       1)   Report to local health authority: In selected endemic areas; in most countries not a reportable disease, Class 3C (see Preface).

2) Isolation: None; prevent access of sandflies to infected individuals for the first few days of illness by very fine screening or mosquito bed nets (10-12 mesh/cm or 25-30 mesh/inch, aperture size not more than 0.085 cm or 0.035 inch) and by spraying quarters with insecticide.

3) Concurrent disinfection: None; destroy sandflies in the dwelling.

4) Quarantine: None.

5) Immunization of contacts: Not currently available.

6) Investigation of contacts and source of infection: In Old World, search for breeding areas of sandflies around dwellings, especially in rubble heaps, masonry cracks, and under stones.

7) Specific treatment: None.

C. *Epidemic measures:*

1) Educate the public on conditions leading to infection, and importance of preventing bites of sandflies by use of repellents while in infected areas, particularly after sundown.

2) Use insecticides to destroy sandflies in and about human habitations, community-wide.

D. *Disaster implications:* None.

E. *International measures:* WHO Collaborating Centres (see Preface).

ARTHROPOD-BORNE VIRAL HEMORRHAGIC FEVERS

I. MOSQUITO-BORNE DISEASES:
Dengue hemorrhagic fever and yellow fever are presented separately.

II. TICK-BORNE DISEASES:
II A. CRIMEAN-CONGO HEMORRHAGIC FEVER   ICD-9 065.0
(Central Asian hemorrhagic fever)

1. **Identification**—A viral disease with sudden onset of fever, malaise, weakness, irritability, headache, severe pain in limbs and loins, and

marked anorexia. Vomiting, abdominal pain and diarrhea occur occasionally. Flush on face and chest, and conjunctival injection develop early. Hemorrhagic enanthem of soft palate, uvula and pharynx, and a fine petechial rash spreading from the chest and abdomen to the body, are generally associated with the disease; occasionally, large purpuric areas are observed. There may be some bleeding from gums, nose, lungs, uterus and intestine, but in large amounts only in serious or fatal cases, and often associated with severe liver damage. Hematuria and albuminuria are common but usually not massive. Fever is constantly elevated for 5-12 days or may be biphasic; it falls by lysis. Convalescence is prolonged. Other findings are leukopenia, with lymphopenia more marked than neutropenia. Thrombocytopenia is common. The reported case fatality rate ranges from 2 to 50%. In the USSR, there are estimated to be five infections for each hemorrhagic case.

Diagnosis is made by isolation of virus from blood by inoculation of cell cultures or suckling mice. Serologic diagnosis is by ELISA, reverse passive hemagglutination inhibition, IFA, CF, immunodiffusion or plaque reduction neutralization test. Specific IgM may be present during the acute phase; convalescent sera often have low neutralization antibody titers.

2. **Infectious agent**—The Crimean-Congo hemorrhagic fever virus, genus *Nairovirus*.

3. **Occurrence**—Observed in the steppe regions of the western Crimea, on the Kersch Peninsula, in Kazakstan and Uzbekistan, in the Rostov-Don and Astrakhan regions of the USSR, as well as in Yugoslavia, Bulgaria, Iraq, the Arabian Peninsula, Pakistan, western China, tropical Africa and South Africa. Most patients are animal husbandry workers or medical personnel. Seasonal occurrence is from June to September, the period of vector activity. Virus or antibodies in man have been observed in several areas of Central and East Africa; hemorrhagic fever cases have been reported from South Africa.

4. **Reservoir**—In nature, believed to be hares, birds and *Hyalomma* spp. of ticks in the USSR and South Africa; reservoir hosts remain undefined in tropical Africa, but *Hyalomma* and *Boophilus* ticks, and insectivores and rodents may be involved. Domestic animals (sheep, goats and cattle) may act as amplifying hosts during epizootics.

5. **Mode of transmission**—By bite of infective adult *Hyalomma marginatum* or *H. anatolicum*. Immature ticks are believed to acquire infection from the animal hosts and by transovarian transmission. Nosocomial transmission from patients to medical workers after exposure to blood and secretions has been important in recent outbreaks; infection is also associated with butchering infected animals.

6. **Incubation period**—Three to 12 days.

7. **Period of communicability**—Usually not directly transmitted from person to person; however, nosocomial infections are common after exposure to blood and secretions. An infected tick probably remains so for life.

8. **Susceptibility and resistance**—Immunity for at least one year.

9. **Methods of control**—

A. *Preventive measures:* See Lyme disease, 9A, for preventive measures against ticks. No vaccine is available in the USA.

B. *Control of patient, contacts and the immediate environment:*

1) Report to local health authority: In selected epidemic areas; in most countries, not a reportable disease, Class 3B (see Preface).
2) Isolation: Blood and body fluid precautions.
3) Concurrent disinfection: Bloody discharges may be infective; decontaminate by heat or chlorine disinfectants.
4) Quarantine: None.
5) Immunization: None.
6) Investigation of contacts and source of infection: Search for missed cases and the presence of infective animals and possible vectors.
7) Specific treatment: Convalescent plasma with a high neutralizing antibody titer is reported to be useful.

C. *Epidemic measures:* See Lyme disease, 9C.

D. *Disaster implications:* None.

E. *International measures:* WHO Collaborating Centres (see Preface).

II B. OMSK HEMORRHAGIC FEVER   ICD-9 065.1
KYASANUR FOREST DISEASE   ICD-9 065.2

1. **Identification**—These two diseases have marked similarities: Onset is sudden, with chills, headache, fever, pain in lower back and limbs, and severe prostration; often associated with conjunctivitis, diarrhea and vomiting by the third or fourth day. A papulovesicular eruption on the soft palate, cervical lymphadenopathy and conjunctival suffusion are usually present. Confusion and encephalopathic symptoms may occur in patients with Kyasanur Forest Disease (KFD); often there is a biphasic course of illness and fever, and the CNS abnormalities develop after an afebrile period of one to two weeks. Severe cases are associated with hemorrhages but with no cutaneous rash. Bleeding occurs from gums, nose, GI tract, uterus and lungs (but rarely from the kidneys), sometimes

for many days and, when serious, results in shock and death; shock may also occur without manifest hemorrhage. Estimated case fatality rate is from 1 to 10%. Leukopenia and thrombocytopenia are marked. Febrile period ranges from 5 days to 2 weeks, at times with a secondary rise in the third week. Convalescence tends to be slow and prolonged.

Diagnosis is made by isolation of virus from blood in suckling mice or cell cultures for as long as 10 days following onset, or by serologic tests.

2. **Infectious agents**—The Omsk hemorrhagic fever (OHF) and KFD viruses are closely related; they belong to the tick-borne encephalitis-louping ill complex of flaviviruses and are similar antigenically to the other viruses in the complex.

3. **Occurrence**—In the Kyasanur Forest of the Shimoga and Kanara districts of Karnataka, India, principally in young adult males exposed in the forest during the dry season, from November to June. In 1983, there were 1155 cases with 150 deaths, the largest epidemic of KFD ever reported. OHF occurs in the entire forest steppe regions of western Siberia, within the Omsk, Novosibirsk, Kurgan and Tumen regions. Seasonal occurrence in each area coincides with vector activity. Laboratory infections are common with both viruses.

4. **Reservoir**—In KFD, probably rodents, shrews and monkeys; in OHF, rodents, muskrats and possibly ticks, since transovarian passage has been reported for other viruses of this complex.

5. **Mode of transmission**—By bite of infective ticks (especially nymphal ticks), probably *Haemaphysalis spinigera* in KFD. In OHF, infective ticks possibly are *Dermacentor reticulatus (pictus)* and *D. marginatus;* recent data implicate direct transmission from muskrat to man and from contaminated water to man, suggesting that ticks may not be the principal vectors.

6. **Incubation period**—Usually 3-8 days.

7. **Period of communicability**—Not directly transmitted from person to person. Infected ticks remain so for life.

8. **Susceptibility and resistance**—All ages and sexes are probably susceptible; previous infection leads to immunity.

9. **Methods of control**—See Tick-borne encephalitis and Lyme disease, sections 9. A formalinized mouse-brain virus vaccine has been reported for OHF; an experimental vaccine has been used to prevent KFD in endemic areas of India.

ASCARIASIS   ICD-9 127.0
(Roundworm infection, Ascaridiasis)

1. **Identification**—A helminthic infection of the small intestine generally associated with few or no symptoms. Live worms, passed in stools or occasionally from the mouth or nose, are often the first recognized sign of infection. Some patients have pulmonary manifestations (pneumonitis, Löffler's syndrome) caused by larval migration (mainly during reinfections) and characterized by wheezing, coughing, fever, blood eosinophilia and pulmonary infiltration. Heavy parasite burdens may aggravate nutritional deficiency. Serious complications, sometimes fatal, include bowel obstruction by a bolus of worms, particularly in children; or obstruction of a hollow viscus, such as bile duct, pancreatic duct and appendix, by one or more adult worms.

Diagnosis is made by identifying eggs in feces or adult worms passed from the anus, mouth or nose. Intestinal worms may be visualized by radiologic techniques; pulmonary involvement may be confirmed by identifying *Ascaris* larvae in the sputum or gastric washings.

2. **Infectious agent**—*Ascaris lumbricoides,* the large intestinal roundworm of man. *A. suum,* a similar parasite of pigs, rarely, if ever, develops to maturity in man, although it may cause larva migrans.

3. **Occurrence**—Common and worldwide, with greatest frequency in moist tropical countries where prevalence often exceeds 50%. The prevalence and intensity of infection are usually highest in children between 3-8 years. The distribution of *Ascaris* in the USA is limited to the southeastern states.

4. **Reservoir**—Man; ascarid eggs in soil.

5. **Mode of transmission**—By ingestion of infective eggs from soil contaminated with human feces or from uncooked produce contaminated with soil containing infective eggs, but not directly from person to person or from fresh feces. Transmission takes place mainly in the vicinity of the home, where children, in the absence of sanitary facilities, fecally pollute the area; heavy infections in children are frequently the result of ingesting soil. Contaminated soil may be carried long distances on feet or footwear into houses and conveyances; transmission of infection by dust is also possible.

Eggs reach the soil in the feces and then undergo development (embryonation); at summer temperatures they become infective after 2-3 weeks and may then remain infective for several months or years in favorable soil. The ingested embryonated eggs hatch in the intestinal lumen; the larvae penetrate the gut wall and reach the lungs via the circulatory system. Larvae grow and develop in the lungs; 9-10 days after infection they pass into the alveoli, ascend the trachea, and are swallowed to reach the small intestine 14-20 days after infection, where they grow to maturity, mate and begin egg-laying 45-60 days after ingestion. Eggs passed by gravid females are discharged in feces.

6. **Incubation period**—The life cycle requires 4-8 weeks to be completed; feces contain fertile eggs about 60 days after ingestion of embryonated eggs.

7. **Period of communicability**—As long as mature fertilized female worms live in the intestine. Usual life span of adult worms is 12 months; maximum may be up to 24 months. The female worm can produce more than 200,000 eggs a day. Under favorable conditions, embryonated eggs can remain viable in soil for years.

8. **Susceptibility and resistance**—Susceptibility is general.

9. **Methods of control**—

Λ. *Preventive measures:*

1) Educate the public in the use of toilet facilities.
2) Provide adequate facilities for proper disposal of feces and prevent soil contamination in areas immediately adjacent to houses, particularly in children's play areas.
3) In rural areas, construct privies which prevent dissemination of ascarid eggs through overflow, drainage, or otherwise. Treating human feces by composting for later use as fertilizer may not kill all eggs.
4) Encourage satisfactory hygienic habits on the part of children; in particular, train them to wash hands before eating and handling food.
5) In endemic areas, protect food from dirt. Food that has been dropped on the floor should not be eaten unless washed or reheated.

B. *Control of patient, contacts and the immediate environment:*

1) Report to local health authority: Official report not ordinarily justifiable, Class 5 (see Preface).
2) Isolation: None.
3) Concurrent disinfection: Sanitary disposal of feces.
4) Quarantine: None.
5) Immunization of contacts: None.
6) Investigation of contacts and source of infection: Determine others who should be treated. Environmental sources of infection should be sought, particularly on premises of affected families.
7) Specific treatment: Mebendazole (Vermox®) and albendazole (Zentel®) (also efficacious against *Trichuris trichiura* and hookworm, see each), but both are contraindicated during pregnancy. Erratic migration of ascarid

worms has been reported following mebendazole therapy; however, this may also occur with other medications, or spontaneously in heavy infections.

Pyrantel pamoate (Antiminth®, Combantrin®) is also effective in a single dose (also against hookworm, but not against *T. trichiura*). Piperazine is effective (and also against *Enterobius vermicularis,* see also). Finally, levamisole may also be used for infections with *Ascaris* only.

C. *Epidemic measures:* Survey for prevalence in highly endemic areas, educate in environmental sanitation and in personal hygiene, and provide treatment facilities.

D. *Disaster implications:* None.

E. *International measures:* None.

ASPERGILLOSIS   ICD-9 117.3

1. **Identification**—A fungal disease which may present with a variety of clinical syndromes produced by several of the *Aspergillus* species. Patients with asthma and allergy to the aspergilli may develop bronchial damage and intermittent bronchial plugging, a condition called "allergic bronchopulmonary aspergillosis." Saprophytic endobronchial colonization in patients with bronchitis or bronchiectasis may cause clumps of hyphae to form within ectatic bronchi, or a large mass of hyphae may fill a previously existing cavity (fungus ball or aspergilloma). An *Aspergillus* species may appear as a concomitant organism in a bacterial lung abscess or empyema. Pneumonic aspergillosis may occur, particularly in patients receiving cytotoxic or immunosuppressive therapy; it may disseminate to the brain, kidneys and other organs and is usually fatal. Invasion of blood vessels with thrombosis and infarction is characteristic of pneumonic and disseminated infection.

The organisms may infect the implantation site of a cardiac prosthetic valve. *Aspergillus* species are the most common causes of otomycosis; the fungi may colonize or cause invasive infection of the paranasal sinuses. Growing on certain foods, many isolates of *A. flavus* (and occasionally other species) will produce aflatoxins or other mycotoxins; these cause disease in animals and fish and are highly carcinogenic for experimental animals. An association between high aflatoxin levels in foods and hepatocellular cancer has been noted in Africa and SE Asia.

Among findings that suggest a diagnosis of allergic aspergillosis are wheal-and-flare response to scratch or intradermal test with *Aspergillus* antigens, episodes of bronchial plugging, eosinophilia, serum precipitating antibodies against *Aspergillus,* elevated serum concentration of IgE and transient pulmonary infiltrates. Saprophytic endobronchial colonization is diagnosed by culture or microscopic demonstration of *Aspergillus* mycelia in sputum or in plugs of expectorated hyphae. Serum precipitins to *Aspergillus* species antigens usually are present. Fungus ball of the lung can usually be diagnosed by chest x-ray and medical history. Diagnosis of invasive aspergillosis depends on microscopic demonstration of the *Aspergillus* mycelia in infected tissue; confirmation by culture is desirable.

2. **Infectious agents**—*Aspergillus fumigatus, A. niger* and *A. flavus* are the most common causes of aspergillosis, although other species have also been implicated. *A. fumigatus* causes most cases of fungus ball; *A. niger* is the usual cause of otomycosis.

3. **Occurrence**—Worldwide; uncommon and sporadic; no distinctive differences in incidence by race or sex.

4. **Reservoir**—Compost piles undergoing fermentation and decay are prominent reservoirs and sources of infection. Aspergilli are also found in hay which had been stored when damp, in decaying vegetation, in cereal grains (especially stored rice and corn) and in a variety of other foodstuffs stored under conditions which permit them to heat.

5. **Mode of transmission**—Inhalation of airborne conidia.

6. **Incubation period**—Probably a few days to weeks.

7. **Period of communicability**—Not transmitted from person to person.

8. **Susceptibility and resistance**—The ubiquity of *Aspergillus* species and the usual occurrence of the disease as a secondary infection suggest a high degree of resistance by healthy persons. Susceptibility is increased by immunosuppressive or cytotoxic therapy.

9. **Methods of control**—

   A. *Preventive measures:* Levels of aflatoxins in foods should be monitored and foods with high levels condemned.

   B. *Control of patient, contacts and the immediate environment:*

      1) Report to local health authority: Official report not ordinarily justifiable, Class 5 (see Preface).
      2) Isolation: None.
      3) Concurrent disinfection: Ordinary cleanliness. Terminal cleaning.
      4) Quarantine: None.
      5) Immunization of contacts: None.
      6) Investigation of contacts: Not ordinarily indicated.

7) Specific treatment: Amphotericin B (Fungizone®) should be tried in tissue invasive forms. Immunosuppressive therapy should be discontinued or reduced as much as possible. Endobronchial colonization should be treated by measures to improve bronchopulmonary drainage.

C. *Epidemic measures:* Not generally applicable; a sporadic disease. Clusters of cases may occur on cancer therapy wards, in which case environmental studies should be carried out to find the source of the spores.

D. *Disaster implications:* None.

E. *International measures:* None.

BABESIOSIS   ICD-9 088.8

1. **Identification**—A relatively rare but potentially severe and sometimes fatal disease of man caused by infection with a protozoan parasite of RBCs. The clinical presentation may include fever, fatigue and hemolytic anemia lasting from several days to a few months. Asymptomatic infections occur, but their proportion is not known. Cases caused by parasite strains found in Europe have been more likely to be severe and fatal than those caused by the strains prevalent in the USA.

Diagnosis is made by identification on a thick and thin blood film of the parasite within RBCs, with confirmation of the presence of specific antibodies by serologic studies (IFA), or by isolation in appropriate animals. Differentiation from *Plasmodium falciparum* on blood film examination may be difficult in patients who have been in malarious areas or who may have acquired infection by blood transfusion; if diagnosis is uncertain, manage as if it were a case of malaria and send thick and thin blood films to an appropriate reference laboratory.

2. **Infectious agents**—*Babesia microti* and other *Babesia* spp., especially *B. divergens* in Europe.

3. **Occurrence**—In the USA, the geographic distribution of *B. microti* infection increases in parallel with the widening range of the tick vector, *Ixodes dammini*. Babesiosis is endemic on Nantucket and other islands in Massachusetts, and Shelter Island and along the coast of Long Island Sound. Infection has been reported also from Connecticut and Wisconsin. Human cases due to species other than *B. microti* have been identified in the USA (California and Georgia) and Mexico. In Europe, human infections caused by *B. divergens* have been reported from France,

Ireland, Scotland, the USSR and Yugoslavia.

4. **Reservoir**—Presumably rodents for *B. microti,* and cattle for *B. divergens.*

5. **Mode of transmission**—*B. microti* is transmitted during the sum-mer months by the bite of nymphal *Ixodes* ticks (*I. dammini*) carried by voles (*Microtus pennsylvanicus*) or deer mice (*Peromyscus leucopus*). The adult tick is normally found on deer (which are not infected by the parasite), but may also parasitize and be spread by a variety of mammalian and avian hosts. The vector of *B. divergens* in Europe appears to be *I. ricinus.* Occasionally cases have been reported to be transmitted by blood transfusion.

6. **Incubation period**—Variable; one week to 12 months reported.

7. **Period of communicability**—Not transmitted from person to person except by blood transfusion.

8. **Susceptibility and resistance**—Susceptibility to *B. microti* is as-sumed to be universal; asplenic persons are at particular risk of having symptomatic infections. Other members of the family Babesiidae have been known to attack immunocompromised, elderly and asplenic persons.

9. **Methods of control**—

   A. *Preventive measures:* Control rodents around human habita-tions and use tick repellents. Educate the public in mode of transmission and means for personal protection.

   B. *Control of patient, contacts and the immediate environment:*

      1) Report to local health authority: Report new suspected cases by telephone, particularly in areas not previously known to be endemic, Class 3B (see Preface).
      2) Isolation: Blood/body fluid precautions.
      3) Concurrent disinfection: None.
      4) Quarantine: None.
      5) Protection of contacts: None, but family members possi-bly exposed at the same time as the patient should be evaluated for infection and observed for fever.
      6) Investigation of contacts and source of infection: Cases occurring in a new area deserve careful study. Blood donors in transfusion-related cases should be investigated promptly.
      7) Specific treatment: The combination of clindamycin and quinine has been effective in experimental animal studies and in most patients with *B. microti* infections who have received this drug combination. Infection does not re-

spond to chloroquine. Pentamidine in combination with co-trimoxazole has been effective in one reported case of *B. divergens.* Exchange transfusion may be required in asplenic patients with a high proportion of parasitized RBCs.

C.   *Epidemic measures:* None.

D.   *Disaster implications:* None.

E.   *International measures:* None.

BALANTIDIASIS   ICD-9 007.0
(Balantidiosis, Balantidial dysentery)

1. **Identification**—A protozoan infection of the colon characteristically producing diarrhea or dysentery, accompanied by abdominal colic, tenesmus, nausea and vomiting. Occasionally the dysentery resembles that due to amebiasis, with stools containing much blood and mucus but relatively little pus. Peritoneal or urogenital invasion is rare.

Diagnosis is made by identifying the trophozoites or cysts of *Balantidium coli* in fresh feces, or trophozoites in material obtained by sigmoidoscopy.

2. **Infectious agent**—*Balantidium coli,* a large ciliated protozoan.

3. **Occurrence**—Worldwide; the incidence of human disease is low. Waterborne epidemics occasionally occur in areas of poor environmental sanitation. Environmental contamination with swine feces may result in a higher incidence. A large epidemic occurred in frontier areas of Ecuador in 1978.

4. **Reservoir**—Swine, and possibly other animals such as rats and nonhuman primates.

5. **Mode of transmission**—Via ingestion of cysts from feces of infected hosts; in epidemics, mainly by fecally contaminated water. Sporadic transmission is by transfer of feces to mouth by hands, contaminated water, or fecally contaminated food.

6. **Incubation period**—Unknown; may be only a few days.

7. **Period of communicability**—As long as the infection persists.

8. **Susceptibility and resistance**—People appear to have a high natural resistance. In individuals debilitated from other diseases the infection may be serious and even fatal.

9. **Methods of control—**

A. *Preventive measures:*

1) Educate the general public in personal hygiene.
2) Educate and supervise foodhandlers via health agencies.
3) Dispose of feces in a sanitary manner.
4) Avoid contact with hog feces.
5) Protect public water supplies against fecal contamination. Diatomaceous earth and sand filters remove all cysts, but ordinary water chlorination does not destroy cysts. Small quantities of water are best treated by boiling.

B. *Control of patient, contacts and the immediate environment:*

1) Report to local health authority: Official report not ordinarily justifiable, Class 5 (see Preface).
2) Isolation: None.
3) Concurrent disinfection: Sanitary disposal of feces.
4) Quarantine: None.
5) Immunization of contacts: Not applicable.
6) Investigation of contacts and source of infection: Microscopic examination of feces of household members and suspected contacts. Also investigate contact with hogs.
7) Specific treatment: Tetracyclines eliminate infection; metronidazole (Flagyl®) may also be effective.

C. *Epidemic measures:* Any grouping of several cases in an area or institution requires prompt epidemiologic investigation, especially of environmental sanitation.

D. *Disaster implications:* None.

E. *International measures:* None.

BARTONELLOSIS ICD-9 088.0
(Oroya fever, Verruga peruana, Carrion's disease)

1. **Identification**—A bacterial infection with two markedly different clinical forms, a febrile anemia (Oroya fever) and a dermal eruption (verruga peruana). Oroya fever is characterized by irregular fever, severe anemia (macrocytic and usually hypochromic), generalized lymphadenopathy, and often delirium. Verruga peruana has a pre-eruptive stage characterized by shifting pain in muscles, bones and joints; the pain, often severe, lasts minutes to several days at any one site. The dermal eruption

may be miliary with widely disseminated, small, hemangioma-like nodules, or nodular with fewer, but larger, deep-seated lesions, most prominent on the extensor surfaces of the limbs. Individual nodules, particularly near joints, may develop into tumor-like masses with an ulcerated surface. Verruga peruana is often preceded by Oroya fever, with an interval of weeks to months between the two stages. The case fatality rate of untreated Oroya fever ranges from 10 to 40%; death is often associated with *Salmonella* septicemia. Verruga peruana has a prolonged course but seldom results in death.

Diagnosis is made by demonstration of the infectious agent adherent to or within RBCs during the acute stage, in sections of skin lesions during the eruptive stage, or by blood culture on special media during either stage. Antigens from the organism have been used in modern test methods and appear promising.

2. **Infectious agent**—*Bartonella bacilliformis*.

3. **Occurrence**—Limited to mountain valleys of Peru, Ecuador and southwest Colombia, between altitudes of 2500 to 8000 ft (750 to 2500 m) above sea level, where the sandfly vector is present; no special predilection for age, race or sex.

4. **Reservoir**—Man; with the agent present in the blood. In endemic areas the asymptomatic carrier rate may reach 5%. There is no known animal reservoir.

5. **Mode of transmission**—By bite of sandflies of the genus *Lutzomyia*. Species are not identified for all areas; *Lutzomyia verrucarum* is important in Peru. These insects feed only from dusk to dawn. Blood transfusion, particularly during the Oroya fever stage, may transmit infection.

6. **Incubation period**—Usually 16-22 days, but occasionally 3-4 months.

7. **Period of communicability**—Not directly transmitted from person to person, other than by transfused blood. Man is infectious for the sandfly for a long period; the agent may be present in blood weeks before and up to several years after actual illness. Duration of infectivity of the sandfly is unknown.

8. **Susceptibility and resistance**—Susceptibility is general, but the disease is milder in children than in adults. Inapparent infections and carriers are known. Recovery from untreated Oroya fever almost invariably gives permanent immunity to this form; the verruga stage may recur.

9. **Methods of control**—

    A. *Preventive measures:*

        1) Control sandflies (see Leishmaniasis, Cutaneous).

2) Avoid known endemic areas after sundown; otherwise apply insect repellent to exposed parts of the body.

B. *Control of patient, contacts and the immediate environment:*

1) Report to local health authority: In selected endemic areas; in most countries not a reportable disease, Class 3B (see Preface).

2) Isolation: Blood/body fluid precautions. The infected individual should be protected from bites of phlebotomines (see 9A, above).

3) Concurrent disinfection: None.

4) Quarantine: None.

5) Immunization of contacts: None.

6) Investigation of contacts and source of infection: Identification of sandflies, particularly in localities where the infected person was exposed after sundown during the preceding 3-8 weeks.

7) Specific treatment: Penicillin, streptomycin, chloramphenicol and tetracyclines are all effective in reducing fever and bacteremia. Ampicillin and chloramphenicol are the drugs of choice; they work directly against Bartonella, but more importantly, also against the frequent secondary salmonellosis.

C. *Epidemic measures:* Intensification of case finding and systematic spraying of houses with a residual insecticide.

D. *Disaster implications:* Only if refugee centers are established in an endemic locus.

E. *International measures:* None.

BLASTOMYCOSIS
ICD-9 116.0
(North American blastomycosis, Gilchrist's disease)

1. **Identification**—Blastomycosis is a granulomatous mycosis, primarily of the lungs and skin. Pulmonary blastomycosis may be acute or chronic. Acute infection is rarely recognized but presents with the sudden onset of fever, cough and a pulmonary infiltrate on chest x-ray. The acute disease resolves spontaneously after 1-3 weeks of illness. During or after the resolution of the pneumonia, some patients exhibit extrapulmonary infection. More commonly, there is an indolent onset, evolving into the chronic disease. Cough and chest aching may be mild or absent so that

patients may present with infection already spread to other sites, particularly skin, and less often to bone, prostate or epididymis. Skin lesions begin as erythematous papules which become verrucous, crusted or ulcerated. Most commonly, lesions are located on the face and distal extremities. Weight loss, weakness and low grade fever are often present. Pulmonary lesions may cavitate. The course of untreated disseminated or chronic pulmonary blastomycosis is eventual progression and, usually, death.

Direct microscopic examination of unstained smears of sputum and material from lesions shows characteristic "broad based" budding forms of the fungus, which can be cultured. Serologic test results can be misleading because of cross reactions with histoplasmosis; CF tests are often negative in cases with active disease.

2. Infectious agent—*Blastomyces dermatitidis (Ajellomyces dermatitidis)*, a dimorphic fungus that grows as a yeast in the tissues and in enriched culture media at 37°C (98.6°F), and as a mold at room temperature (25°C/77°F).

3. Occurrence—Uncommon. Occurs sporadically in central and southeastern USA, Canada, Africa (Zaire, Tanzania, South Africa), India, Israel and Saudi Arabia. Rare in children; more frequent in males than females. Disease in dogs is frequent; it has also been reported in cats, a horse, a captive African lion and a sea lion.

4. Reservoir—Probably soil.

5. Mode of transmission—Conidia, typical of the mold or saprophytic growth form, probably are inhaled in spore-laden dust.

6. Incubation period—Indefinite; probably a few weeks or less to months.

7. Period of communicability—Not transmitted directly from people or animals to people.

8. Susceptibility and resistance—Unknown. Inapparent pulmonary infections are probable but of undetermined frequency. There is no information on immunity; the rarity of the natural disease and of laboratory-acquired infections suggests people are relatively resistant.

9. Methods of control—

    A. Preventive measures: Unknown.

    B. Control of patient, contacts and the immediate environment:

        1) Report to local health authority: Official report not ordinarily justifiable, Class 5 (see Preface).
        2) Isolation: None.

3) Concurrent disinfection: Sputum, discharges and all contaminated articles. Terminal cleaning.
4) Quarantine: None.
5) Immunization of contacts: None.
6) Investigation of contacts and source of infection: Not profitable.
7) Specific treatment: Ketoconazole is the drug of choice, but amphotericin B (Fungizone®) is indicated in patients severely ill or with brain lesions.

C. *Epidemic measures:* Not applicable, a sporadic disease.

D. *Disaster implications:* None.

E. *International measures:* None.

BOTULISM
BOTULISM, INFANT

ICD-9 005.1
ICD-9 008.49

1. Identification—There are three forms of botulism—the classical form, a form known as infant botulism which was first recognized as a distinct clinical entity in 1976, and wound botulism in which the organism proliferates within a wound.

Classical botulism is a severe intoxication resulting from ingestion of toxin preformed in contaminated food. The illness is characterized by clinical manifestations relating primarily to the nervous system. Visual difficulty (blurred or double vision), dysphagia, and dry mouth are often the first complaints. These symptoms may be followed by descending symmetrical flaccid paralysis in an alert person. Vomiting and constipation or diarrhea may be present initially. Fever is absent unless a complicating infection occurs. With good respiratory care and specific antitoxin, the case fatality rate in the USA during the last decade has generally been under 15%. Recovery may be slow (months and rarely years).

In **wound botulism** the same clinical picture has been seen after the causative organism contaminated a wound in which anaerobic conditions developed; rare.

Infant botulism is the most common form of botulism; it results from colonization and subsequent outgrowth and in vivo toxin production in the intestine by the botulinal bacillus. It affects infants under 1 year of age almost exclusively, but can affect adults who have altered GI anatomy and microflora. The illness typically begins with constipation, followed by lethargy, listlessness, poor feeding, ptosis, difficulty in swallowing, loss of head control, hypotonia and generalized weakness (the "floppy" baby) and, in some cases, respiratory insufficiency and arrest. Infant botulism has a wide spectrum of clinical severity, ranging from mild illness to sudden infant death; various studies suggest that it may cause an estimated 5% of cases of Sudden Infant Death Syndrome (SIDS). The case fatality rate of hospitalized cases in the USA is 2%; without access to hospitals with pediatric intensive care units, more would die.

Diagnosis of classical botulism is supported by demonstration of the specific toxin in serum, stool or incriminated food, or by culture of *Clostridium botulinum* from stool in a clinical case. Wound botulism is diagnosed by serum toxin or positive wound culture. Identification of organisms in a suspected food is helpful but not diagnostic since botulinum spores are so ubiquitous; the presence of toxin is more significant. The diagnosis may be accepted in a person with the clinical syndrome who had consumed a food item incriminated in a laboratory-confirmed case.

The diagnosis of infant botulism is established by identification of *Clostridium botulinum* organisms and/or toxin in patients' feces or in autopsy specimens. With few exceptions, toxin has not been detected in the sera of patients. Electromyography may be useful in corroborating the clinical diagnosis.

2. **Infectious agent**—Classical botulism is caused by toxins produced by *Clostridium botulinum,* a spore-forming obligate anaerobic bacillus. Most human outbreaks are due to types A, B and E, with rare cases due to types F and G. Type E outbreaks are usually related to fish, seafood and meat from marine mammals. Toxin is produced in improperly processed, canned, low-acid or alkaline foods, and in pasteurized and lightly cured foods held without refrigeration, especially in airtight packaging. The toxin is destroyed by boiling; inactivation of spores requires much higher temperatures. Type E toxin can be produced slowly at temperatures as low as 3°C (37.4°F), which is lower than that of ordinary refrigeration. Most cases of infant botulism have been caused by types A or B. A few cases (toxin types E and F) have been reported due to neurotoxigenic clostridial species other than *C. botulinum.*

3. **Occurrence**—Worldwide; sporadic cases, family and general outbreaks occur where food products are prepared or preserved by methods that do not destroy the spores and permit toxin formation. Cases rarely result from contaminated commercially processed products; outbreaks have occurred from contamination after processsing through damaged cans.

Cases of infant botulism have been reported from five continents: Asia, Australia, Europe, and N and S America. The actual incidence and distribution of infant botulism remains to be determined. As of January 1990, over 700 cases had been reported in the USA.

4. **Reservoir**—Spores are ubiquitous in soil; they are frequently recovered from agricultural products. They are also found in marine sediment and the intestinal tract of animals, including fish.

5. **Mode of transmission**—Classical botulism is acquired by ingestion of food in which toxin has been formed, predominantly after inadequate heating during canning and without subsequent adequate cooking. Most poisonings in the USA are due to home-canned vegetables and fruits; meat is an infrequent vehicle. Cases associated with baked potatoes and improperly handled commercial potpies have been reported. One recent outbreak was attributed to sautéed onions, two others to minced garlic in oil. Newer varieties of some garden foods such as tomatoes, formerly considered too acidic to support growth of *C. botulinum,* may no longer be low-hazard foods for home canning. In Canada, outbreaks have been associated with seal meat, smoked salmon and fermented salmon eggs. In Europe, most cases are due to sausages and smoked or preserved meats; in Japan, to seafood. These differences have been attributed in part to the greater use in the USA of sodium nitrite for preserving meats. Most cases of wound botulism are secondary to contamination of the wounds by ground-in soil or gravel; several cases have been reported among chronic drug abusers (skin infection in "skin poppers" and sinusitis in cocaine "sniffers").

Infant botulism arises from ingestion of botulinum spores rather than preformed toxin. Possible sources of spores for infants are multiple, including foods and dust. Honey, a food item fed to infants, often contains *C. botulinum* spores.

6. **Incubation period**—Neurologic symptoms of classical botulism usually appear within 12-36 hours, sometimes several days, after eating contaminated food. In general, the shorter the incubation period, the more severe the disease and the higher the case fatality rate. The incubation period of infant botulism is unknown, since it cannot be determined precisely when the infant ingested the causal botulinum spores.

7. **Period of communicability**—Despite excretion of *C. botulinum* toxin and organisms at high levels (ca. 10^6 organisms/ g) in patients' feces for weeks to months after onset of illness, no instances of secondary person-to-person transmission have been documented.

8. **Susceptibility and resistance**—Susceptibility is general. All patients hospitalized to date with infant botulism have been between 2 weeks and 1 year of age; 94% were 6 months of age or less, and the median age at onset was 13 weeks. Cases of infant botulism have occurred in all major racial and ethnic groups. Adults with special bowel problems leading to unusual GI flora may be susceptible to "infant-type" botulism.

9. Methods of control—

A. *Preventive measures:*

1) Ensure effective control of processing and preparation of commercially canned and preserved foods.

2) Educate housewives and others concerned with home canning and other food preservation techniques regarding the proper time, pressure and temperature required to destroy spores, the need for adequately refrigerated storage of incompletely processed foods, and the effectiveness of boiling, with stirring, home-canned vegetables for at least 3 minutes to destroy botulinum toxins.

3) *C. botulinum* may or may not cause container lids to bulge and the contents to have "off-odors." Other contaminants can also cause cans or bottle lids to bulge. Bulging containers should not be opened, and foods with "off-odors" should not be eaten or "taste tested." Commercial cans with bulging lids should be returned unopened to the vendor.

4) While *C. botulinum* spores are ubiquitous, identified sources, such as honey, should not be fed to infants.

B. *Control of patient, contacts and the immediate environment:*

1) Report to local health authority: Case report of suspected and confirmed cases obligatory in most states (USA) and countries, Class 2A (see Preface); immediate telephone report indicated.

2) Isolation: Not required, but handwashing is indicated after handling soiled diapers.

3) Concurrent disinfection: The implicated food(s) should be detoxified by boiling before discarding, or the containers broken and buried deeply in soil to prevent ingestion by animals. Contaminated utensils should be sterilized by boiling or by chlorine disinfection to inactivate any remaining toxin. Usual sanitary disposal of feces from infant cases. Terminal cleaning.

4) Quarantine: None.

5) Management of contacts: None for simple direct contacts. Those who are known to have eaten the incriminated food should be purged with cathartics, given gastric lavage and high enemas, and kept under close medical observation. The decision to provide presumptive treatment with polyvalent antitoxin to asymptomatic individuals should be weighed carefully, balancing the potential protection when antitoxin is administered early (within

1-2 days after eating the implicated meal) against the risk of adverse reactions and sensitization to horse serum.

6) Investigation of contacts and source of toxin: Study recent food history of those ill, and recover all suspected foods for appropriate testing and disposal. Search for other cases of botulism to rule out foodborne botulism.

7) Specific treatment: Intravenous and intramuscular administration as soon as possible of trivalent botulinum antitoxin (types A, B and E), available from CDC, Atlanta, through state health departments (see Preface) is considered a part of routine treatment. Blood serum should be collected to identify the specific toxin before antitoxin is administered, but antitoxin should not be withheld pending test results. Most important is immediate access to an intensive care unit so that respiratory failure, the usual cause of death, can be anticipated and managed promptly. For wound botulism, in addition to antitoxin, the wound should be debrided and/or drainage established, and appropriate antibiotics (e.g., penicillin) administered.

In infant botulism, meticulous supportive care is essential. Botulinum antitoxin (an equine product) is not used because of the hazard of sensitization and anaphylaxis. Antibiotics have not been shown to effect the course of the disease; they should be used only to treat secondary infections. Assisted respiration may be required.

C. *Epidemic measures:* Suspicion of a single case of botulism should immediately raise the question of a group outbreak involving a family or others who have shared a common food. Home-preserved foods should be the prime suspect until ruled out, although widely distributed commercially preserved foods are occasionally identified as the source of intoxication and pose a far greater threat to the public health. In addition, since recent outbreaks have implicated unusual food items, even theoretically unlikely foods should be considered. When any food is implicated by epidemiologic or laboratory findings, immediate recall of the product is necessary, as is immediate search for persons who shared the suspected food and for any remaining food from the same source that may be similarly contaminated; such food, if found, should be submitted for laboratory examination. Sera and stools from patients and (when indicated) from others exposed but not ill, should be collected and forwarded immediately to a reference laboratory before administration of antitoxin.

D. *Disaster implications:* None.

E. *International measures:* Commercial products may have been distributed widely; international efforts may be required to recover and test implicated foods.

BRUCELLOSIS   ICD-9 023
(Undulant fever, Malta fever, Mediterranean fever)

1. **Identification**—A systemic bacterial disease with acute or insidious onset, characterized by continued, intermittent or irregular fever of variable duration, headache, weakness, profuse sweating, chills, arthralgia, depression, weight loss and generalized aching. Localized suppurative infections may occur; subclinical and unrecognized infections are frequent. The disease may last for several days, months, or occasionally for a year or more.

Osteoarticular complications are common; vertebral osteomyelitis and, more rarely, prepatellar bursitis are characteristic features. Genitourinary involvement is reported in 2-20% of cases, with orchitis and epididymitis most common. The case fatality rate without treatment is ≤2%; higher for *Brucella melitensis* infections. Recovery is usual but disability is often pronounced. Part or all of the original syndrome may reappear as relapses, especially on re-exposure. A neurotic symptom complex is sometimes attributed to chronic brucellosis. In the USA, the disease is very rare in children and is usually mild when it does occur.

Laboratory diagnosis is made by appropriate isolation of the infectious agent from blood, bone marrow or other tissues, or from discharges of the patient. Serologic tests in experienced laboratories are valuable, especially when paired sera show a rise in antibody titer. Interpretation of serologic tests in chronic and recurrent cases is especially difficult since titers are usually low. Tests measuring IgG antibody may be useful, particularly in chronic cases, since active infection is associated with a rise. Specific serologic techniques are needed for *B. canis* antibodies.

2. **Infectious agents**—*Brucella abortus,* biovars 1-6 and 9; *B. melitensis,* biovars 1-3; *B. suis,* biovars 1-5; and *B. canis.*

3. **Occurrence**—Worldwide, especially in Mediterranean countries of Europe and North and East Africa, India, central Asia, Mexico, Central and S America. The sources of infection and the responsible organism vary according to geographic area. It is predominantly an occupational disease of those working with infected animals or their tissues, especially farm workers, veterinarians and abattoir workers, hence more frequent

among males. Sporadic cases and outbreaks occur among consumers of unpasteurized milk and milk products (especially cheese) from cows, sheep and goats. Isolated cases of infection with *B. canis* occur in animal handlers from contact with dogs. Currently reported incidence in the USA is <100 cases annually; worldwide, the disease is often unrecognized and unreported.

4. **Reservoir**—Of human infection in the USA: cattle and swine; outside the USA: goats and sheep. It may occur in dogs, coyotes and caribou. *B. canis* is a problem in laboratory dog colonies and kennels; a small percentage of pet dogs and a higher proportion of strays have positive *B. canis* antibody titers.

5. **Mode of transmission**—By contact with tissues, blood, urine, vaginal discharges, aborted fetuses and especially placentas (through breaks in the skin), and by ingestion of raw milk and dairy products (cheese) from infected animals. Airborne infection of animals occurs in pens and stables, and of man in laboratories and abattoirs. A small number of cases result from accidental self-inoculation of strain 19 *Brucella* vaccine; the same risk is present when Rev-I vaccine is handled.

6. **Incubation period**—Highly variable and difficult to ascertain; usually 5-60 days, 1 to 2 months commonplace, occasionally several months.

7. **Period of communicability**—No evidence of communicability from person to person.

8. **Susceptibility and resistance**—Severity and duration of clinical illness are subject to wide variation. Duration of acquired immunity is uncertain.

9. **Methods of control**—Ultimate control of human brucellosis rests on the elimination of the disease among domestic animals.

   A. *Preventive measures:*

   1) Educate the public not to drink untreated milk nor eat products made from unpasteurized or otherwise untreated milk.
   2) Educate farmers and workers in slaughter houses, packing plants and butchers' shops as to the nature of the disease and the risk in the handling of carcasses and products of potentially infected animals, and the proper operation of abattoirs to reduce exposure.
   3) Search for infection among livestock by serologic testing and by ring test of cows' milk; eliminate infected animals by segregation and/or slaughter. Infection among swine usually requires slaughter of the herd. In areas of high prevalence, immunize young goats and sheep with live

attenuated Rev-I strain of *B. melitensis;* and calves and sometimes adult animals with strain 19, *B. abortus.*

4) Persons inadvertently inoculated with strain 19 or Rev-I vaccines should be given doxycycline, 200 mg, combined with rifampin, 600-900 mg daily for 10 days.

5) Pasteurize milk and dairy products from cows, sheep and goats. Boiling milk is effective when pasteurization is impossible.

6) Exercise care in handling and disposal of placenta, discharges and fetus from an aborted animal. Disinfect contaminated areas.

B. *Control of patient, contacts and the immediate environment:*

1) Report to local health authority: Case report obligatory in most states (USA) and countries, Class 2B (see Preface).

2) Isolation: Draining/secretion precautions if there are draining lesions; otherwise none.

3) Concurrent disinfection: Of purulent discharges.

4) Quarantine: None.

5) Immunization of contacts: None.

6) Investigation of contacts and source of infection: Trace infection to the common or individual source, usually infected domestic goats, swine or cattle, or unpasteurized milk or dairy products from cows and goats. Test suspected animals, remove reactors.

7) Specific treatment: A combination of rifampin (RIF), 600-900 mg and doxycycline, 200 mg daily, for at least 6 weeks is the treatment of choice. Tetracycline should be avoided, if possible, in children less than 7 years old. Co-trimoxazole is effective but relapses are common. In severely ill patients, steroids may be administered to decrease systemic toxicity. Relapses occur in about 5% of treated patients and are not due to resistant organisms; they should be retreated with the original regimen. Arthritis may occur in recurrent cases and may benefit from the use of corticosteroids.

C. *Epidemic measures:* Search for common vehicle of infection, usually unpasteurized milk or milk products, especially cheese, from an infected herd. Recall incriminated products; stop production and distribution unless pasteurization is instituted.

D. *Disaster implications:* None.

E. *International measures:* Control of domestic animals and animal products in international trade and transport. WHO Collaborating Centres (see Preface).

CAMPYLOBACTERIOSIS
ICD-9 027.9
DIARRHEA CAUSED BY
ICD-9 008.49
CAMPYLOBACTER
(Campylobacter enteritis, Vibrionic enteritis)

1. **Identification**—An acute enteric bacterial disease of variable severity characterized by diarrhea, abdominal pain, malaise, fever, nausea and vomiting. The illness is frequently over within 2 to 5 days and usually lasts no more than 10 days. Prolonged illness may occur in adults; relapses can occur. Gross or occult blood in association with mucus and WBCs is often present in the liquid stools. A typhoid-like syndrome, reactive arthritis, and rarely, febrile convulsions and meningitis may occur. Some cases mimic acute appendicitis. Many infections are asymptomatic.

Diagnosis is based on isolation of the organisms from stool using selective media, reduced oxygen tension, and an incubation temperature of 43°C (109.4°F). Visualization of motile and curved, spiral or S-shaped rods similar to those of *Vibrio cholerae* by phase-contrast or darkfield microscopy of stool can provide rapid presumptive evidence for campylobacter enteritis.

2. **Infectious agents**—*Campylobacter jejuni (C. fetus,* subsp. *jejuni)* and (rarely) *C. coli* are the usual causes of campylobacter diarrhea in man. A variety of biotypes and serotypes occurs; their identification may be helpful for epidemiologic purposes. A number of other *Campylobacters,* including *C. laridis* and *C. fetus,* subsp. *fetus,* have been associated with diarrhea in normal hosts. *C. cinaedi, C. fennelliae* and other *Campylobacter* spp. have been associated with diarrhea in homosexual men.

3. **Occurrence**—These organisms are an important cause of diarrheal illness in all parts of the world and all age groups, causing 5-14% of diarrhea worldwide. In developed countries, children and young adults have the highest incidence of illness, while in developing countries, illness is confined largely to children below 2 years of age. Common-source outbreaks have occurred, most often associated with foods, especially chicken and unpasteurized milk, and unchlorinated water. The largest number of cases in temperate areas occurs in the warmer months. These organisms are an important cause of travelers' diarrhea.

4. **Reservoir**—Animals, most frequently cattle and poultry. Puppies,

kittens, other pets, swine, cattle, sheep, rodents and birds may also be sources of human infection.

5. **Mode of transmission**—By ingestion of the organisms in food or in unpasteurized milk or water; from contact with infected pets (especially puppies and kittens), wild animals, or infected infants. Contamination of milk most frequently occurs from carrier cattle; foods are contaminated from poultry handled on common cutting boards, etc. Infected children may transmit infection to puppies or kittens, which may then expose other children.

6. **Incubation period**—Three to 5 days, with a range of 1-10 days.

7. **Period of communicability**—Throughout the course of infection; usually from several days to several weeks. Individuals not treated with antibiotics excrete organisms for as long as 2-7 weeks. The temporary carrier state is probably of little epidemiologic importance, except in infants and others who are incontinent of stool. Chronic infection of poultry and other animals constitutes the primary source of infection.

8. **Susceptibility and resistance**—Universal susceptibility when enough organisms (>500) are ingested. Immune mechanisms are not well understood, but lasting immunity to serologically related strains follows infection. In developing countries, most people develop immunity in the first year of life.

9. **Methods of control**—

   A. *Preventive measures:*

      1) Thoroughly cook all foodstuffs derived from animal sources, particularly poultry. Avoid recontamination from uncooked foods within the kitchen after cooking is completed.
      2) Pasteurize all milk and chlorinate all water supplies.
      3) Recognize, prevent and control campylobacter infections among domestic animals and pets. Puppies and kittens with diarrhea are possible sources of infection; erythromycin may be used to treat their infections, reducing risk of transmission to children. Stress handwashing after animal contact.
      4) Minimize contact with poultry and their feces; wash hands when this cannot be avoided.

   B. *Control of patient, contacts and the immediate environment:*

      1) Report to local health authority: Obligatory case report, Class 2B (see Preface).
      2) Isolation: Enteric precautions for hospitalized patients. Exclude symptomatic individuals from foodhandling, care

of people in hospitals, custodial institutions and day-care centers; exclusion of asymptomatic convalescent stool-positive individuals is indicated only for those with questionable handwashing habits. Stress proper handwashing.

3) Concurrent disinfection: Of feces and articles soiled therewith. In communities with a modern and adequate sewage disposal system, feces can be discharged directly into sewers without preliminary disinfection. Terminal cleaning.

4) Quarantine: None.

5) Immunization of contacts: No immunization available.

6) Investigation of contacts and source of infection: Useful only to detect outbreaks; investigate outbreaks to identify the implicated food, water or raw milk to which others may have been exposed.

7) Specific treatment: None generally indicated except rehydration and electrolyte replacement (see Cholera, 9B7). A short course of antibiotic therapy may be given to patients with severe illness, or when prompt termination of fecal excretion of *C. jejuni* or *C. coli* is desired. Antimicrobial treatment may be helpful if given at the outset of the disease, but does not shorten the duration of clinical illness when given later. *C. jejuni* or *C. coli* organisms are susceptible in vitro to a number of antimicrobial agents, including erythromycin, tetracyclines and quinolones.

C. **Epidemic measures:** Groups of cases, such as in classrooms, should be reported immediately to local health authority, with search for vehicle and mode of spread.

D. **Disaster implications:** A risk when mass feeding and poor sanitation coexist.

E. **International measures:** WHO Collaborating Centres (see Preface).

GASTRITIS CAUSED BY ICD-9 535
CAMPYLOBACTER-LIKE ORGANISMS

Bacteria which were originally designated *Campylobacter pylori* but now classified as *Helicobacter pylori,* are found in biopsy specimens of the gastric antral mucosa from patients with active chronic gastritis and duodenal peptic ulcer. Clinical manifestations include dyspepsia and excessive "burping"; there is typical pain in those with ulcers. One volunteer with biopsy-confirmed normal gastric mucosa who ingested 10^9 *H. pylori* organisms developed colonization of the gastric epithelium associated with hypochlorhydria, halitosis and mild GI disturbance after about eight days; symptoms were terminated on the 14th day when tinidazole therapy was instituted. In a group of volunteers who developed *H. pylori* infections while undergoing studies of gastric acidity, mild to moderate epigastric pain, nausea and vomiting lasting 1-4 days were followed by hypochlorhydria.

Infected individuals have elevated specific IgG antibodies by ELISA testing, and elevated pepsinogen I and gastrin levels; these fall after treatment with colloidal bismuth subcitrate (given over a four-week period) and amoxicillin or tinidazole (given for six weeks). These two antibiotics have been used together with good results. No antibacterial regime is established as the treatment of choice. The organisms elaborate urease, so diagnosis can be made by a positive urease test directly on the biopsy tissue, as well as by culturing biopsy material obtained endoscopically from areas of gastritis.

The source of these organisms has not been identified. However, in one study, antibody levels were significantly higher among abattoir workers in contact with animal viscera, suggesting a zoonotic association, at least in some cases. These observations suggest a possible bacterial etiology for gastritis and peptic ulcer disease.

CANDIDIASIS   ICD-9 112
(Moniliasis, Thrush, Candidosis)

1. **Identification**—A mycosis usually confined to the superficial layers of skin or mucous membranes, presenting clinically as oral thrush, intertrigo, vulvovaginitis, paronychia or onychomycosis. Ulcers or pseudomembranes may be formed in the esophagus, GI tract or bladder. Hematogenous dissemination may produce lesions in other organs, such as kidney, spleen, lung, liver, endocardium, eye, meninges, brain, or around prosthetic cardiac valves.

Diagnosis requires evaluation of both laboratory and clinical evidence of candidiasis. The single most valuable laboratory test is microscopic demonstration of pseudohyphae and/or yeast cells in infected tissue or body fluids. Culture confirmation is important, but isolation from sputum, bronchial washings, stool, urine, mucosal surfaces, skin or wounds is not proof of a causal relationship to the disease. Confirmed infection in an adult calls for additional studies to exclude HIV infection as the basic problem.

2. **Infectious agents**—*Candida albicans, C. tropicalis,* and occasionally, other species of *Candida. Torulopsis (Candida) glabrata* is distin-

guished from other causes of candidiasis by lack of pseudohyphae formation in tissue.

3. **Occurrence**—Worldwide. The fungus *(C. albicans)* is often part of the normal human flora.

4. **Reservoir**—Man.

5. **Mode of transmission**—By contact with secretions or excretions of mouth, skin, vagina, and especially feces, from patients or carriers; by passage from mother to infant during childbirth; and by endogenous spread. Disseminated candidiasis may originate from mucosal lesions, unsterile narcotic injections, percutaneous intravenous catheters, and indwelling urinary catheters.

6. **Incubation period**—Variable, 2-5 days for thrush in infants.

7. **Period of communicability**—Presumably while lesions are present.

8. **Susceptibility and resistance**—The frequent isolation of *Candida* species from sputum, throat, feces and urine, in the absence of clinical evidence of infection, suggests a low level of pathogenicity or widespread immunity. Oral thrush is a common, usually benign condition during the first few weeks of life. Clinical disease occurs when host defense is low. Local factors contributing to superficial candidiasis include interdigital intertrigo and paronychia on hands with excessive water exposure (as with housewives and bartenders) and intertrigo in moist skin folds of obese individuals. Repeated clinical skin or mucosal eruptions are common.

Prominent among systemic factors predisposing to candidiasis are general debilitation, diabetes mellitus, therapy with broad-spectrum antibiotics or supraphysiologic doses of adrenal corticosteroids, parenteral hyperalimentation, cancer chemotherapy and certain immune deficiencies (see AIDS). Most adults and older children have a delayed dermal hypersensitivity to the fungus and possess humoral antibodies.

9. **Methods of control**—

   A. *Preventive measures:*

      1) Detect and treat vaginal candidiasis during third trimester of pregnancy to prevent neonatal thrush.

      2) Detect early, and treat locally, infection in the mouth, esophagus or urinary bladder of those with predisposing systemic factors (see 8, above) to prevent systemic spread.

   B. *Control of patient, contacts and the immediate environment:*

      1) Report to local health authority: Official report not ordinarily justifiable, Class 5 (see Preface).

2) Isolation: None.
3) Concurrent disinfection: Of secretions and contaminated articles.
4) Quarantine: None.
5) Immunization of contacts: None.
6) Investigation of contacts and source of infection: Not profitable in sporadic cases.
7) Specific treatment: Ameliorating the underlying causes of candidiasis often facilitates cure, e.g., removal of indwelling venous catheters. Topical nystatin or an imidazole (miconazole, clotrimazole, ketoconazole) is useful in many forms of superficial candidiasis. Oral clotrimazole (Mycelex®) troches or nystatin suspension is effective for treatment of oral thrush. Oral ketoconazole is effective in candidiasis of the skin and mucous membranes of the mouth, esophagus and vagina. Vaginal infection may be treated with topical clotrimazole, miconazole, butoconazole, terconazole or nystatin. Amphotericin B (Fungizone®) IV, with or without 5-fluorocytosine, is the drug of choice for visceral or invasive candidiasis.

C. **Epidemic measures:** Epidemics are largely limited to contaminated intravenous solutions and thrush in newborn nurseries. Concurrent disinfection and terminal cleaning should be practiced with care comparable to that used for epidemic diarrhea in hospital nurseries (see Diarrhea, III9A).

D. **Disaster implications:** None.

E. **International measures:** None.

CAPILLARIASIS

Three types of nematodes of the superfamily Trichuroidea, genus *Capillaria*, produce disease in man.

I. CAPILLARIASIS DUE TO   ICD-9 127.5
CAPILLARIA PHILIPPINENSIS
(Intestinal capillariasis)

1. **Identification**—A clinical syndrome first described on Luzon, Philippines, in 1963. Clinically, the disease is an enteropathy with massive protein loss and a malabsorption syndrome which lead to

progressive weight loss and extreme emaciation. Fatal cases are characterized by the presence of large numbers of parasites in the small intestine together with ascites and pleural transudate. Case fatality rates of 10% have been reported. Subclinical cases also occur, but usually become symptomatic in time.

Diagnosis is made on clinical findings plus the identification of eggs, or larval or adult parasites in the stool. The eggs resemble those of *Trichuris trichiura*. Jejunal biopsy may reveal the worms in the mucosa.

2. **Infectious agent**—*Capillaria philippinensis*.

3. **Occurrence**—Intestinal capillariasis is endemic in the northern Philippine Islands; it has been found in Thailand and a few cases have been reported from Japan. Single cases are reported from Iran and Egypt. It has reached epidemic proportions on Luzon where more than 1,800 cases have been seen since 1967. In some villages, one-third of the population was found to be infected. Males between the ages of 20 and 45 appear to be particularly at risk.

4. **Reservoir**—Unknown; thought to be aquatic birds. Fish are considered to serve as intermediate hosts.

5. **Mode of transmission**—Experimentally, infective larvae develop in the intestine of freshwater fish which ingest eggs; monkeys, Mongolian gerbils and some birds fed these fish become infected and the parasite matures within their intestines. A history of ingestion of raw or inadequately cooked small fish eaten whole is usually obtained from patients.

6. **Incubation period**—Unknown in man; in animal studies, about a month or more.

7. **Period of communicability**—Not transmitted directly from person to person.

8. **Susceptibility and resistance**—Susceptibility appears to be general in those geographic areas in which the parasite is prevalent. Attack rates are often high.

9. **Methods of control**—

    A. *Preventive measures:*

        1) Do not eat uncooked fish and other aquatic animal life in known endemic areas.

        2) Provide adequate facilities for the disposal of feces.

    B. *Control of patient, contacts and the immediate environment:*

        1) Report to local health authority: Case report by most practicable means, Class 3B (see Preface).

        2) Isolation: None.

        3) Concurrent disinfection: None. Sanitary disposal of feces.

4) Quarantine: None.
5) Immunization of contacts: None.
6) Investigation of contacts and source of infection: Fecal examination of all members of family group and others with common exposure to raw or undercooked fish, with treatment of infected individuals.
7) Specific treatment: Mebendazole (Vermox®) or albendazole (Zentel®) is the drug of choice.

C. *Epidemic measures:* Prompt investigation of cases and contacts with treatment of cases as indicated. Education on the need to cook all fish.

D. *Disaster implications:* None.

E. *International measures:* None.

II. CAPILLARIASIS DUE TO ICD-9 128.8 *CAPILLARIA HEPATICA* (Hepatic capillariasis)

1. **Identification**—An uncommon and occasionally fatal disease in humans due to the presence of adult *Capillaria hepatica* in the liver. The picture is that of an acute or subacute hepatitis with marked eosinophilia resembling the picture of visceral larva migrans; the organism can disseminate to the lungs and other viscera.

Diagnosis is made by demonstrating eggs or the parasite in a liver biopsy or at necropsy.

2. **Infectious agent**—*Capillaria hepatica (Hepaticola hepatica).*

3. **Occurrence**—Since its first recognition in 1924, about 25 cases of human disease have been reported from N America, India, Turkey, Czechoslovakia, Italy, Africa, Hawaii, Mexico and Brazil.

4. **Reservoir**—Primarily an infection of rats (as many as 86% infected in some reports) and other rodents, but also seen in a large variety of domestic and wild mammals. The adult worms live and produce eggs in the liver.

5. **Mode of transmission**—The adult worms produce fertilized eggs which remain in the liver until the death of the animal. When infected liver is eaten, the eggs are freed by digestion, reach the soil in the feces and develop to the infective stage in 2 to 4 weeks. When a suitable host ingests these embryonated eggs, they hatch in the intestine, the larvae migrate through the wall of the gut and are transported via the portal system to the liver where they mature and produce eggs. "Spurious infection" of human beings may be detected when eggs are found in the stool after infected liver, raw or cooked, has been eaten; since these eggs

are not embryonated, infection cannot be established.

6. **Incubation period**—Three to 4 weeks.

7. **Period of communicability**—Not directly transmitted from person to person.

8. **Susceptibility and resistance**—Susceptibility is universal; malnourished children are more often infected.

9. **Methods of control**—

A. *Preventive measures:*

1) Avoid ingestion of dirt directly (pica) or in contaminated food or water or on hands.
2) Protect water supplies and food from soil contamination.

B. *Control of patient, contacts and the immediate environment:*

1) Report to local health authority: Official report not ordinarily justifiable, Class 5 (see Preface).
2) Isolation: None.
3) Concurrent disinfection: None.
4) Quarantine: None.
5) Immunization of contacts: None.
6) Investigation of contacts and source of infection: Not applicable.
7) Specific treatment: Thiabendazole (Mintezol®) or albendazole (Zentel®) is probably effective. Sodium antimony gluconate may have some effect.

C. *Epidemic measures:* Not applicable.

D. *Disaster implications:* None.

E. *International measures:* None.

PULMONARY CAPILLARIASIS   ICD-9 128.8

A pulmonary disease manifested by fever, cough and asthmatic breathing, caused by *Capillaria aerophila (Thominx aerophila)*, a nematode parasite of cats, dogs and other carnivorous mammals. Pneumonitis may be severe and heavy infections may be fatal. The worms live in tunnels in the epithelial lining of the trachea, bronchi and bronchioles; fertilized eggs are sloughed into the air passages, coughed up, swallowed and discharged from the body in the feces. In the soil, larvae develop in the eggs and remain infective for a year or longer. Infection is acquired by people, mostly children, by ingesting infective eggs in soil or in soil-contaminated food or water. Eggs may appear in the sputum in 4 weeks; symptoms may appear earlier or later. Human cases have been recorded from USSR (8 cases), Morocco and Iran (1 each); animal infection has been reported in N and S America, Europe, Asia and Australia.

CARDITIS, COXSACKIE   ICD-9 074.2
(Viral carditis, Enteroviral carditis)

1. **Identification**—An acute or subacute viral myocarditis or pericarditis, which occurs as a manifestation (occasionally associated with other manifestations) of infection with enteroviruses, especially group B coxsackievirus.

The myocardium is particularly affected in neonates, in whom fever and lethargy may be followed rapidly by heart failure with pallor, cyanosis, dyspnea, tachycardia and enlargement of heart and liver. Heart failure may be progressive and fatal, or recovery may take place over a few weeks; some cases run a relapsing course over months and may show residual heart damage. In adults, pericarditis is the more common manifestation, with acute chest pain, disturbance of heart rate and rhythm, and often dyspnea. The disease may be associated with epidemic myalgia (see Myalgia, Epidemic). A similar clinical picture can be produced infrequently by infection with other viral agents. A diagnosis is usually made by serologic studies or by isolation of the virus from feces, but such results are not conclusive. Virus is rarely isolated from pericardial fluid, myocardial biopsy, or postmortem heart tissue; such an isolation provides a definitive diagnosis.

2. **Infectious agents**—Group B coxsackievirus (types 1-5); occasionally group A coxsackievirus (types 1, 4, 9, 16, 23) and other enteroviruses.

3. **Occurrence**—An uncommon disease, mainly sporadic but increased during epidemics of group B coxsackievirus infection. Institutional outbreaks, with high case fatality rates in newborns, have been described in maternity units.

4., 5., 6., 7., 8., and 9. **Reservoir, Mode of transmission, Incubation period, Period of communicability, Susceptibility and resistance,** and **Methods of control**—Same as Epidemic Myalgia (q.v.).

CAT-SCRATCH DISEASE   ICD-9 078.3
(Cat-scratch fever, Benign lymphoreticulosis)

1. **Identification**—A subacute, usually self-limited disease character-

ized by malaise, granulomatous lymphadenitis and variable patterns of fever. It is often preceded by a cat scratch which produces a pustular lesion, followed by involvement of a regional lymph node, usually within 2 weeks, which may progress to suppuration. A red papule usually appears at the inoculation site; in most (50-90%) cases, an inoculation site is found. Recurrent and chronic forms occur. Complications such as encephalitis, osteolytic lesions, hepatic granulomata and Parinaud's oculoglandular syndrome have been reported.

Cat-scratch disease can be clinically confused with other diseases which cause regional lymphadenopathies such as tularemia, brucellosis, tuberculosis and pasteurellosis (see below); these diseases must be excluded before consideration of cat-scratch disease.

Diagnosis is based on a consistent clinical picture and histopathologic characteristics of involved lymph nodes. Pus obtained from lymph nodes is bacteriologically sterile by conventional techniques. Skin-test antigens, derived from infected human lymph nodes, are not recommended for general use because of the danger of transmitting other agents.

2. Infectious agent—Pleomorphic, Gram-negative, silver-staining bacilli have been consistently described in involved lymph nodes early in the course of infection. Bacteria meeting this description have been isolated on biphasic brain-heart infusion broth from lymph nodes of 10 of 19 patients; specific antibodies against this organism were demonstrated in the sera of convalescent patients by the IF technique. When inoculated intradermally into skin of an armadillo, the cultured organisms produced lesions identical to early lesions in human skin.

3. Occurrence—Worldwide but uncommon. Sexes are equally affected; more frequent in children and young adults. Familial clustering occurs. Majority of cases are seen during late summer, fall and winter months.

4. Reservoir—Unknown. Cats are carriers; there is no evidence of clinical infection.

5. Mode of transmission—Most patients (over 90%) give a history of scratch, bite, lick, or other exposure to a healthy, usually young, cat (often a kitten). Dog scratch or bite, and monkey bite prior to the syndrome have been reported, but cat involvement was not excluded.

6. Incubation period—Variable, usually 3-14 days from inoculation to primary lesion.

7. Period of communicability—Unknown. Not directly transmitted from person to person.

8. Susceptibility and resistance—Unknown.

9. **Methods of control—**

A. *Preventive measures:* Thorough cleansing of cat scratches and bites.

B. *Control of patient, contacts and the immediate environment:*

1) Report to local health authority: Official report not ordinarily justifiable, Class 5 (see Preface).
2) Isolation: None.
3) Concurrent disinfection: Of discharges from purulent lesions.
4), 5), and 6) Quarantine, Immunization of contacts, and Investigation of contacts and source of infection: None.
7) Specific treatment: There are reports of response to intravenous gentamicin; isolated organisms were susceptible to cefoxitin, cefotaxime, aminoglycosides and mezlocillin in vitro. Surgical drainage of suppurative lymphadenitis may be required.

C. *Epidemic measures:* Not applicable.

D. *Disaster implications:* None.

E. *International measures:* None.

OTHER INFECTIONS ASSOCIATED WITH ANIMAL SALIVA

Other diseases resulting from animal bites include pasteurellosis *(Pasteurella multocida* and *P. haemolytica)* from cat and (more rarely) dog bites; B-virus (cercopithecine herpesvirus 1) from monkey bites (see under Herpes simplex); encephalitis, especially due to other rhabdoviruses such as Duvenhage virus; also tularemia, rat-bite fever, plague, tetanus, rabies and pyogenic infections.

Pasteurellosis (ICD-9 027.2) is caused by *Pasteurella multocida,* an organism which is a frequent resident of the respiratory tract of healthy cats, dogs and other animals. It causes cellulitis, swelling, and pain out of proportion to the visible lesion, with onset usually <24 hours after an animal contact, such as a cat scratch or dog bite; lymphadenopathy and sepsis can occur. The majority of these exposures has been to cats. Chronic respiratory tract disease also occurs among elderly patients with underlying disease. The organism is susceptible to penicillin, the drug of choice; a tetracycline or a cephalosporin is an effective alternative therapeutic agent.

Capnocytophaga (CDC Group DF-2) Infections (ICD-9 027.8): A group of cases of febrile illness has occurred after having been licked, bitten or scratched by dogs (2 cases were associated with cats). Cellulitis, fever, septicemia, purulent meningitis, endocarditis and septic arthritis appear after 1 to 5 days; case fatality rates reported in various groups vary from 4% to 27%. Splenectomy and chronic alcoholism are predisposing factors; the incidence is higher in men and those over 40. Diagnosis is made by finding Gram-negative bacilli within neutrophils and by isolating the etiologic organism. This had been designated at CDC as Dysgonic fermenter 2 (DF2), the name *Capnocytophaga canimorsus* has been proposed for this organism, and *C. cynodegmi* has been proposed for a related organism isolated from wound infections which followed dog bites or cat scratch. Both of these organisms are frequently present in the mouths of healthy dogs and cats. Penicillin G is the antibiotic of choice for treating these infections; it should be given prophylactically to asplenic or chronic alcoholic individuals bitten by a dog or cat.

CHANCROID

ICD-9 099.0

(Ulcus molle, Soft chancre)

1. **Identification**—An acute bacterial infection localized in the genital area and characterized clinically by single or multiple painful, necrotizing ulcers at the site of infection, frequently accompanied by painful inflammatory swelling and suppuration of regional lymph nodes. Minimally symptomatic lesions may occur on the vaginal wall or cervix; asymptomatic infections may occur in women. Extragenital lesions have been reported. Chancroid ulcers, like other genital ulcers, are associated with increased risk of HIV infection.

Diagnosis is made by isolation of the organism from lesion exudate on a selective medium which incorporates vancomycin into chocolate, rabbit, or horse-blood agar enriched with fetal calf serum.

2. **Infectious agent**—*Haemophilus ducreyi*, the Ducrey bacillus.

3. **Occurrence**—More frequently seen in men, with no particular differences in incidence according to age or race except as determined by sexual habits. Most prevalent in tropical and subtropical regions of the world, where the incidence may be higher than that of syphilis and may approach that of gonorrhea in men. The disease is much less common in temperate zones but may occur in small outbreaks.

4. **Reservoir**—Man.

5. **Mode of transmission**—By direct sexual contact with discharges from open lesions and pus from buboes. Autoinoculation to non-genital

sites may occur in infected persons. Non-sexual transmission is rare. Sexual promiscuity and uncleanliness favor transmission.

6. **Incubation period**—From 3-5 days, up to 14 days.

7. **Period of communicability**—As long as the infectious agent persists in the original lesion or discharging regional lymph nodes; usually until healed, in most instances a matter of weeks.

8. **Susceptibility and resistance**—Susceptibility is general; no evidence of natural resistance.

9. **Methods of control**—

    A. *Preventive measures:*

        1) Preventive measures are those for syphilis (q.v.).
        2) Follow up all patients with genital ulcerations serologically for syphilis.

    B. *Control of patient, contacts and the immediate environment:*

        1) Report to local health authority: Case report obligatory in many states (USA) and countries, Class 2B (see Preface).
        2) Isolation: None; avoid sexual contact until all lesions are healed.
        3) Concurrent disinfection: None; stress personal cleanliness.
        4) Quarantine: None.
        5) Immunization of contacts: None.
        6) Investigation of contacts and source of infection: Search for sexual contacts of 2 weeks before and after onset. Women without visible signs may be carriers. Sexual contacts without signs should receive prophylactic treatment.
        7) Specific treatment: Ceftriaxone or erythromycin is the recommeded drug, with co-trimoxazole, amoxicillin or ciprofloxacin as alternatives. Fluctuant inguinal nodes should be aspirated to prevent spontaneous rupture.

    C. *Epidemic measures:* Persisting occurrence or an increased incidence is an indication for more rigid application of measures outlined in 9A or 9B, above. When compliance with the treatment schedule (9B7) is a problem, consideration should be given to a single dose of ceftriaxone. Empirical therapy to high-risk groups with or without lesions, including prostitutes, clinic patients reporting prostitute contact, and clinic patients with darkfield-negative findings may be required to control an outbreak.

D. **Disaster implications:** None.

E. **International measures:** See Syphilis, 9E.

CHICKENPOX-HERPES ZOSTER   ICD-9 052 & 053
(Varicella - Shingles)

1. **Identification**—Chickenpox (varicella) is an acute, generalized viral disease with sudden onset of slight fever, mild constitutional symptoms and a skin eruption which is maculopapular for a few hours, vesicular for 3-4 days, and leaves a granular scab. Lesions commonly occur in successive crops, with several stages of maturity present at the same time; they tend to be more abundant on covered than on exposed parts of the body. They may appear on the scalp, high in the axilla, on mucous membranes of the mouth and upper respiratory tract and on the conjunctivae; they tend to occur in areas of irritation, such as sunburn, diaper rash, etc. They may be so few as to escape observation. Mild, atypical and inapparent infections occur. Occasionally, especially in adults, the fever and constitutional disturbance may be severe.

The disease is rarely fatal. The most common cause of death in adults is primary viral pneumonia, among children, it is septic complications and encephalitis. Children with acute leukemia, including those in remission after chemotherapy, are at increased risk of disseminated disease, fatal in 5 to 10%. Neonates developing varicella between ages 5 and 10 days, and those whose mothers develop the disease 5 days prior to or within 2 days after delivery, are at increased risk of developing severe generalized chickenpox, with a case fatality rate of up to 30%. Infection early in pregnancy may rarely be associated with congenital malformations. Clinical chickenpox has been a frequent antecedent of Reye syndrome.

Herpes zoster (shingles) is a local manifestation of recurrent, recrudescent or reactivation infection with the virus that causes chickenpox. Vesicles with an erythematous base are restricted to skin areas supplied by sensory nerves of a single or associated group of dorsal root ganglia. Lesions may appear in crops in irregular fashion along nerve pathways, are usually unilateral, deeper seated and more closely aggregated than those of chickenpox; histologically they are identical. Severe pain and paresthesia are common. Zoster occurs mainly in older adults, although there is some evidence that almost 10% of children being treated for a malignant neoplasm are prone to develop zoster; persons with HIV infection are also at increased risk of zoster. In the immunosuppressed and those with diagnosed malignancies, extensive chickenpox-like lesions may appear outside the dermatome; this may also occur in otherwise normal individuals with fewer lesions. Intrauterine infection and varicella before 2 years of age are also associated with zoster at an early age. Occasionally , a varicelliform eruption follows some days after zoster, and rarely there is a secondary eruption of zoster after chickenpox.

Laboratory tests, such as visualization of the virus by EM, isolation of virus in cell cultures, or the demonstration of a rise in serum antibodies, are not routinely required but are useful in complicated cases and in epidemiologic studies. A number of antibody assays are now commercially available; in contrast, a promising skin test is not yet commercially available. Multinucleated giant cells may be detected in Giemsa-stained scrapings from the base of a lesion; these are not found in vaccinia lesions but do occur in herpes simplex lesions.

2. Infectious agent—Human (alpha) herpesvirus 3 (varicella-zoster virus, V-Z virus), a member of the *Herpesvirus* group.

3. Occurrence—Worldwide. Infection with human (alpha) herpesvirus 3 is nearly universal. In metropolitan communities, at least 90% of the population has had chickenpox by age 15 and at least 95% by young adulthood. Zoster occurs more commonly in older people. In temperate zones, chickenpox occurs most frequently in winter and early spring.

4. Reservoir—Man.

5. Mode of transmission—From person to person by direct contact, droplet, or airborne spread of secretions of the respiratory tract of chickenpox cases or of the vesicle fluid of patients with herpes zoster; indirectly through articles freshly soiled by discharges from vesicles and mucous membranes of infected persons. In contrast to vaccinia and variola, scabs from varicella lesions are not infective. Chickenpox is one of the most readily communicable of diseases, especially in the early stages of the eruption; zoster has a much lower rate of transmission (the contact develops chickenpox).

6. Incubation period—From 2 to 3 weeks; commonly 13-17 days; may be prolonged after passive immunization against varicella (see 9A2, below) and in the immunodeficient.

7. Period of communicability—As long as 5 but usually 1-2 days before onset of rash, and not more than 5 days after the appearance of the first crop of vesicles. Contagiousness may be prolonged in patients with altered immunity. Patients with zoster may be sources of infection for a week after the appearance of their vesiculopustular lesions. Susceptible individuals should be considered infectious 10-21 days following exposure.

8. Susceptibility and resistance—Susceptibility to chickenpox is universal among those not previously infected; ordinarily a more severe disease of adults than of children. Infection confers long immunity;

second attacks are rare. Infection apparently remains latent and may recur years later as herpes zoster in a proportion of older adults, sometimes in children.

Neonates whose mothers are not immune, and patients with leukemia may suffer severe, prolonged or fatal chickenpox. Adults with cancer, especially of lymphoid tissue, with or without steroid therapy, immunodeficient patients and those on immunosuppressive therapy, may have an increased frequency of severe zoster, both localized and disseminated.

9. Methods of control—

   A. *Preventive measures:*

      1) Protect high risk individuals such as nonimmune neonates and the immunodeficient from exposure.

      2) Varicella-Zoster Immune Globulin (VZIG), prepared from the plasma of normal blood donors with high antibody titer to varicella-zoster virus, is effective in modifying or preventing disease if given within 96 hours after exposure (see 9B5, below).

      3) A live attenuated varicella virus vaccine has been shown to protect children with leukemia exposed to siblings with chickenpox. An efficacy trial of this vaccine among normal children has shown a very high level of protection; in adults, the vaccine provides protection from severe infection, but breakthrough infections are not uncommon. The vaccine is not yet available commercially in the USA; a similar vaccine has been licensed in Japan.

   B. *Control of patient, contacts and the immediate environment:*

      1) Report to local health authority: In many states (USA) and countries, not a reportable disease, Class 3C (see Preface).

      2) Isolation: Exclude children from school for at least 5 days after the eruption first appears or until vesicles become dry; avoid contact with susceptibles. In the hospital, strict isolation is appropriate because of the risk of serious varicella in immunocompromised susceptible patients.

      3) Concurrent disinfection: Articles soiled by discharges from the nose and throat and from lesions.

      4) Quarantine: Usually none. However, in a hospital where susceptible children with known recent exposure must remain for medical reasons, the risk of spread to steroid-treated or immunologically compromised patients may justify quarantine of known contacts for a period of at least 10-21 days after exposure (up to 28 days if VZIG has been given).

5) Protection of contacts: VZIG given within 96 hours of exposure may prevent or modify disease in susceptible close contacts of cases. VZIG is available from regional offices of the American Red Cross for certain high-risk individuals exposed to chickenpox. It is indicated for newborns of mothers who develop chickenpox within 5 days prior to or within 48 hours after delivery. There is no assurance that administration of VZIG to a pregnant woman will prevent fetal infection.

6) Investigation of contacts and source of infection: Of no practical importance.

7) Specific treatment: While both vidarabine (adenine arabinoside, Ara-A®) and acyclovir (Zovirax®) are effective in treating varicella-zoster infections, the latter is generally considered the antiviral agent of choice.

C. **Epidemic measures:** None.

D. **Disaster implications:** Outbreaks of chickenpox may occur among children when crowded together in emergency housing situations.

E. **International measures:** None.

CHLAMYDIAL INFECTIONS

As laboratory techniques improve, chlamydial organisms are increasingly implicated as causes of human disease. Chlamydiae are obligate intracellular bacteria, which differ from viruses and rickettsiae but, like the latter, have been sensitive to broad-spectrum antimicrobials. They have been classified into two species: *Chlamydia psittaci,* the etiologic agent of psittacosis (q.v.), and *C. trachomatis,* including several serotypes which cause trachoma (q.v.), genital infections, chlamydial conjunctivitis (q.v.) and infant pneumonia (q.v.); others cause lymphogranuloma venereum (q.v.). Chlamydiae are now recognized as important pathogens responsible for an increasingly apparent number of sexually transmitted infections, with eye and lung infections in infants the consequences of genital infections in their mothers. *C. pneumoniae* has been proposed as the species name for a newly recognized agent, identified as TWAR, which has been associated with outbreaks of respiratory disease in Taiwan, Scandinavia, the USA and the Philippines (see under Pneumonia).

GENITAL INFECTIONS, CHLAMYDIAL   ICD-9 099.8

1. **Identification**—Sexually transmitted genital infections, manifested in males primarily as a urethritis, and in females by mucopurulent cervicitis. Clinical manifestations of urethritis are usually indistinguishable from gonorrhea and include an opaque discharge of moderate or scanty quantity, urethral itching, and burning on urination. Asymptomatic infection occurs in men; infection may be found in 1-10% of sexually active men. Possible complications or sequelae of male urethral infections include epididymitis, infertility and Reiter's syndrome. In homosexual men, receptive anorectal intercourse may result in chlamydial proctitis.

In the female, the clinical manifestations may be similar to those of gonorrhea, frequently presenting as a mucopurulent endocervical discharge, with edema, erythema and easily induced endocervical bleeding, caused by inflammation of the endocervical columnar epithelium. However, most women with endocervical or urethral infections are asymptomatic. Complications and sequelae are salpingitis with subsequent risk of infertility or ectopic pregnancy. Asymptomatic, chronic infections of the endometrium and fallopian tubes may lead to the same outcome. Less frequent manifestations include bartholinitis, urethral syndrome with dysuria and pyuria, perihepatitis (Fitz-Hugh-Curtis syndrome) and proctitis. Infection during pregnancy may result in conjunctival and pneumonic infection of the newborn. It is not yet clear whether these infections contribute significantly to low birth weight, prematurity, or postpartum endometritis. Endocervical chlamydial infection has been associated with increased risk of acquiring human immunodeficiency virus (HIV) infection.

Chlamydial infections may be acquired concurrently with gonorrhea and persist after the gonorrhea has been successfully treated. Because gonococcal and chlamydial cervicitis are often difficult to distinguish clinically, treatment for both organisms is recommended when one is suspected.

Diagnosis of nongonococcal urethritis (NGU) or cervicitis is usually based on the failure to demonstrate *Neisseria gonorrhoeae* by smear and culture; chlamydial etiology is confirmed by examination of intraurethral or endocervical swab material by direct IF test with monoclonal antibody, EIA, or cell culture. The intracellular organisms are less readily recoverable from the discharge itself. For other agents, see Urethritis, Nongonococcal, below.

2. **Infectious agent**—*Chlamydia trachomatis,* immunotypes D through K, has been identified in approximately 35-50% of cases of NGU in the USA.

3. **Occurrence**—Common worldwide; in the USA, Canada, Australia and Europe, recognition has increased steadily in the last two decades.

4. **Reservoir**—Man.

5. **Mode of transmission**—Sexual intercourse.

6. **Incubation period**—Poorly defined, probably 7-14 days or longer.

7. **Period of communicability**—Unknown. Relapses are probably common.

8. **Susceptibility and resistance**—Susceptibility is general. No acquired immunity has been demonstrated.

9. **Methods of control**—

A. *Preventive measures:* Health and sex education; same as for syphilis (q.v.), with emphasis on use of a condom during sexual intercourse.

B. *Control of patient, contacts and the immediate environment:*

1) Report to local health authority: Case report is required in some states in the USA, Class 2B (see Preface).
2) Isolation: Drainage/secretion precautions for hospitalized patients. Appropriate antibiotic therapy renders discharges noninfectious; patients should refrain from sexual intercourse until treatment is completed.
3) Concurrent disinfection: Care in disposal of articles contaminated with urethral and vaginal discharges.
4) Quarantine: None.
5) Immunization of contacts: Not applicable.
6) Investigation of contacts and source of infection: Prophylactic treatment of sexual partners is recommended. As a minimum, concurrent treatment of regular consorts is a practical approach to management. If neonates born to infected mothers have not received systemic treatment, chest x-ray at 3 weeks may be considered to exclude subclinical chlamydial pneumonia.
7) Specific treatment: Tetracycline, 2 g/day for 7 days, or doxycycline, 100 mg twice daily for 7 days. Erythromycin is an alternative drug and is the drug of choice for the newborn and for women with a known or suspected pregnancy.

C. *Epidemic measures:* None.

D. *Disaster implications:* None.

E. *International measures:* None.

URETHRITIS, NONGONOCOCCAL AND NONSPECIFIC   ICD-9 099.4
(NGU, NSU)

While chlamydiae are the most frequently isolated etiologic agents in cases of gonococcus-negative urethritis, other agents are involved in a significant number of cases. *Ureaplasma urealyticum* is considered the etiologic agent in approximately 10-20% of NGU cases; *Herpesvirus* type 2 and *Trichomonas vaginalis* have rarely been implicated. If laboratory facilities for demonstration of chlamydia are not available, all cases of NGU (together with their sexual partners) are best managed as though their infections were chlamydial, especially since many chlamydia-negative cases also respond to the antibiotic therapy.

CHOLERA   ICD-9 001

1. **Identification**—An acute bacterial enteric disease with sudden onset, profuse painless watery stools, occasional vomiting, rapid dehydration, acidosis and circulatory collapse. Asymptomatic infection is much more frequent than clinical illness, especially with organisms of the eltor biotype; mild cases with only diarrhea are common, particularly among children. In severe untreated cases, death may occur within a few hours and the case fatality rate may exceed 50%; with proper treatment, the rate is below 1%.

Diagnosis is confirmed by culturing *Vibrio cholerae* of the serogroup O1 from feces. Visualization by darkfield or phase microscopy of the characteristic vibrio motility inhibited by preservative-free serotype-specific antiserum, or demonstration of a significant rise in titer of antitoxic and vibriocidal antibodies help in presumptive diagnosis. In newly invaded areas, the isolated organisms should be confirmed by appropriate biochemical and serologic reactions and, if possible, by testing whether the organisms produce toxin.

2. **Infectious agent**—*Vibrio cholerae* serogroup O1 includes two biovars (biotypes)—cholerae (classical) and eltor—each of which includes organisms of Inaba and Ogawa serotypes. A similar enterotoxin is elaborated by these organisms so that the clinical pictures are similar. In any single epidemic, one particular type tends to be dominant; presently the eltor biotype is predominant, except in Bangladesh, where the classical biotype has reappeared. *V. mimicus* is a closely related species which can cause diarrhea; some strains elaborate an enterotoxin indistinguishable from that produced by *V. cholerae*.

Vibrios that are biochemically indistinguishable but do not agglutinate in *V. cholerae* serogroup O1 antiserum were formerly known as non-agglutinable vibrios (NAGs) or non-cholera vibrios (NCVs). They are now included in the species *V. cholerae*. Some strains elaborate the enterotoxin but most do not. Non-O1 strains have caused sporadic cases and rare outbreaks of diarrheal disease, but have not been associated with large epidemics or pandemics. In the USA, most sporadic cases follow eating raw or inadequately cooked seafood. The reporting of non-O1 *V. cholerae* infections as cholera is inaccurate and leads to confusion.

3. **Occurrence**—During the 19th century, pandemic cholera repeatedly spread from the Gangetic delta of India to most of the world. During the first half of the 20th century, the disease was confined largely to Asia, except for a severe epidemic in Egypt in 1947.

Since 1961, *V. cholerae* of the eltor biotype has spread from Indonesia through most of Asia into eastern Europe and Africa, and from North Africa to the Iberian Peninsula and into Italy in 1973. In 1977 and 1978, there were small outbreaks in Japan and, for the first time in this pandemic, cholera occurred in the S Pacific. Disease has continued in Africa, with 13 countries reporting cases in 1983. In Asia, 11 countries reported cholera, with both the classical and eltor biotypes occurring in Bangladesh; large outbreaks occurred in the Truk Islands in 1982 and 1983.

In 1988, thirty countries reported a total of 44,120 cases; there was a large outbreak in rural areas of China. Sporadic imported cases have continued to occur among travelers returning to western Europe, Canada, the USA and Australia.

Except for two laboratory-acquired cases, there was no known indigenous cholera in the Western Hemisphere between 1911 and 1973, when a case due to *V. cholerae* eltor Inaba occurred in Texas with no known source. In 1978, there were sporadic *V. cholerae* O1 eltor Inaba infections in Louisiana with 8 cases and 3 asymptomatic infections, and in 1981, an outbreak due to the identical *V. cholerae* strain occurred involving 16 persons on a Texas floating oil rig. Cases have continued to occur, with 16 indigenous cases in 1986, four in 1987, and eight in 1988 associated with consumption of raw oysters harvested in the Gulf of Mexico. (There were no cases reported for 1989.) Indigenous cases also occur in Queensland, Australia.

4. **Reservoir**—People; recent observations in the USA and Australia suggest that environmental reservoirs exist, apparently in association with copepods or other zooplankton.

5. **Mode of transmission**—Primarily through ingestion of water contaminated with feces or vomitus of patients, or, to a lesser extent, feces of carriers; or ingestion of unrefrigerated food which has been contaminated by dirty water, feces, soiled hands, or perhaps flies. Eltor organisms can

persist in water for long periods. Raw or undercooked seafood from polluted waters has caused outbreaks or epidemics in Guam, Portugal, Italy and Kiribati. The Louisiana cases have been traced to eating home-prepared crabs taken from lake and estuary waters contaminated with *V. cholerae*, serotype Inaba.

6. **Incubation period**—From a few hours to 5 days, usually 2-3 days.

7. **Period of communicability**—Presumably for the duration of the stool-positive stage, usually only a few days after recovery. However, occasionally the carrier state may persist for several months. Effective antibiotics, e.g., tetracycline, shorten the period of communicability. Rarely, chronic biliary infection, lasting for years, has been observed in adults, associated with intermittent shedding of vibrios in the stool.

8. **Susceptibility and resistance**—Variable; gastric achlorhydria increases risk of disease and breastfed infants are protected. Clinical cholera usually is confined to the lowest socioeconomic groups. Cholera gravis due to the eltor biotype occurs significantly more often in individuals of blood group O. Even in severe epidemics, attack rates rarely exceed 2%. Infection results in a rise in agglutinating, vibriocidal and antitoxic antibodies, and increased resistance to reinfection which lasts longer against the homologous serotype. In endemic areas, most persons acquire antibodies by early adulthood.

9. **Methods of control**—

    A. *Preventive measures:*

        1) See Typhoid fever, 9A1-7.
        2) Active immunization with the current killed whole-cell vaccine given parenterally is of no practical value in epidemic control or management of contacts of cases. These vaccines have been shown to provide partial protection (50%) of short duration (3-6 months) in highly endemic areas and do not prevent asymptomatic infection; these are not ordinarily recommended. Oral vaccines are under study.
        3) Measures that inhibit or otherwise compromise the movement of people, foods, or other goods are not justified unless specifically indicated on epidemiologically proven grounds.

    B. *Control of patient, contacts and the immediate environment:*

        1) Report to local health authority: Case report universally required by International Health Regulations (1969), Third Annotated Edition, 1983, WHO, Geneva; Class 1 (see Preface).

2) Isolation: Hospitalization with enteric precautions is desirable for severely ill patients; strict isolation is not necessary. Less severe cases can be managed on an outpatient basis with oral rehydration and tetracycline. Crowded cholera wards can be operated without hazard to staff and visitors when effective handwashing and basic procedures of cleanliness are practiced. Fly control should be practiced.

3) Concurrent disinfection: Of feces and vomitus and of linens and articles used by patients; by heat, carbolic acid or other disinfectant. In communities with a modern and adequate sewage disposal system, feces can be discharged directly into the sewers without preliminary disinfection. Terminal cleaning.

4) Quarantine: None.

5) Management of contacts: Surveillance of contacts for 5 days from last exposure. Mass chemoprophylaxis is not helpful, but for household members, chemoprophylaxis with tetracycline (1 g/day for 5 days in adults and 50 mg/kg/day for children over 9 years of age) is recommended. Doxycycline (single dose of 200 mg for adults and 4-6 mg/kg for children) or furazolidone (Furoxone®, 100 mg every 6 hours for 3 days for adults and 5 mg/kg/day for children) may also be used. Co-trimoxazole (8 and 40 mg/kg/day) may also be used in children. Immunization of contacts is not indicated.

6) Investigation of contacts and source of infection: Investigate possibilities of infection from polluted drinking water and contaminated food. A search by stool culture for unreported cases is recommended only among household members or those exposed to a possible common source in a previously uninfected area.

7) Specific treatment: Prompt fluid therapy with volumes of electrolyte solution adequate to correct dehydration, acidosis and hypokalemia is the keystone of cholera therapy. Most patients with mild or moderate fluid loss can be treated entirely with oral rehydration using solutions which contain glucose 20 g/l (or sucrose 40 g/l or cooked rice powder 50 g/l); NaCl (3.5 g/l); KCl (1.5 g/l); and $NaHCO_3$ (2.5 g/l) or trisodium citrate dihydrate (2.9 g/l).

Mild and moderate volume depletion should be corrected with oral solutions by replacing, over 4-6 hours, a volume matching the estimated fluid loss (approximately 5% of body weight for mild and 7% for moderate dehydration). Continuing losses are replaced by giving over 4 hours, a volume of oral solution 1-1/2 times the stool volume lost in the previous 4 hours.

Patients in shock should be given rapid intravenous rehydration with a balanced multi-electrolyte solution containing approximately 130 meq/l of Na^+; 25-48 meq/l of bicarbonate, acetate or lactate ions; and 10-15 meq/l of K^+. Useful solutions include: "Dacca solution" (5 g NaCl, 4 g $NaHCO_3$, and 1 g KCl/l), which can be prepared locally in an emergency; and Ringer's lactate or WHO "diarrhea treatment solution" (4 g NaCl, 1 g KCl, 6.5 g sodium acetate and 8 g glucose/l). After circulatory collapse has been effectively reversed, most patients can be switched to oral rehydration to complete the 10% initial fluid deficit replacement and to match continuing fluid loss.

Tetracycline and other antimicrobial agents shorten the duration of the diarrhea and reduce the volume of rehydration solutions required, as well as shortening the duration of vibrio excretion. Adults are given 2 g daily, either as a single daily dose or as 500 mg every 6 hours; children are given co-trimoxazole, furazolidone or tetracyline at 40 mg/kg. Where organisms are tetracycline-resistant (occasionally in East Africa and in Bangladesh), alternate medications include co-trimoxazole, furazolidone, erythromycin and chloramphenicol.

C. *Epidemic measures:*

1) Educate the population at risk concerning the need to seek appropriate treatment without delay.
2) Provide effective treatment facilities.
3) Adopt emergency measures to assure a safe water supply; chlorinate or boil water used for drinking, cooking, and for washing dishes and food containers unless the water supply is adequately chlorinated and protected from contamination thereafter.
4) Assure careful supervision of food and drink preparation. After cooking or boiling, protect against contamination by flies and unsanitary handling. Food served at funerals of cholera victims may be particularly hazardous and should be discouraged during epidemics.
5) Initiate a thorough investigation designed to find the vehicle and circumstances (time, place, person) of transmission and plan control measures accordingly.
6) Provide appropriate safe facilities for sewage disposal.
7) Vaccine is inappropriate in the epidemic situation.

D. **Disaster implications:** Risk of outbreaks is high in areas where cholera is endemic if large groups of people are crowded together without adequate food handling or sanitary facilities.

E. **International measures:**

1) Telegraphic notification by governments to WHO and adjacent countries of the first imported, first transferred or first nonimported case of cholera in an area previously free of the disease.

2) Measures applicable to ships, aircraft and land transport arriving from cholera areas are specified in International Health Regulations (1969), Third Annotated Edition, 1983, WHO, Geneva.

3) International travelers: Immunization is not recommended by WHO for travel from country to country in any part of the world and is not required by the USA. However, a few countries continue to require vaccination and vaccination certificates. International Health Regulations state that "a person on an international voyage, who has come from an infected area within the incubation period of cholera and who has symptoms indicative of cholera, may be required to submit to stool examination."

4) WHO Collaborating Centres (see Preface).

CHROMOBLASTOMYCOSIS   ICD-9 117.2
(Chromomycosis, Dermatitis verrucosa)

1. **Identification**—A chronic spreading mycosis of the skin and subcutaneous tissues, usually of a lower extremity. Progression to contiguous tissues is slow, over a period of years, with eventual large verrucous or even cauliflower-like masses and lymphatic stasis. Rarely a cause of death. Hematogenous spread to the brain has been reported.

Microscopic examination of scrapings or biopsies from lesions reveals characteristic large, brown, thick-walled, rounded cells that divide by fission in two planes. Confirmation of the diagnosis should be made by biopsy, and cultures of the fungus attempted.

2. **Infectious agents**—*Phialophora verrucosa, Fonsecaea (Rhinocladiella, Phialophora) pedrosoi, F. compacta, Cladosporium carrionii,* and *Rhinocladiella aquaspersa.*

3. **Occurrence**—Worldwide; sporadic cases in widely scattered areas, but mainly Central America, Caribbean Islands, southern USA, S America, S Pacific Islands, Australia, Japan, Madagascar and Africa. Primarily a disease of rural, barefooted agricultural workers in tropical regions, probably because of more frequent penetrating wounds of feet and limbs not protected by shoes or clothing. The disease is most common in men aged 30 to 50 years; women are rarely infected.

4. **Reservoir**—Wood, soil, and decaying vegetation.

5. **Mode of transmission**—Minor penetrating trauma, usually a sliver with contaminated wood or other materials.

6. **Incubation period**—Unknown; probably months.

7. **Period of communicability**—Not transmitted from person to person.

8. **Susceptibility and resistance**—Unknown, but rarity of disease and absence of laboratory-acquired infections suggest that people are relatively resistant.

9. **Methods of control**—

   A. *Preventive measures:* Protect against small puncture wounds by wearing shoes or protective clothing.

   B. *Control of patient, contacts, and the immediate environment:*

      1) Report to local health authority: Official report not ordinarily justifiable, Class 5 (see Preface).
      2) Isolation: None.
      3) Concurrent disinfection: Of discharges from lesions and articles soiled therewith.
      4) Quarantine: None.
      5) Immunization of contacts: Not applicable.
      6) Investigation of contacts and source of infection: Not indicated.
      7) Specific treatment: Oral 5-fluorocytosine benefits most patients and cures some. Large lesions respond better when 5-fluorocytosine is combined with amphotericin B (Fungizone®) IV. Oral ketoconazole has marginal efficacy when used alone. Small lesions are sometimes cured by excision.

   C. *Epidemic measures:* Not applicable, a sporadic disease.

   D. *Disaster implications:* None.

   E. *International measures:* None.

CLONORCHIASIS   ICD-9 121.1
(Chinese or oriental liver fluke disease)

1. **Identification**—A trematode disease of the bile ducts. Clinical complaints may be slight or absent in light infections; symptoms result from local irritation of bile ducts by the flukes. Loss of appetite, diarrhea, and a sensation of abdominal pressure are common early symptoms. Rarely, bile duct obstruction producing jaundice, may be followed by cirrhosis, enlargement and tenderness of the liver and progressive ascites and edema. A chronic disease, sometimes of 30 years or longer duration, but not often a direct or contributing cause of death and often completely asymptomatic. However, it is a significant risk factor for development of cholangiocarcinoma.

Diagnosis is made by finding the characteristic eggs in feces or duodenal drainage fluid; to be differentiated from those of other flukes. Serologic diagnosis by ELISA can be performed.

2. **Infectious agent**—*Clonorchis sinensis,* the Chinese liver fluke.

3. **Occurrence**—Highly endemic in SE China, but present throughout the country except in the northwest; occurs in Japan, Taiwan, Korea, Laos, Cambodia (Kampuchea) and Vietnam, principally in the Mekong (Red) River delta. In other parts of the world, imported cases may be recognized in immigrants from Asia. In endemic areas highest prevalence is among those over the age of 40.

4. **Reservoir**—Man, cats, dogs, swine and other animals.

5. **Mode of transmission**—People are infected by eating raw or undercooked freshwater fish or crayfish (reported from China) containing encysted larvae. During digestion, larvae are freed from cysts and migrate via the common bile duct to biliary radicles. Eggs deposited in the bile passages are evacuated in feces. Eggs in feces contain fully developed miracidia; when ingested by a susceptible operculate snail (i.e., *Bulinus, Semisulcospira,* etc.), they hatch in its intestine, penetrate the tissues and asexually generate larvae (cercariae) that emerge into the water. On contact with a second intermediate host (about 80 species of freshwater fish belonging mostly to the family Cyprinidae or several species of crayfish), cercariae penetrate the host fish and encyst, usually in muscle, occasionally on the underside of scales. The complete life cycle, from person to snail to fish to person, requires at least 3 months.

6. **Incubation period**—Unpredictable as it varies with the number of worms present; flukes reach maturity within 1 month after encysted larvae are ingested.

7. **Period of communicability**—Infected individuals may pass viable eggs for as long as 30 years. Not directly transmitted from person to person.

8. **Susceptibility and resistance**—Susceptibility is universal.

9. **Methods of control**—

   A. *Preventive measures:*

      1) Thoroughly cook all freshwater fish. Freezing at -10°C (14°F) for at least 5 days, or storage for several weeks in a saturated salt solution has been recommended but remains unproven.

      2) In endemic areas, educate the public to the dangers of eating raw or improperly treated fish and the necessity for sanitary disposal of feces to avoid contaminating sources of food fish. Prohibit use of nightsoil in fishponds.

   B. *Control of patient, contacts and the immediate environment:*

      1) Report to local health authority: Official report not ordinarily justifiable, Class 5 (see Preface).

      2) Isolation: None.

      3) Concurrent disinfection: Sanitary disposal of feces.

      4) Quarantine: None.

      5) Immunization of contacts: Not applicable.

      6) Investigation of contacts and source of infection: Of the individual case, not usually indicated. A community problem (see 9C, below).

      7) Specific treatment: The drug of choice is praziquantel (Biltricide®).

   C. *Epidemic measures:* Locate source of infected fish. Shipments of dried or pickled fish are the likely source in nonendemic areas.

   D. *Disaster implications:* None.

   E. *International measures:* Control of fish or fish products imported from endemic areas.

OPISTHORCHIASIS   ICD-9 121.0

Opisthorchiasis is caused by small liver flukes of cats and some other fish-eating mammals. *Opisthorchis felineus* occurs in Europe and Asia, and *O. viverrini* is endemic in SE Asia, especially Thailand. The biology of these flatworms, the characteristics of the disease and methods of control are essentially the same as those for clonorchiasis, given above. Eggs cannot be easily distinguished from those of *Clonorchis*.

COCCIDIOIDOMYCOSIS   ICD-9 114
(Valley fever, San Joaquin fever, Desert fever, Desert rheumatism,
Coccidioidal granuloma)

1. **Identification**—A systemic mycosis which generally begins as a respiratory infection. The primary infection may be entirely asymptomatic or resemble an acute influenzal illness with fever, chills, cough and (rarely) pleural pain. About one-fifth of clinically recognized cases (an estimated 5% of all primary infections) develop erythema nodosum, most frequently in white females, and rarest in black males. Primary infection may heal completely without detectable residuals, or may leave fibrosis, calcification of pulmonary lesions, a persistent thin-walled cavity, or, most rarely, progress to the disseminated form of the disease.

Disseminated coccidioidomycosis is a progressive, frequently fatal but uncommon, granulomatous disease, characterized by lung lesions and abscesses throughout the body, especially in subcutaneous tissues, skin, bone, peritoneum, testes, thyroid and the CNS. Coccidioidal meningitis resembles tuberculous meningitis but runs a more chronic course. An estimated 1/1000 cases of symptomatic coccidioidomycosis become disseminated. Dissemination is more common in blacks, Filipinos and other Asians, pregnant women, and in patients with AIDS or other forms of immunosuppression.

Diagnosis is made by demonstrating the fungus by microscopic examination or culture of sputum, pus, urine or CSF. (Handling cultures is extremely hazardous and must be carried out in a BSL 2 or 3 safety hood.) A positive skin test to coccidioidin or spherulin appears from 2-3 days to 3 weeks after onset of symptoms. Precipitin and CF tests are usually positive within the first 3 months of clinical disease. Serial skin and serologic tests may be necessary to confirm a recent infection or indicate dissemination; skin tests are often negative in disseminated disease, and serologic tests may be negative in the immunocompromised.

2. **Infectious agent**—*Coccidioides immitis,* a dimorphic fungus. It grows in soil and culture media as a saprophytic mold that reproduces by arthroconidia; in tissues and under special conditions of culture, the parasitic form grows as spherical cells (spherules) which reproduce by endospore formation.

3. **Occurrence**—Primary infections are common in arid and semiarid areas of the Western Hemisphere only: in the USA, from California to southern Texas; in northern Argentina, Paraguay, Colombia, Venezuela, Mexico and Central America. Elsewhere, dusty fomites from endemic areas can transmit infection; disease has occurred in persons who have merely traveled through endemic areas. The disease affects all ages, both sexes, and all races. More than half of patients with symptomatic infection are between 15 and 25 years of age; males are affected much more frequently than females, probably because of occupational exposure.

Infection is most frequent in summer, especially after wind and dust storms. It is an important disease among migrant workers, archeologists and military personnel from nonendemic areas who move into endemic areas.

4. **Reservoir**—Soil; especially in and around Indian middens and rodent burrows, in regions with appropriate temperature, moisture and soil requirements ("Lower Sonoran Life Zone"); infects man, cattle, cats, dogs, horses, burros, sheep, swine, wild desert rodents, coyotes, chinchillas, llamas and other animal species.

5. **Mode of transmission**—Inhalation of the infective arthroconidia from soil and in laboratory accidents from cultures. While the parasitic form is normally not infective, accidental inoculation of infected pus or culture suspension into the skin or bone can result in granuloma formation.

6. **Incubation period**—One to 4 weeks in primary infection. Dissemination may develop insidiously, sometimes without recognized symptoms of primary pulmonary infection and years after the primary infection.

7. **Period of communicability**—Not directly transmitted from man or animal to man. *C. immitis* on casts and dressings may rarely change from the parasitic to the infective saprophytic form after 7 days.

8. **Susceptibility and resistance**—A general susceptibility to primary infection is indicated by the high prevalence of positive coccidioidin or spherulin reactors in endemic areas; recovery is generally followed by solid, lifelong immunity. However, reactivation can occur in those who become immunosuppressed therapeutically or by HIV infection. Susceptibility to dissemination is much greater in blacks, Filipinos and other Asians, pregnant women and those with AIDS or other types of immunosuppression; isolated coccidioidal meningitis is more common in Caucasian males.

9. **Methods of control**—

  A. *Preventive measures:*

    1) In endemic areas: plant grass, oil unpaved airfields, and use other dust control measures (including use of face masks and air conditioned cabs, wetting soil, etc.).
    2) Individuals from nonendemic areas should preferably not be recruited to dusty occupations, such as road building. Skin testing could be used to screen out susceptibles.

  B. *Control of patient, contacts and the immediate environment:*

    1) Report to local health authority: Case report of recognized cases, especially outbreaks, in selected endemic

areas (USA); in many countries not a reportable disease, Class 3B (see Preface).

2) Isolation: None.
3) Concurrent disinfection: Of discharges and soiled articles. Terminal cleaning.
4) Quarantine: None.
5) Immunization of contacts: None.
6) Investigation of contacts and source of infection: Not recommended except in cases appearing in nonendemic areas, where residence, work exposure and travel history should be obtained.
7) Specific treatment: Amphotericin B (Fungizone®) is beneficial in severe and disseminated infections and is currently the agent of choice for meningeal infection (given by intrathecal or intraventricular injection). Ketoconazole has been useful in chronic, nonmeningeal coccidioidomycosis.

C. *Epidemic measures:* Outbreaks occur only when groups of susceptibles are infected by airborne conidia. Dust control measures should be instituted where practicable (see 9A1, above).

D. *Disaster implications:* Possible hazard if large groups of susceptibles are forced to move through or to live under dusty conditions in areas where the fungus is prevalent.

E. *International measures:* None.

CONJUNCTIVITIS
I. ACUTE BACTERIAL CONJUNCTIVITIS

ICD-9 372.0
ICD-9 372.03

(Pink-eye, Brazilian purpuric fever)

1. Identification—A clinical syndrome beginning with lacrimation, irritation and hyperemia of the palpebral and bulbar conjunctivae of one or both eyes, followed by edema of lids, photophobia and mucopurulent discharge. In severe cases, ecchymoses of the bulbar conjunctiva and marginal infiltration of the cornea may occur. A nonfatal disease (except as noted below), the clinical course may last from 2 days to 2-3 weeks;

many patients have no more than hyperemia of the conjunctivae and slight exudate for a few days.

Occasional cases of systemic disease have occurred among children in several communities in Brazil, 1-3 weeks after conjunctivitis due to *Haemophilus influenzae* biogroup *aegyptius*. This severe clinical illness, Brazilian purpuric fever (BPF), with a 70% case fatality rate in the fewer than 60 cases recognized, may be clinically indistinguishable from meningococcemia. The etiologic agent has been isolated from conjunctival, pharyngeal and blood cultures.

Confirmation of clinical diagnosis by microscopic examination of a stained smear or bacteriologic culture of the discharge is required to differentiate bacterial from allergic conjunctivitis, or infection by adenovirus or echovirus. Inclusion conjunctivitis (see below), trachoma and gonococcal conjunctivitis are described separately.

2. Infectious agents—*Haemophilus influenzae*, biogroup *aegyptius* (Koch-Weeks bacillus), and *Streptococcus pneumoniae* appear to be the most important; *H. influenzae* serovar b, *Moraxella lacunata* and *Corynebacterium diphtheriae* may also produce the disease. Staphylococci, streptococci and *Pseudomonas aeruginosa* may produce the disease in newborn infants.

3. Occurrence—Widespread and common throughout the world, particularly in warmer climates; frequently epidemic. In the USA, infection with *H. aegyptius* is confined largely to southern rural areas extending from Georgia to California, primarily during summer and early autumn; in North Africa and the Middle East, it occurs as seasonal epidemics. Infection due to other organisms occurs throughout the world, often in association with acute viral respiratory disease during cold seasons. BPF has been restricted essentially to Brazil; two cases which occurred in Australia were similar clinically, but the organism differed from the Brazilian strain.

4. Reservoir—Man. Carriers of *H. aegyptius* and *H. influenzae* are common in many areas during interepidemic periods.

5. Mode of transmission—Contact with discharges from the conjunctivae or upper respiratory tracts of infected persons, from contaminated fingers, clothing and other articles, including shared eye makeup applicators, multiple-dose eye medications and inadequately sterilized instruments such as tonometers. The organisms may be mechanically transmitted by eye gnats or flies in some areas, but their importance as vectors is undetermined and probably differs from area to area.

6. Incubation period—Usually 24 to 72 hours.

7. Period of communicability—During the course of active infection.

8. Susceptibility and resistance—Children under 5 are most often affected; incidence decreases with age. The very young, the debilitated and the aged are particularly susceptible to staphylococcal infections. Immunity after attack is low-grade and varies with the infectious agent.

9. Methods of control—

A. *Preventive measures:* Personal hygiene, hygienic care and treatment of affected eyes.

B. *Control of patient, contacts and the immediate environment:*

   1) Report to local health authority: Obligatory report of epidemics; no case report for classical disease, Class 4; for systemic disease, Class 2A (see Preface).
   2) Isolation: Drainage/secretion precautions. Children should not attend school during the acute stage.
   3) Concurrent disinfection: Of discharges and soiled articles. Terminal cleaning.
   4) Quarantine: None.
   5) Immunization of contacts: None.
   6) Investigation of contacts and source of infection: Usually not profitable for conjunctivitis; should be undertaken for BPF.
   7) Specific treatment: Local application of an ointment or drops containing tetracycline, erythromycin, chloramphenicol, gentamicin or a sulfonamide such as sodium sulfacetamide, depending on the infecting organism. For BPF, systemic treatment is required; isolates are sensitive to both ampicillin and chloramphenicol and resistant to co-trimoxazole. Oral rifampin (20 mg/kg/day for 2 days) may be more effective than local chloramphenicol in eradication of the BPF clone, and may be useful in the prevention of BPF among children with BPF clone conjunctivitis.

C. *Epidemic measures:*

   1) Prompt and adequate treatment of patients and their close contacts.
   2) In areas where insects are suspected of mechanically transmitting infection, measures to prevent access of eye gnats or flies to eyes of sick and well persons.
   3) Insect control, according to the suspected vector.

D. *Disaster implications:* None.

E. *International measures:* None.

II. ADENOVIRAL HEMORRHAGIC   ICD-9 077.2
CONJUNCTIVITIS
(Pharyngoconjunctival fever)
ENTEROVIRAL HEMORRHAGIC   ICD-9 077.4
CONJUNCTIVITIS
(Apollo 11 disease, Acute hemorrhagic conjunctivitis)

1. **Identification**—In adenoviral conjunctivitis, lymphoid follicles usually develop, the conjunctivitis lasts 7-15 days and there are frequently small subconjunctival hemorrhages. In one adenoviral syndrome, pharyngoconjunctival fever (PCF), there is upper respiratory disease and fever with minor degrees of corneal epithelial inflammation (epithelial keratitis).

In enteroviral acute hemorrhagic conjunctivitis (AHC), onset is sudden with redness, swelling and pain often in both eyes; the course of the inflammatory disease is 4-6 days, during which time subconjunctival hemorrhages appear on the bulbar conjunctiva as petechiae which enlarge to form confluent subconjunctival hemorrhages. The large hemorrhages gradually resolve over a 7-12 day period. In large outbreaks of enteroviral AHC, there has been a low incidence of polio-like paralysis, including cranial nerve palsies, lumbosacral radiculomyelitis and lower motor neuron paralysis. The neurologic complications start a few days to a month after the conjunctivitis and often leave some residual weakness.

Laboratory confirmation of adenovirus infections is made by isolation of the virus from conjunctival swabs in cell culture, by detection of viral antigens by IF, by identification of viral nucleic acid with a DNA probe, and by a rising antibody titer. Enterovirus infection is diagnosed by isolation of the agent or by demonstration of a rising antibody titer.

2. **Infectious agents**—Adenoviruses and picornaviruses. Most adenoviruses can cause PCF, but types 3, 4 and 7 are the most common causes; adenovirus type 3 outbreaks have occurred from poorly chlorinated swimming pools.

The most prevalent picornavirus type has been designated as enterovirus 70; this and a variant of coxsackievirus A24 have caused large outbreaks of AHC.

3. **Occurrence**—PCF occurs during outbreaks of adenovirus-associated respiratory disease or as summer epidemics associated with swimming pools. AHC was first recognized in Ghana in 1969 and Indonesia in 1970; since then numerous epidemics have occurred in many tropical areas of Asia, Africa, Central and S America, the Pacific Islands, and parts of Florida and Mexico. An outbreak in American Samoa in 1986 due to coxsackie A24 variant was estimated to have attacked 48% of the population. Smaller outbreaks have occurred in some European countries, usually associated with eye clinics. Cases also have occurred among

SE Asian refugees arriving in the USA and travelers returning to the USA from areas with AHC epidemics.

4. **Reservoir**—Man.

5. **Mode of transmission**—By direct or indirect contact with discharge from infected eyes. Person-to-person transmission is most noticeable in families, where high attack rates often occur. Adenovirus can be transmitted in poorly chlorinated swimming pools and has been reported as "swimming pool conjunctivitis"; it is also transmitted by respiratory droplets. The large epidemics of AHC in developing countries are associated with overcrowding and low hygienic standards. School children have been implicated in the rapid dissemination of AHC throughout a community.

6. **Incubation period**—Adenovirus infection: 4 to 12 days (mean=8 days). For picornavirus infection: 12 hours to 3 days.

7. **Period of communicability**—Adenovirus infections may be communicable up to 14 days after onset, picornavirus at least 4 days after onset.

8. **Susceptibility and resistance**—Infection can occur at all ages. Reinfections and/or relapses have been reported. The role and duration of the immune response are not yet clear.

9. **Methods of control**—

A. *Preventive measures:* Personal hygiene, including no sharing of towels; avoid overcrowding. Strict asepsis in eye clinics; wash hands before examining each patient. Closing schools may be indicated. Adequately chlorinate swimming pools.

B. *Control of patient, contacts and the immediate environment:*

1) Report to local health authority: Obligatory report of epidemics; no case report, Class 4 (see Preface).
2) Isolation: Drainage/secretion precautions; desirable to restrict contact with cases while disease is active; e.g., children should not attend school.
3) Concurrent disinfection: Of conjunctival discharges and articles soiled by them. Terminal cleaning.
4) Quarantine: None.
5) Immunization of contacts: None.
6) Investigation of contacts and source of infection: Locate other cases to determine whether a common source of infection is involved.
7) Specific treatment: None.

C. *Epidemic measures:*

1) Organize adequate facilities for the diagnosis and symptomatic treatment of cases.
2) Improve standard of hygiene and limit overcrowding wherever possible.

D. *Disaster implications:* None.

E. *International measures:* WHO Collaborating Centres (see Preface).

iII. CHLAMYDIAL CONJUNCTIVITIS   ICD-9 077.0
(Inclusion conjunctivitis, Paratrachoma, Neonatal inclusion blennorrhea, "Sticky eye")

1. **Identification**—In the newborn, an acute conjunctivitis with purulent discharge, with usual onset 5-12 days after birth; the acute stage usually subsides spontaneously in a few weeks, but inflammation of the eye may persist for as long as a year or more if untreated, and result in mild scarring of the conjunctivae and infiltration of the cornea (micropannus). Chlamydial pneumonia (q.v.) occurs in some infants with concurrent nasopharyngeal infection. All cases of neonatal conjunctivitis require definitive testing to rule out gonococcal infection, which may rapidly lead to blindness.

In children and adults, an acute follicular conjunctivitis is seen with preauricular lymphadenopathy on the involved side, conjunctival follicles, hyperemia, infiltration and a slight mucopurulent discharge; often with superficial corneal involvement. In adults, there may also be a chronic phase with scant discharge and symptoms which sometimes persist for a year or longer if untreated. The agent may infect the urethral epithelium in men and women, and the cervix in women; the conjuntivitis is sometimes associated with a urethritis or cervicitis.

Laboratory confirmation is made by specific IF staining, by EIA methods, and by isolation of the agent in cell culture from conjunctival scrapings.

2. **Infectious agent**—*Chlamydia trachomatis* of serovars D through K.

3. **Occurrence**—Sporadic eye cases are reported throughout the world in sexually promiscuous adults. Neonatal conjunctivitis due to *C. trachomatis* is common, occurring in 35-50% of newborns exposed to maternal infection. Among adults with genital chlamydial infection, 1 in 300 develops chlamydial eye disease.

4. **Reservoir**—Man.

5. **Mode of transmission**—The agent is transmitted during sexual intercourse; the genital discharges of infected persons are infectious. Eye infection in the newborn is usually by direct contact with infected birth passages; in utero infection may occur. The eyes of adults become infected by the transmission of genital secretions to the eye, usually by the fingers or by oral-genital sexual activities. Occasionally older children may acquire eye infection from infected newborns in the household, and gynecologists during operating procedures. Outbreaks reported among swimmers in nonchlorinated pools have not been confirmed by culture.

6. **Incubation period**—Five to 12 days with a range from 3 days to 6 weeks in newborns; 6 to 19 days for adults.

7. **Period of communicability**—While genital or ocular infection persists. Ocular carriage has been observed as long as 2 years after birth.

8. **Susceptibility and resistance**—There is no evidence of resistance to reinfection, although the severity of the disease may be decreased.

9. **Methods of control**—

   A. *Preventive measures:* Difficult to apply in view of the frequent clinically inapparent nature of the genital infections.

   1) General preventive measures are those for other sexually transmitted diseases (see Syphilis, 9A).
   2) Routine prophylaxis for gonoccocal ophthalmia neonatorum should be practiced. The method of choice is either a single application into the eyes of the newborn of tetracycline 1% eye ointment, erythromycin 0.5% eye ointment or silver nitrate 1% eye drops within 1 hour after delivery. All methods give comparable results in preventing gonococcal conjunctivitis. Controversy exists whether any of these methods is effective in preventing chlamydial ophthalmia. In addition, ocular prophylaxis does not prevent nasopharyngeal colonization and risk of subsequent chlamydial pneumonia. Penicillin is ineffective against chlamydia.
   3) Identification of infection in pregnant women by culture or antigen detection is critical. Treatment of cervical infection in pregnant women will prevent subsequent transmission to the infant. Erythromycin, 500 mg four times daily for 14 days, is usually effective.

   B. *Control of patient, contacts and the immediate environment:*

   1) Report to local health authority: Case report of neonatal

cases obligatory in many states (USA) and countries, Class 2B (see Preface).

2) Isolation: Drainage/secretion precautions for the first 96 hours after starting treatment.

3) Concurrent disinfection: Aseptic techniques and handwashing by personnel appear to be adequate to prevent nursery transmission.

4) Quarantine: None.

5) Immunization of contacts: Not applicable.

6) Investigation of contacts and source of infection: All sexual consorts of adult cases, and mothers and fathers of neonatally infected infants, should be examined and treated. Infected adults should also be investigated for gonorrhea and syphilis.

7) Specific treatment: For ocular and genital infections of adults, the tetracyclines, erythromycin or sulfonamides are effective when given by mouth for 1 week. Oral treatment of neonatal ocular infections with erythromycin, 40 mg/kg/day in 4 doses for 2 weeks, is recommended to eliminate the risk of chlamydial pneumonia also.

C. *Epidemic measures:* Sanitary control of swimming pools; ordinary chlorination suffices.

D. *Disaster implications:* None.

E. *International measures:* WHO Collaborating Centres (see Preface).

COXSACKIEVIRUS DISEASES ICD-9 074

The coxsackieviruses, which are members of the enterovirus group of the family Picornaviridae, are the causal agents of a group of diseases discussed here, and also epidemic myalgia, coxsackie carditis, epidemic hemorrhagic conjunctivitis and meningitis (see each disease under its individual listing). They cause disseminated disease in newborns, and there is evidence suggesting their involvement in the etiology of juvenile-onset, insulin-dependent diabetes.

ENTEROVIRAL VESICULAR   ICD-9 074.0
PHARYNGITIS
(Herpangina, Aphthous pharyngitis)
ENTEROVIRAL VESICULAR   ICD-9 074.3
STOMATITIS WITH EXANTHEM
(Hand, foot, and mouth disease)
ENTEROVIRAL LYMPHONODULAR   ICD-9 074.8
PHARYNGITIS
(Acute lymphonodular pharyngitis, Vesicular pharyngitis, Vesicular
stomatitis with exanthem)

1. **Identification**—Vesicular pharyngitis (herpangina) is an acute, self-limited, viral disease characterized by sudden onset, fever, sore throat, and small (1-2 mm), discrete, grayish, papulovesicular pharyngeal lesions on an erythematous base, which gradually progress to slightly larger ulcers. These lesions, which usually occur on the anterior pillars of the tonsillar fauces, soft palate, uvula and tonsils, may be present for 4 to 6 days after the onset of illness. No fatalities have been reported. In one series, febrile convulsions occurred in 5% of cases.

Vesicular stomatitis with exanthem differs from vesicular pharyngitis in that oral lesions are more diffuse and may occur on the buccal surfaces of the cheeks and gums and on the sides of the tongue. Papulovesicular lesions, which may persist from 7 to 10 days, also occur commonly as an exanthem, especially on the palms, fingers and soles; occasionally maculopapular lesions appear on the buttocks. Although usually self-limited, rare cases in infants have been fatal.

Acute lymphonodular pharyngitis also differs from vesicular pharyngitis in that the lesions are firm, raised, discrete, whitish to yellowish nodules, surrounded by a 3- to 6-mm zone of erythema. They occur predominantly on the uvula, anterior tonsillar pillars and posterior pharynx, with no exanthem.

Stomatitis due to herpes simplex virus requires differentiation; it has larger, deeper, more painful ulcerative lesions, commonly located in the front of the mouth. These diseases are not to be confused with vesicular stomatitis caused by the vesicular stomatitis virus, normally of cattle and horses, which in man usually occurs in dairy workers, animal husbandrymen and veterinarians. Foot-and-mouth disease of cattle, sheep and swine rarely affects laboratory workers handling the virus; however, man can be a mechanical carrier of the virus and the source of animal outbreaks. A virus not serologically differentiable from coxsackievirus B-5 causes vesicular disease in swine, which may be transmitted to man.

Differentiation of the related but distinct coxsackie syndromes is facilitated during epidemics. Virus may be isolated from lesions and nasopharyngeal and stool specimens in suckling mice and/or tissue culture. Since many serotypes may produce the same syndrome and common antigens are lacking, serologic diagnostic procedures are not routinely available unless virus is isolated for use in the serologic tests.

2. **Infectious agents**—Coxsackievirus, group A: types 1-6, 8, 10 and 22 for vesicular pharyngitis; type 16 predominantly, and types 4, 5, 9, 10 and enterovirus 71 less often, for vesicular stomatitis; and type 10 for acute lymphonodular pharyngitis. Other enteroviruses have occasionally been associated with these diseases.

3. **Occurrence**—Probably worldwide for vesicular pharyngitis and vesicular stomatitis, both sporadically and in epidemics, with greatest incidence in summer and early autumn; occurs mainly in children under 10 years, but adult cases (especially in young adults) are not unusual. Isolated outbreaks of acute lymphonodular pharyngitis, predominantly in children, may occur in summer and early fall. These diseases frequently occur in outbreaks among groups of children in nursery schools, child-care centers, etc.

4. **Reservoir**—Man.

5. **Mode of transmission**—Direct contact with nose and throat discharges and feces of infected persons (who may be asymptomatic) and by aerosol droplet spread; no reliable evidence of spread by insects, water, food or sewage.

6. **Incubation period**—Usually 3-5 days for vesicular pharyngitis and vesicular stomatitis; 5 days for acute lymphonodular pharyngitis.

7. **Period of communicability**—During the acute stage of illness and perhaps longer, since these viruses persist in stool for several weeks.

8. **Susceptibility and resistance**—Susceptibility to infection is universal. Immunity to the specific etiologic virus is probably acquired by clinical or inapparent infection; duration unknown. Second attacks may occur with group A coxsackievirus of a different serologic type.

9. **Methods of control**—

A. *Preventive measures:* Reduce person-to-person contact, where practicable, by measures such as crowd reduction and ventilation. Promote handwashing and other hygienic measures in the home.

B. *Control of patient, contacts and the immediate environment:*

1) Report to local health authority: Obligatory report of epidemics; no case report, Class 4 (see Preface).
2) Isolation: Enteric precautions.
3) Concurrent disinfection: Of nose and throat discharges. Wash or discard articles soiled therewith. Give careful

attention to prompt handwashing when handling discharges, feces and articles soiled therewith.

4) Quarantine: None.

5) Immunization of contacts: None.

6) Investigation of contacts and source of infection: Of no practical value except to detect other cases in groups of preschool children.

7) Specific treatment: None.

C. **Epidemic measures:** General notice to physicians of increased incidence of the disease, together with a description of onset and clinical characteristics. Isolation of diagnosed cases and all children with fever, pending diagnosis, with special attention to respiratory secretions and feces.

D. **Disaster implications:** None.

E. **International measures:** WHO Collaborating Centres (see Preface).

CRYPTOCOCCOSIS   ICD-9 117.5
(Torulosis, European blastomycosis)

1. **Identification**—A mycosis, usually presenting as a subacute or chronic meningitis. Infection of lungs, kidneys, prostate, bone and liver may occur. The skin may show acneiform lesions, ulcers or subcutaneous tumor-like masses. Occasionally, *Cryptococcus neoformans* may act as an endobronchial saprophyte in patients with lung disease of other origin. Untreated meningitis terminates fatally within several months.

Diagnosis of cryptococcal meningitis is aided by visualizing encapsulated budding forms on microscopic examination of CSF mixed with India ink; urine or pus may also contain these forms. Tests for antigen in serum and CSF are often helpful. Diagnosis is confirmed by histopathology or by culture (media containing cycloheximide inhibit *C. neoformans* and should not be used).

2. **Infectious agents**—*Cryptococcus neoformans* var. *neoformans* and *C. neoformans* var. *gattii*. The perfect states are called *Filobasidiella neoformans* and *F. bacillispora*.

3. **Occurrence**—Sporadic cases occur in all parts of the world. Mainly adults are infected; males twice as frequently as females. Approximately 8% of AIDS patients in the USA and Africa have developed cryptococ-

cosis. Infection also occurs in cats, dogs, horses, cows, monkeys and other animals.

4. **Reservoir**—Saprophytic growth in the external environment. The infectious agent can be isolated consistently from old pigeon nests and pigeon droppings and from soil in many parts of the world.

5. **Mode of transmission**—Presumably by inhalation.

6. **Incubation period**—Unknown. Pulmonary disease may precede brain infection by months or years.

7. **Period of communicability**—Not transmitted directly from person to person, or between animals and people.

8. **Susceptibility and resistance**—All races are susceptible; however, the frequency of *C. neoformans* in the external environment and the rarity of disease suggest that people have appreciable resistance. Susceptibility is increased during corticosteroid therapy, immune deficiency disorders (especially AIDS), and in disorders of the reticuloendothelial system, particularly Hodgkin's disease and sarcoidosis.

9. **Methods of control**—

A. *Preventive measures:* While there have been no case clusters traced to exposure of same, the ubiquity of *C. neoformans* in weathered pigeon droppings suggests that removal of large accumulations should be preceded by chemical decontamination, such as by an iodophor, or thorough wetting with water or oil to prevent aerosolization of the agent.

B. *Control of patient, contacts and the immediate environment:*

1) Report to local health authority: Official report required in some jurisdictions as a possible manifestation of AIDS, Class 2B (see Preface).
2) Isolation: None.
3) Concurrent disinfection: Of discharges and contaminated dressings. Terminal cleaning.
4) Quarantine: None.
5) Immunization of contacts: None.
6) Investigation of contacts and source of infection: Important only if the patient has HIV infection (see AIDS).
7) Specific treatment: Amphotericin B (Fungizone®) IV is effective in many cases; 5-fluorocytosine is less effective alone, but is useful in combination with low-dose amphotericin B. The combination is often the therapy of choice but has substantial toxicity. Cryptococcosis in

AIDS patients has proven very difficult to cure; flucona-
zole is useful to prevent relapse after amphotericin B
therapy.

C. *Epidemic measures:* None.

D. *Disaster implications:* None.

E. *International measures:* None.

CRYPTOSPORIDIOSIS   ICD-9 136.8

1. **Identification**—A parasitic infection of medical and veterinary
importance, which infects epithelial cells of the GI, biliary and respiratory
tracts of man as well as other vertebrates, including poultry and other
birds, fish, reptiles, small mammals (rodents, cats, dogs) and large
mammals (particularly cattle and sheep). The major symptom in human
patients is diarrhea, which may be profuse and watery, preceded by
anorexia and vomiting in children. The diarrhea is associated with
cramping abdominal pain. General malaise, fever, anorexia, nausea and
vomiting occur less often. Infection may be asymptomatic. Symptoms
usually wax and wane, but remit in fewer than 30 days in most
immunologically healthy persons. Immunodeficient persons, especially
AIDS patients, may be unable to clear the parasite and the disease has a
prolonged and fulminant clinical course, contributing to death. Symptoms
of cholecystitis may occur in biliary tract infections; the relationship
between respiratory tract infections and clinical symptoms is unclear.

Diagnosis is made by identification of oocysts in fecal smears or of life
cycle stages of the parasites in intestinal biopsy sections. Oocysts are small
(4-6 μ) and may be confused with yeast unless appropriately stained.
Oocysts are best identified after concentration from feces by a technique
such as Sheather's sucrose flotation method. Most commonly used stains
include auramine-rhodamine, a modified acid-fast, and safranin-
methylene blue. A fluorescein-tagged monoclonal antibody is useful for
detecting oocysts in stool or environmental samples. Infection with this
organism is not easily detected unless looked for specifically. Serologic
assays may be helpful in epidemiologic studies, but when the antibody
appears and how long it lasts after infection are not known.

2. **Infectious agent**—*Cryptosporidium* spp., a coccidian protozoan.

3. **Occurrence**—Worldwide. *Cryptosporidium* oocysts have been identified in human fecal specimens from more than 50 countries on six
continents. In developed areas such as the USA and Europe, prevalence

of infection was found in from <1% to 4.5% of individuals surveyed. In developing regions, the prevalence is significantly higher, ranging from 3 to 20%. Children over 2 years of age, animal handlers, travelers, homosexual men, and close personal contacts of infected individuals (families, health care and day-care workers) may be particularly likely to be infected. More than a dozen outbreaks have been reported in day-care centers around the world. Two major waterborne outbreaks have been documented, and several suspected waterborne outbreaks have been reported.

4. **Reservoir**—Man, cattle and other domestic animals.

5. **Mode of transmission**—Fecal-oral, with person-to-person, animal-to-person, and waterborne transmission important. The parasite infects intestinal epithelial cells, multiplying initially by schizogony, followed by a sexual cycle resulting in oocysts which pass out in the feces where they can survive under adverse environmental conditions for long periods of time. One or more autoinfectious cycles may occur in man.

6. **Incubation period**—Not precisely known; 1 to 12 days is the likely range, with an average of about 7 days.

7. **Period of communicability**—Oocysts, the infectious stage, appear in the stool at the onset of symptoms and continue to be excreted in the stool for several weeks after symptoms resolve; outside the body, they may remain infective for 2-6 months in a moist environment.

8. **Susceptibility and resistance**—People with intact immune function may have asymptomatic or self-limited symptomatic infections; it is not clear whether reinfection and latent infection with reactivation can occur. Individuals with impaired immunity generally clear their infections when the causes of immunosuppression (including malnutrition or inter-current viral infections such as measles) are removed. In those with acquired immunodeficiency syndrome (see AIDS), even though the clinical course may vary and asymptomatic periods may occur, the infection persists throughout the illness; approximately 4% of AIDS patients reported to CDC are infected with cryptosporidiosis when AIDS is diagnosed, and hospital experience indicates that 10-20% develop infection at some time during their illness.

9. **Methods of control**—

  A. *Preventive measures:*

   1) Educate the public in personal hygiene.
   2) Dispose of feces in a sanitary manner; use care in handling animal excreta.
   3) Careful handwashing by those in contact with calves and other animals with diarrhea (scours).

4) Filter or boil drinking water supplies; chemical disinfectants are not effective against oocysts.

B. *Control of patient, contacts, and the immediate environment:*

1) Report to local health authority: Case report by most practicable means, Class 3B (see Preface).
2) Isolation: For hospitalized patients, enteric precautions in the handling of feces, vomitus and contaminated clothing and bed linen; exclusion of symptomatic individuals from foodhandling and from direct care of hospitalized and institutionalized patients; release to return to work in sensitive occupations when asymptomatic. Stress proper handwashing.
3) Concurrent disinfection: Of feces and articles soiled therewith. In communities with modern and adequate sewage disposal systems, feces can be discharged directly into sewers without preliminary disinfection. Terminal cleaning. Heating to 45° C (113°F) for 5 to 20 minutes or chemical disinfection with 10% formalin or 5% ammonia solutions are effective.
4) Quarantine: None.
5) Immunization of contacts: None.
6) Investigation of contacts and source of infection: Microscopic examination of feces of household members and other suspected contacts, especially those who are symptomatic. Contact with cattle or domestic animals would warrant investigation.
7) Specific treatment: No treatment other than rehydration, when indicated, has been proven to be effective. If the individual is taking immunosuppressive drugs, these should be stopped if possible.

C. *Epidemic measures:* Epidemiologically investigate clustered cases in an area or institution to determine source of infection and mode of transmission; search for a common vehicle, such as water or raw milk; and institute applicable prevention or control measures. Control of person-to-person or animal-to-person transmission requires special emphasis on personal cleanliness and sanitary disposal of feces.

D. *Disaster implications:* None.

E. *International measures:* None.

CYTOMEGALOVIRUS INFECTIONS

Infection with cytomegalovirus (CMV) rarely produces symptomatic disease; when it does, the manifestations vary depending on the age and immunocompetence of the individual at the time of infection.

CONGENITAL CYTOMEGALOVIRUS INFECTION
ICD-9 771.1

CYTOMEGALOVIRUS DISEASE
ICD-9 078.5

1. **Identification**—The most severe form of disease occurs in the perinatal period, following congenital or acquired infection, with signs and symptoms of severe generalized infection, especially involving the CNS and liver. Lethargy, convulsions, jaundice, petechiae, purpura, hepatosplenomegaly, chorioretinitis, intracerebral calcifications and pulmonary infiltrates occur in varying degrees. Survivors may exhibit mental retardation, microcephaly, motor disabilities, hearing loss and evidence of chronic liver disease. Death may occur in utero; neonatal case fatality rate is high for severely affected infants. Although neonatal CMV infection occurs in 0.3-1% of births, most of these are inapparent; however, about 10% of asymptomatic congenital infections eventually manifest some degree of neurosensory disability. Fetal infection may occur during either primary or reactivated maternal infections; primary infections carry a higher risk but are much less common than reactivated infections.

Infection acquired later in life is generally inapparent, but may cause a syndrome clinically and hematologically similar to EBV mononucleosis, but distinguishable by virologic or serologic tests, or by the absence of heterophile antibodies. CMV causes up to 10% of all cases of "mononucleosis" seen among university students and hospitalized adults in the 25-34 year age group. A similar syndrome may follow blood transfusion, although many post-transfusion infections are clinically inapparent. Disseminated infection, with pneumonitis, retinitis and hepatitis, occurs in immunodeficient and immunosuppressed patients; this is a serious manifestation of AIDS.

Diagnosis is based on isolation of the virus from urine, saliva, cervical secretions, semen, breast milk, or tissue in human fibroblast cell cultures, by demonstration of typical "cytomegalic" cells in sediments of body fluids or tissues and by significant rises in serum antibody titers. Rapid diagnosis permits early institution of therapy, especially for patients with retinitis.

2. **Infectious agent**—Human (beta) herpesvirus 5 (human cytomegalovirus), a member of the subfamily Betaherpesvirus of the family Herpesviridae; includes several antigenically related strains.

3. **Occurrence**—Worldwide. Infection is acquired early in life in

developing countries. The prevalence of serum antibodies in adults varies from 40% in highly developed countries to almost 100% in developing countries; it is inversely related to socioeconomic status within the USA and is higher in women than in men. In the UK, prevalence of antibodies is related to race rather than social class. In various population groups, from 8 to 60% of infants begin shedding virus in the urine during their first year of life.

4. **Reservoir**—Man is the only known reservoir of human CMV; strains found in many animal species are not infectious for man.

5. **Mode of transmission**—Intimate exposure by mucosal contact with infectious tissues, secretions and excretions. CMV is excreted in urine, saliva, breast milk, cervical secretions and semen during primary and reactivated infections. The fetus may be infected in utero from either a primary or reactivated maternal infection; serious fetal infection with manifest disease at birth occurs most commonly during a mother's primary infection, but infection (usually without disease) may develop even when maternal antibodies existed prior to conception. Postnatal infection occurs more commonly in infants born of mothers shedding CMV in cervical secretions at delivery; thus, transmission of the virus from the infected cervix at delivery is a common means of infection in early life. Virus can be transmitted to infants through infected breast milk, an important source of infection. Viremia may be present in asymptomatic persons, and the virus may be transmitted by blood transfusion, probably associated with leukocytes. CMV is the most common cause of post-transfusion mononucleosis.

6. **Incubation period**—Information is inexact. Illness following transfusion with infected blood begins 3-8 weeks following the transfusion. Infections acquired during birth are first demonstrable 3-12 weeks after delivery.

7. **Period of communicability**—Virus is excreted in urine and saliva for many months and may persist or be episodic for several years following primary infection. After neonatal infection, virus may be excreted for 5-6 years. Adults appear to excrete virus for shorter periods, but the virus persists as a latent infection. Fewer than 3% of healthy adults are pharyngeal excretors. Excretion recurs with immunodeficiency and immunosuppression.

8. **Susceptibility and resistance**—Infection is nearly universal. Fetuses, patients with debilitating diseases, those on immunosuppressive drugs, and especially organ allograft recipients (kidney, heart, bone marrow) are more susceptible to overt and severe disease.

9. **Methods of control—**

   A. *Preventive measures:*
   1) Care in handling diapers, and handwashing after diaper changes and toilet care of newborns.
   2) Women of childbearing age who work in hospitals (especially delivery and pediatric wards) should use universal precautions; in preschools (especially those with mentally retarded populations) observe strict standards of hygiene such as handwashing.
   3) Wet nurses for babies born of mothers known to be antibody-free should be checked serologically to ensure freedom from infectivity.
   4) Avoid transfusing neonates of seronegative mothers with blood from CMV seropositive donors.
   5) Avoid transplanting organ tissues from CMV seropositive donors to seronegative recipients. If unavoidable, hyperimmune IG may be helpful.

   B. *Control of patient, contacts and the immediate environment:*
   1) Report to local health authority: Official report not ordinarily justifiable, Class 5 (see Preface).
   2) Isolation: None. Secretion precautions may be applied while in the hospital for patients known to be excreting virus.
   3) Concurrent disinfection: Discharges from hospitalized patients and articles soiled therewith.
   4) Quarantine: None.
   5) Immunization of contacts: None available.
   6) Investigation of contacts and source of infection: None, because of the high prevalence of asymptomatic shedders in the population.
   7) Specific treatment: Gancyclovir has been approved for the treatment of CMV retinitis in immunocompromised persons.

   C. *Epidemic measures:* None.
   D. *Disaster implications:* None.
   E. *International measures:* None.

DENGUE FEVER
(Breakbone fever)

ICD-9 061

1. **Identification**—An acute febrile viral disease characterized by

sudden onset, fever for 3-5 days (rarely more than 7, and often diphasic) intense headache, myalgia, arthralgia, retro-orbital pain, anorexia, GI disturbances and rash. Early generalized erythema occurs in some cases. A generalized maculopapular rash usually appears about the time of defervescence. Dengue infections with increased vascular permeability, unusual bleeding manifestations and involvement of specific organs are presented below under dengue hemorrhagic fever. Minor bleeding phenomena, such as petechiae, epistaxis or menometrorrhagia may occur at any time during the febrile phase. Dark-skinned races frequently have no visible rash. Recovery may be associated with prolonged fatigue and depression. Lymphadenopathy and leukopenia with relative lymphocytosis are usual; thrombocytopenia (<100,000/cu mm) and elevated transaminases occur less frequently. Epidemics are explosive, but fatalities in the absence of dengue hemorrhagic fever are rare.

Differential diagnosis includes all epidemiologically relevant diseases listed under arthropod-borne viral fevers, measles, rubella, and other systemic febrile illnesses.

HI, CF, ELISA, IgG and IgM antibody-capture and neutralization tests are diagnostic aids. Virus is isolated from blood by inoculation of mosquitoes, or by mosquito or vertebrate cell culture techniques, then identified with type-specific monoclonal antibodies.

2. **Infectious agent**—The viruses of dengue fever include immunologic types 1, 2, 3, and 4 (dengue-1, etc.); they are flaviviruses. The same viruses are responsible for dengue hemorrhagic fever (see below).

3. **Occurrence**—Dengue viruses of multiple types are now endemic in most countries in the tropics. In Asia, dengue viruses are highly endemic in southern China and Hainan, Vietnam, Laos, Cambodia (Kampuchea), Thailand, Myanmar (Burma), India, Sri Lanka, Indonesia, the Philippines, Malaysia and Singapore; with lower endemicity in New Guinea, Bangladesh, Nepal, Taiwan, and much of Polynesia. Dengue viruses of several types have circulated in northern Australia since 1983.

All four serotypes are now endemic in Africa. In large areas of West Africa, dengue viruses are probably transmitted epizootically in monkeys; urban dengue involving man is also common in this area. In recent years, limited outbreaks of dengue fever have occurred on the east coast of Africa from Mozambique to Somalia and on off-shore islands, such as the Seychelles.

In the American region: After the successive introduction or emergence of all four types in the Caribbean and Middle America since 1977 and extension into Texas in 1980, presently one or more dengue viruses are endemic in Mexico, most of the Caribbean, much of Central America, Venezuela, Colombia and Equador. Since 1986, large outbreaks in Brazil have radiated to Bolivia and Paraguay. In 1981, a major epidemic occurred in Cuba affecting 400,000 people. Epidemics may occur wherever vectors are present and virus is introduced, whether in urban or rural areas.

4. **Reservoir**—Man, together with the mosquito; the monkey-mosquito complex may be a reservoir in SE Asia and West Africa. Dengue virus may be transmitted transovarially in several species of *Aedes* mosquitoes.

5. **Mode of transmission**—By the bite of infective mosquitoes, principally *Aedes aegypti*. This is a day-biting species with increased biting activity for two hours after sunrise and two hours before sunset. Both *Ae. aegypti* and *Ae. albopictus* are effective vectors, often found in urban settings, and both are present within the USA.

In much of tropical Asia, *Ae. albopictus* may contribute to transmission of dengue virus in rural areas, while in Polynesia, one of the *Ae. scutellaris* complex may serve as the vector. In Malaysia, *Ae. niveus* complex, and in West Africa, *Ae. furcifer-taylori* complex and *Ae. aegypti* mosquitoes are involved in enzootic monkey-mosquito transmission.

6. **Incubation period**—Three to 14 days, commonly 7-10 days.

7. **Period of communicability**—Not directly transmitted from person to person. Patients are usually infective for mosquitoes from the day before to the end of the febrile period, an average of about 5 days. The mosquito becomes infective 8-12 days after the blood meal and remains so for life.

8. **Susceptibility and resistance**—Susceptibility is apparently universal, but children usually have a milder disease than adults. Recovery from infection with one serotype provides homologous immunity of long duration, but does not provide protection against another serotype, and instead may exacerbate the second infection (see dengue hemorrhagic fever, below).

9. **Methods of control**—

   A. *Preventive measures:*

      1) Educate the public on personal measures for destroying breeding sites and protecting against day-biting mosquitoes, including use of screening, protective clothing and repellents (see Malaria, 9A3 and 9A4).
      2) Community survey to determine density of vector mosquitoes, to identify breeding places (which for *Ae. aegypti* is usually in artificial or natural containers holding clear water close to or within human habitations, e.g., in old tires, etc.) and to promote and implement plans for their elimination.

B. **Control of patient, contacts and the immediate environment:**

1) Report to local health authority: Obligatory report of epidemics; no case report, Class 4 (see Preface).
2) Isolation: Blood precautions. Prevent access of day-biting mosquitoes to patients until fever subsides, by screening the sickroom, or by spraying quarters with a knockdown adulticide or residual insecticide, or by a bed net, preferrably insecticide impregnated.
3) Concurrent disinfection: None.
4) Quarantine: None.
5) Immunization of contacts: None. If dengue occurs near possible jungle foci of yellow fever, immunize the population for yellow fever because the urban vector for the two diseases is the same.
6) Investigation of contacts and source of infection: Determine place of residence of patient during the fortnight before onset and search for unreported or undiagnosed cases.
7) Specific treatment: None.

C. **Epidemic measures:**

1) Search for and destroy *Aedes* species of mosquitoes in places of human habitation, and eliminate or apply larvicide to all potential breeding sites of *Ae. aegypti*.
2) Use mosquito repellents for persons exposed through occupation to bites of vector mosquitoes.
3) Fogging and airplane spraying with suitable insecticides may help abort epidemics.

D. **Disaster implications:** Epidemics can be extensive, especially as a consequence of hurricanes or tropical storms.

E. **International measures:** Enforce international agreements designed to prevent spread of the disease by man, monkey and mosquito, and transfer of *Ae. aegypti* via ships, airplanes and land transport from areas where infection exists. WHO Collaborating Centres (see Preface).

DENGUE HEMORRHAGIC FEVER/ DENGUE SHOCK SYNDROME (DHF/DSS)　　　　ICD-9 065.4

1. **Identification**—A severe illness endemic in most of SE Asia, characterized by abnormal vascular permeability, hypovolemia and abnormal blood clotting mechanisms. Recognized principally in children; in adults with severe or fatal dengue, bleeding is the principal pathophysi-

ologic defect. Illness is biphasic, beginning abruptly with fever, and, in children, with mild upper respiratory complaints, often anorexia, facial flush and mild GI disturbances. Coincident with defervescence, the patient's condition suddenly worsens with profound weakness, severe restlessness, facial pallor and often profound diaphoresis and circumoral cyanosis. Extremities are cool, skin blotchy, pulse rapid and weak; patients may be hypotensive with a narrow pulse pressure.

Hemorrhagic phenomena are seen frequently and include scattered petechiae, a positive tourniquet test, easy bruisability, and less frequently, epistaxis, bleeding at venipuncture sites, a petechial rash, and gum bleeding. Gastrointestinal hemorrhage, while infrequent, is an ominous prognostic sign and may follow a prolonged period of shock. The liver may be enlarged, usually 2 or more days after the hypotensive stage. The presence of hypovolemia, as measured by a 20% or greater increase in the hematocrit, and abnormal hemostasis as evidenced by a platelet count ≤100,000/cu mm, are consistent with a diagnosis of dengue hemorrhagic fever (DHF), even in the absence of manifest bleeding. These findings, plus hypotension for age or a pulse pressure ≤20 mm Hg, are consistent with a diagnosis of the dengue shock syndrome (DSS). In severe cases there is accumulation of fluids in serosal cavities, low serum albumin, elevated transaminases, a prolonged prothrombin time and low levels of C3 complement protein. Case fatality rates in untreated or mistreated shock have been as high as 40-50%; with good physiologic replacement therapy, rates should be <5%.

Liver necrosis, with or without encephalopathy, was observed in some children affected during large outbreaks of dengue-3 in Indonesia and Thailand during the past decade.

Serologic tests show a rise in titer against dengue viruses, usually of the anamnestic (secondary) type (IgG). Primary-type antibody responses are seen commonly in patients less than one year old, and more rarely, in older children. Virus can be isolated from blood during the acute febrile stage by inoculation of mosquitoes or cell cultures. Isolation from organs at autopsy is difficult, but possible by mosquito inoculation.

(Infection with dengue viruses without hemorrhagic manifestations is covered above. The related yellow fever and other hemorrhagic fevers are presented separately.)

2. Infectious agent—See Dengue fever, above. All four dengue serotypes can cause DHF/DSS.

3. Occurrence—Recent outbreaks have occurred in the Philippines, China, Vietnam, Laos, Cambodia (Kampuchea), Thailand, Malaysia, Singapore, Indonesia, Myanmar (Burma) and Cuba. In 1981, 158 deaths occurred in Cuba among 116,000 hospitalized cases of dengue-2, four years after introduction of type 1 virus into the Caribbean; one-half of the deaths occurred among those <15 years old. The largest outbreak reported to date is that in Vietnam in 1987, when 370,000 cases were

reported. In tropical Asia, DHF/DSS is observed almost exclusively among the indigenous population. Occurrence is greatest during the rainy season and in areas of high *Ae. aegypti* prevalence.

4., 5., 6., and 7. Reservoir, Mode of transmission, Incubation period, and **Period of communicability**—See Dengue fever, above.

8. Susceptibility and resistance—Pathogenesis of the acute vascular permeability syndrome is best explained by immune enhancement of infection, in which heterologous dengue antibody, passively or actively acquired from earlier infection, promotes the infection of mononuclear phagocytes by formation of immune complexes. Enhanced virulence of dengue strains and human genetic susceptibility appear to play adjunctive roles. In the 1981 Cuban outbreak, DHF/DSS was observed fivefold less frequently in blacks than whites, when both had equal virus exposure. Orientals, East Indians and whites are fully susceptible. Modal age in SE Asia is 3-6 years, with a range from 4 months to the late teens. Severe disease with bleeding complications probably has a different pathogenesis than the acute vascular permeability syndrome. In endemic areas, prevalence of dengue antibodies is high in older children and adults with attendant immunity.

9. **Methods of control**—

   A. *Preventive measures:* See Dengue fever, above.

   B. *Control of patient, contacts and immediate environment:*

   1), 2), 3), 4), 5) and 6) Report to local health authority, Isolation, Concurrent disinfection, Quarantine, Immunization of contacts, and Investigation of contacts and source of infection: See Dengue fever, above.

   7) Specific treatment: Hypovolemic shock resulting from plasma loss from an acute increase in vascular permeability often responds to oxygen therapy and rapid replacement with fluid and electrolyte solution (lactated Ringer's solution at 10-20 ml/kg/hour). In more severe cases of shock, plasma and/or plasma expanders should be used. The rate of fluid and plasma administration must be judged by estimates of loss, usually by microhematocrit. A continued rise in hematocrit value in the presence of vigorous intravenous fluid administration indicates need for plasma or other colloid. Blood transfusions are indicated only when severe bleeding results in a true falling hematocrit. Heparin may be used when there is severe hemorrhage with specific laboratory evidence of severe and unremitting disseminated intravascular coagulation. Aspirin is contraindicated because of its hemorrhagic potential.

C., D., and *E. Epidemic measures, Disaster implications,* and *International measures:* See Dengue fever, above.

🏛️

DERMATOPHYTOSIS ICD-9 110
(Tinea, Ringworm, Dermatomycosis, Epidermophytosis, Trichophytosis, Microsporosis)

Dermatophytosis and tinea are general terms, essentially synonymous, applied to mycotic disease of keratinized areas of the body (hair, skin and nails). Various genera and species of fungi known collectively as the dermatophytes are causative agents. The dermatomycoses are subdivided according to the site of infection.

I. TINEA CAPITIS ICD-9 110.0
(Ringworm of the scalp and beard, Kerion, Favus)

1. **Identification**—Begins as a small papule and spreads peripherally, leaving scaly patches of temporary baldness. Infected hairs become brittle and break off easily. Occasionally, boggy, raised and suppurative lesions develop, called kerions.

Favus of the scalp (ICD-9 110.9) is a variety of tinea capitis caused by *Trichophyton schoenleinii.* It is characterized by a mousy odor and by formation of small, yellowish, cuplike crusts (scutulae) which look as though they were stuck on the scalp. Affected hairs do not break off but become gray and lusterless and eventually fall out and leave baldness which may be permanent.

Tinea capitis is easily distinguished from piedra, a fungus infection of the hair occurring in S America and some countries of SE Asia and Africa. Piedra is characterized by black, hard "gritty" or white, soft pasty nodules on the hair shafts, caused by *Piedraia hortai* and *Trichosporon beigelii,* respectively.

Examination of the scalp under UV light (Wood's lamp) for yellow-green fluorescence is helpful in diagnosing tinea capitis caused by *Microsporum canis* and *M. audouinii; Trichophyton* species do not fluoresce. Microscopic examination of scales and hair in 10% potassium hydroxide reveals characteristic hyaline ectothrix arthrospores. The fungus should be cultured for confirmation of the diagnosis.

2. **Infectious agents**—Various species of *Microsporum* and *Trichophyton.* Identification of genus and species is important for epidemiologic and prognostic reasons.

3. **Occurrence**—Tinea capitis caused by *M. audouinii* had been wide-

spread in the past, particularly in urban areas; *T. tonsurans* infections are now epidemic in urban areas in eastern USA, Puerto Rico and Mexico. *M. canis* infections occur in both rural and urban areas wherever infected cats and dogs are present and is the primary causative agent in Australia. *T. mentagrophytes* var. *mentagrophytes* and *T. verrucosum* infections occur primarily in rural areas where the disease exists in cattle, horses, rodents and wild animals.

4. **Reservoir**—Man for *M. audouinii, T. schoenleinii* and *T. tonsurans;* animals, especially dogs, cats and cattle, harbor the other organisms noted above.

5. **Mode of transmission**—Direct skin-to-skin or indirect contact, especially from the backs of theater seats, barber clippers, toilet articles such as combs and hairbrushes, or clothing and hats contaminated with hair from infected persons or animals.

6. **Incubation period**—Ten to 14 days.

7. **Period of communicability**—Fungus persists on contaminated materials as long as active lesions are present.

8. **Susceptibility and resistance**—Children below the age of puberty are highly susceptible to *M. canis;* all ages are subject to *Trichophyton* infections. Reinfections are rarely if ever noted.

9. **Methods of control**—

A. *Preventive measures:*

1) Educate the public, especially parents, to the danger of acquiring infection from infected children as well as from dogs, cats and other animals.

2) In the presence of epidemics or in hyperendemic areas involving non-*Trichophyton* species, survey heads of young children by UV light (Wood's lamp) before entering school. Also search for spotty alopecia and well-circumscribed lesions, especially in children with unkempt hair.

3) Vaccine is used in the USSR to protect animals from *Trichophyton* infection, with resultant reduction in human exposure.

B. *Control of patient, contacts and the immediate environment:*

1) Report to local health authority: Obligatory report of epidemics; no individual case report, Class 4 (see Preface). Outbreaks in schools should be reported to school authorities.

2) Isolation: None.

3) Concurrent disinfection: In mild cases, daily washing of the scalp removes loose hair. In severe cases, wash scalp daily and cover hair with a cap. Contaminated caps should be boiled after use.
4) Quarantine: Not practical.
5) Immunization of contacts: None.
6) Investigation of contacts and source of infection: Study household contacts, pets and farm animals for evidence of infection; treat if infected. Some animals, especially cats, may be inapparent carriers.
7) Specific treatment: Griseofulvin (GrisPEG®) by mouth for at least 4 weeks is treatment of choice for many. Topical antifungal medications such as Whitfield's ointment may be used concurrently. Systemic antibacterial agents are useful if ringworm lesions become secondarily infected by bacteria; in the case of kerions, also use a keratolytic cream and a cotton cover for the scalp. Examine weekly and take cultures; when cultures become negative, complete recovery may be assumed.

C. *Epidemic measures:* In epidemics in schools or other institutions, educate children and parents as to mode of spread, prevention and personal hygiene; enlist services of physicians and nurses for diagnosis; carry out follow-up surveys.

D. *Disaster implications:* None.

E. *International measures:* None.

II. TINEA UNGUIUM   ICD-9 110.1
(Ringworm of the nails, Onychomycosis)

1. **Identification**—A chronic fungal disease involving one or more nails of the hands or feet. The nail gradually thickens, becomes discolored and brittle, and an accumulation of caseous-appearing material forms beneath the nail, or the nail becomes chalky and disintegrates.

Diagnosis is made by microscopic examination of potassium hydroxide preparations of the nail and of detritus beneath the nail for hyaline fungal elements. Etiology should be confirmed by culture.

2. **Infectious agents**—*Epidermophyton floccosum,* various species of *Trichophyton* and rarely *Microsporum* species.

3. **Occurrence**—Common.

4. **Reservoir**—Man; rarely animals or soil.

5. **Mode of transmission**—Presumably by direct contact with skin or nail lesions of infected persons, possibly from indirect contact (contam-

inated floors and shower stalls). Low rate of transmission, even to close family associates.

6. **Incubation period**—Unknown.

7. **Period of communicability**—As long as an infected lesion is present.

8. **Susceptibility and resistance**—Injury to nail predisposes to infection. Reinfection is frequent.

9. **Methods of control**—

    A. *Preventive measures:* Cleanliness and use of a fungicidal agent such as cresol for disinfecting floors in common use; frequent hosing and rapid draining of shower rooms.

    B. *Control of patient, contacts and the immediate environment:*

        1) Report to local health authority: Official report not ordinarily justifiable, Class 5 (see Preface).

        2), 3), 4), 5), and 6) Isolation, Concurrent disinfection, Quarantine, Immunization of contacts, and Investigation of contacts and source of infection: Not practical.

        7) Specific treatment: Griseofulvin (GrisPEG®) by mouth is the treatment of choice; should be given until nails grow out (about 6 months for fingernails, 18 months for toenails).

    C., D., and E. *Epidemic measures, Disaster implications* and *International measures:* Not applicable.

III. TINEA CRURIS   ICD-9 110.3
(Ringworm of groin and perianal region)
TINEA CORPORIS   ICD-9 110.5
(Ringworm of the body)

1. **Identification**—A fungal disease of the skin other than of the scalp, bearded areas and feet, characteristically appearing as flat, spreading, ring-shaped lesions. The periphery is usually reddish, vesicular or pustular and may be dry and scaly or moist and crusted. As the lesion progresses peripherally, the central area often clears, leaving apparently normal skin. Differentiation from inguinal candidiasis is necessary, since treatment differs.

Presumptive diagnosis is made by taking scrapings from the advancing lesion margins, clearing in 10% potassium hydroxide and examining microscopically for segmented, branched hyaline filaments of fungus. Final identification is by culture.

2. **Infectious agents**—Most species of *Microsporum* and *Trichophyton;* also *Epidermophyton floccosum.*

3. **Occurrence**—Worldwide and relatively frequent. Males are infected more often than females.

4. **Reservoir**—Man, animals and soil; tinea cruris is almost always in males.

5. **Mode of transmission**—Direct or indirect contact with skin and scalp lesions of infected persons, lesions of animals; contaminated floors, shower stalls, benches and similar articles.

6. **Incubation period**—Four to 10 days.

7. **Period of communicability**—As long as lesions are present and viable fungus persists on contaminated materials.

8. **Susceptibility and resistance**—Susceptibility is widespread, aggravated by friction and excessive perspiration in axillary and inguinal regions, and when environmental temperatures and humidity are high. All ages are susceptible.

9. **Methods of control**—

A. *Preventive measures:* Launder towels and clothing with hot water and/or fungicidal agent; general cleanliness in showers and dressing rooms of gymnasiums, especially repeated washing of benches; frequent hosing and rapid draining of shower rooms. A fungicidal agent such as cresol should be used to disinfect benches and floors.

B. *Control of patient, contacts and the immediate environment:*

1) Report to local health authority: Obligatory report of epidemics; no individual case report, Class 4 (see Preface). Report infections of school children to school authorities.

2) Isolation: While under treatment, infected children should be excluded from gymnasiums, swimming pools and activities likely to lead to exposure of others.

3) Concurrent disinfection: Effective and frequent laundering of clothing.

4) Quarantine: None.

5) Immunization of contacts: None.

6) Investigation of contacts and source of infection: Examine school and household contacts, household pets and farm animals; treat infections as indicated.

7) Specific treatment: Thorough bathing with soap and water, removal of scabs and crusts, and application of an effective topical fungicide such as miconazole, ketocona-

zole, clotrimazole, tolnaftate or ciclopirox may suffice. Griseofulvin (GrisPEG®) by mouth is effective; oral ketoconazole is useful in griseofulvin-resistant ringworm, but hepatotoxicity prevents it from being the drug of choice.

C. *Epidemic measures:* Educate children and parents concerning the nature of the infection, its mode of spread and the need to maintain good personal hygiene.

D. *Disaster implications:* None.

E. *International measures:* None.

IV. TINEA PEDIS ICD-9 110.4
(Ringworm of the foot, Athlete's foot)

1. **Identification**—Scaling or cracking of the skin, especially between the toes, or blisters containing a thin watery fluid are characteristic; commonly called "athlete's foot." In severe cases, vesicular lesions appear on various parts of the body, especially the hands; these dermatophytids do not contain the fungus but are an allergic reaction to fungus products.

Diagnosis is verified by microscopic examination of potassium hydroxide-treated scrapings from lesions between the toes which reveal septate branching filaments. Clinical appearance of lesions is not diagnostic.

2. **Infectious agents**—*Trichophyton rubrum, T. mentagrophytes* var. *interdigitale* and *Epidermophyton floccosum.*

3. **Occurrence**—Worldwide; a common disease. Adults more often affected than children; males more than females. Infections are more frequent and more severe in hot weather.

4. **Reservoir**—Man.

5. **Mode of transmission**—Direct or indirect contact with skin lesions of infected persons or contaminated floors, shower stalls and other articles used by infected persons.

6. **Incubation period**—Unknown.

7. **Period of communicability**—As long as lesions are present and viable spores persist on contaminated materials.

8. **Susceptibility and resistance**—Susceptibility is variable and infection may be inapparent. Repeated attacks are frequent.

9. **Methods of control**—

A. *Preventive measures:* Those for tinea corporis, above. Educate the public to maintain strict personal hygiene; special care in drying areas between toes after bathing. Regular use of a dusting powder containing an effective fungicide on the feet and particularly between the toes. Occlusive shoes may predispose to infection and disease.

B. *Control of patient, contacts and the immediate environment:*

1) Report to local health authority: Obligatory report of epidemics; no individual case report, Class 4 (see Preface). Report high incidence in schools to school authorities.
2) Isolation: None.
3) Concurrent disinfection: Boil socks of heavily infected individuals to prevent reinfection.
4) Quarantine: None.
5) Immunization of contacts: None.
6) Investigation of contacts and source of infection: None.
7) Specific treatment: Topical fungicides such as miconazole, clotrimazole, ketoconazole, ciclopirox or tolnaftate. Expose feet to air by wearing sandals; use dusting powders. Griseofulvin (GrisPEG®) by mouth may be indicated in severe, protracted disease, but is usually less effective than conscientious application of local fungicides.

C. *Epidemic measures:* Thoroughly clean and wash floors of gymnasiums, showers and similar sources of infection, disinfect with a fungicidal agent such as cresol. Educate the public concerning the mode of spread.

D. *Disaster implications:* None.

E. *International measures:* None.

DIARRHEA, ACUTE BACTERIAL

Diarrhea is a clinical syndrome of diverse etiology associated with frequent loose or watery stools, and often vomiting and fever. It is a symptom of infection by bacterial, viral and parasitic enteric agents that cause cholera, shigellosis, salmonellosis, yersiniosis, giardiasis, campylobacteriosis, cryptosporidiosis and viral gastroenteropathy. (See each disease under its individual listing.) It can also be caused by infection with certain categories of *Escherichia coli* strains, non-O1 *Vibrio cholerae* and *Vibrio parahaemolyticus,* other infectious diseases such as malaria and measles, as well as chemical agents. Approximately 70-80% of diarrheal episodes in people visiting treatment facilities in less-developed countries can be diagnosed etiologically if the complete battery of newer laboratory tests were available and utilized. In industrialized countries, the comparable figure is about 45% of cases (except among infants in the winter months in temperate climates, when the percentage is much higher because rotavirus alone accounts for 50-70% of the cases). However, very few laboratories can identify all the newly described pathogens.

From a practical clinical standpoint, diarrheal illnesses can be divided into six clinical presentations:

(1) simple diarrhea, managed by oral rehydration with solutions containing water, glucose and electrolytes (ORS), with its specific etiology not important for management;

(2) dysentery, with scanty stools containing blood and/or mucus, caused by *Shigella* or certain other organisms;

(3) persistent diarrhea that lasts at least 14 days;

(4) severe purging as seen in cholera;

(5) vomiting disease, in which minimal diarrhea is associated with repeated and persistent vomiting typical of viral gastroenteritis; and

(6) hemorrhagic colitis, with watery diarrhea containing gross blood but with no fever or fecal leukocytes. Several of these illnesses may be thought of as a single entity since the basic therapy required to prevent a fatal outcome, fluid and electrolyte replacement, is similar. This chapter will present the varieties of *E. coli* diarrhea.

DIARRHEA CAUSED BY *ESCHERICHIA COLI* ICD-9 008.0

Strains of *Escherichia coli* that cause diarrhea are of five major categories: 1) enterotoxigenic, 2) enteroinvasive, 3) enteropathogenic, 4) enterohemorrhagic and 5) "enteroaggregative." Each category has a different pathogenesis, possesses distinct virulence properties, and comprises a separate set of O:H serotypes. Differing clinical syndromes and epidemiologic patterns may also be seen.

I. DIARRHEA CAUSED BY ENTEROTOXIGENIC STRAINS (ETEC)

1. **Identification**—A major cause of travelers' diarrhea in persons from industrialized countries who visit less-developed countries, it is also an important cause of dehydrating diarrhea in infants and children in less-developed countries. Enterotoxigenic strains may behave more like *Vibrio cholerae* in producing a profuse watery diarrhea without blood or mucus. Abdominal cramping, vomiting, acidosis, prostration and dehydration can occur and low-grade fever may or may not be present; the

symptoms usually last fewer than 3 to 5 days.

ETEC can be identified by demonstrating enterotoxin production by immunoassays, bioassays or DNA probe techniques that identify LT and ST genes (for heat-labile and heat-stable toxins) in colony blots.

2. **Infectious agent**—ETEC elaborate a heat-labile toxin (LT), a heat stable toxin (ST) or both toxins (LT/ST). The most common O serogroups include O6, O8, O15, O20, O25, O27, O63, O78, O80, O114, O115, O128ac, O148, O153, O159 and O167.

3. **Occurrence**—Primarily an infection of developing countries: During the first three years of life, children in developing countries experience multiple ETEC infections; illness in older children and adults occurs less frequently. Infection occurs among travelers from industrialized countries who visit less-developed countries.

4. **Reservoir**—Man ETEC infections are largely species-specific; man constitutes the reservoir for strains causing diarrhea in man.

5. **Mode of transmission**—Contaminated food, and less often, contaminated water. Transmission via contaminated weaning foods may be particularly important in infection of infants. Direct contact transmission by fecally-contaminated hands is believed to be rare.

6. **Incubation period**—Incubations as short as 10-12 hours have been observed in outbreaks and in volunteer studies with certain LT-only and ST-only strains. The incubation of LT/ST diarrhea in volunteer studies has usually been 24-72 hours.

7. **Period of communicability**—For the duration of excretion of the pathogenic ETEC, which may be prolonged.

8. **Susceptibility and resistance**—Epidemiologic studies and rechallenge studies in volunteers clearly demonstrate that serotype-specific immunity is acquired following ETEC infection. Multiple infections with different serotypes are required to develop broad-spectrum immunity against ETEC.

9. **Methods of control**—

  A. *Preventive measures:*

  1) For general measures for prevention of fecal-oral spread of infection, see Typhoid fever, 9A.
  2) For travelers going to high-risk areas where it is not possible to obtain safe food or water, prophylactic antibiotic therapy may be used; norfloxacin, 400 mg daily, has been shown to be effective. However, very early treatment of disease is preferable, beginning with the onset of diarrhea. (See 9B7, below.)

B.   *Control of patient, contacts and the immediate environment:*

1)   Report to local health authority: Obligatory report of epidemics; no individual case report, Class 4 (see Preface).

2)   Isolation: Enteric precautions for known and suspected cases.

3)   Concurrent disinfection: Of all fecal discharges and soiled articles. In communities with a modern and adequate sewage disposal system, feces can be discharged directly into sewers without preliminary disinfection. Thorough terminal cleaning.

4)   Quarantine: None.

5)   Immunization of contacts: None.

6)   Investigation of contacts and source of infection: Not indicated.

7)   Specific treatment: Electrolyte-fluid therapy to prevent or treat dehydration is the most important measure (see Cholera, 9B7). Most cases do not require any other therapy. For severe "travelers' diarrhea," early treatment with co-trimoxazole (160 mg-800 mg) orally twice daily, or doxycycline (100 mg) orally once daily, for 5 days is effective. Preliminary data suggest that oral ciprofloxacin, 500 mg twice daily for 5 days, is a useful alternative. Feeding should be continued, according to the patient's appetite.

C.   *Epidemic measures:* Epidemiologic investigation may be indicated to determine how transmission is occurring.

D.   *Disaster implications:* None.

E.   *International measures:* WHO Collaborating Centres (see Preface).

II. DIARRHEA CAUSED BY ENTEROINVASIVE STRAINS (EIEC)

1. **Identification**—This inflammatory disease of the gut mucosa and submucosa, caused by EIEC strains of *E. coli,* closely resembles that produced by *Shigella.* The organisms possess the same plasmid-dependent ability to invade and multiply within epithelial cells; clinically, they cause dysentery. The O antigens of EIEC may cross-react with *Shigella* O antigens. Illness begins with severe abdominal cramps, malaise, watery stools, tenesmus and fever, and progresses to the passage of multiple, scanty, fluid stools containing blood and mucus.

EIEC may be suspected by the presence of many fecal leukocytes visible in a stained smear of mucus. An immunoassay detects the plasmid-encoded specific outer membrane proteins that are associated with epithelial cell invasiveness; a bioassay (the guinea pig keratoconjunctivitis test) detects epithelial cell invasiveness; DNA probes detect the enteroinvasiveness plasmid.

2. Infectious agent—Strains of *E. coli* shown to possess enteroinvasiveness. The main O serogroups in which EIEC fall include O28ac, O29, O112, O124, O136, O143, O144, O152, O164 and O167.

3. Occurrence—EIEC infections are endemic in less-developed countries, comprising about 1-5% of persons visiting treatment centers for diarrhea. Occasional infections and outbreaks of EIEC diarrhea have been reported in industrialized countries.

4. Reservoir—Man.

5. Mode of transmission—Scanty available evidence suggests that EIEC is transmitted by contaminated food.

6. Incubation period—Incubations as short as 10 and 18 hours have been observed in volunteer studies and outbreaks, respectively.

7. Period of communicability—Duration of excretion of EIEC strains.

8. Susceptibility and resistance—Little is known about susceptibility and immunity to EIEC.

9. Methods of control—Same as for ETEC, above. For the rare cases of severe diarrhea with enteroinvasive strains, oral absorbable or parenteral antibiotics such as ampicillin (50 mg/kg/day) may be given.

III. DIARRHEA CAUSED BY ENTEROPATHOGENIC STRAINS (EPEC)
(Enteropathogenic *E. coli* enteritis)

1. Identification—This is the oldest recognized category of diarrheagenic *E. coli,* implicated in 1940s and 1950s' case-control studies wherein certain O:H serotypes were found to be associated with infant summer diarrhea, outbreaks of diarrhea in infant nurseries, and community epidemics of infant diarrhea. Diarrheal disease in this category is virtually confined to infants less than one year of age, in whom it causes watery diarrhea with mucus, fever and dehydration. EPEC cause dissolution of the microvilli of enterocytes; the diarrhea in infants can be both severe and prolonged, and may be associated with high case fatality.

EPEC can be tentatively identified by agglutination with antisera that detect EPEC O serogroups, but confirmation requires both O and H typing. EPEC organisms also show localized adherence to HEp-2 cells, and the EPEC adherence factor (EAF) can be demonstrated by a DNA probe; there is a 98% correlation between the detection of localized adherence and EAF probe positivity.

2. **Infectious agent**—The major EPEC O serogroups include O55, O86, O111, O119, O125, O126, O127, O128ab and O142.

3. **Occurrence**—Since the late 1960s, EPEC has largely disappeared as an important cause of infant diarrhea in N America and Europe. However, it remains a major agent of infant diarrhea in many developing areas, including S America, southern Africa and Asia.

4. **Reservoir**—Man.

5. **Mode of transmission**—By contaminated infant formula and weaning foods. In infant nurseries, transmission by fomites and by contaminated hands can occur if handwashing techniques are compromised.

6. **Incubation period**—As short as 9-12 hours in adult volunteer studies. It is not known whether the same incubation applies to infants who acquire infection by natural transmission.

7. **Period of communicability**—Limited to the duration of excretion of the pathogenic *E. coli* EPEC, which may be prolonged.

8. **Susceptibility and resistance**—Although susceptibility to clinical infection appears to be confined virtually to young infants in nature, it is not known if this is due to immunity or to age-related, non-specific host factors. Since diarrhea can be induced experimentally in some adult volunteers, specific immunity may be important in determining susceptibility.

9. **Methods of control**—

    A. *Preventive measures:* Prevention of hospital nursery outbreaks depends primarily on adequate handwashing practices, a scrupulously clean nursery, isolation of patients with diarrhea, and culturing stools to establish the etiologic agent.

      1) Breast feed if possible; encourage mother-infant (rooming-in) hospitalization in obstetrical facilities.

      2) If breast feeding is not possible, prepare feeding formulas aseptically: fill the bottle, apply nipple, cover with a cap, sterilize, and refrigerate with nipple and caps on bottles until feeding time; if available, use disposable formula containers. Evaluate sterility by periodic bacteriologic sampling of locally prepared formulas; such sampling of

commercially prepared formula is not necessary except in epidemiologic investigations.

3) Provide nurseries for the healthy newborn and premature infants separate from those for ill infants. Provide each infant with individual equipment, including thermometer, kept at the bassinet; use no common bathing or dressing tables and no bassinet stands for holding or transporting more than one infant at a time.

4) Provide separate isolation facilities for sick infants and older children. Isolate for at least 6 days any infant born to a mother with diarrheal or respiratory illness. Control visitors to minimize spread of infection. Monitor laundry procedures to assure absence of pathogens from materials returned to the nursery.

5) Keep a systematic daily record of number and consistency of stools for each infant.

6) Limit spread of infection (even in the absence of an outbreak) by housing each entire cohort of infants born during different time periods in separate areas throughout their hospitalization. Personnel should not care for more than one cohort of infants.

B. *Control of patient, contacts and the immediate environment:*

1) Report to local health authority: Obligatory report of epidemics; no individual case report, Class 4 (see Preface). Two or more concurrent cases of diarrhea requiring treatment for these symptoms in a nursery or among those recently discharged are to be interpreted as an outbreak requiring investigation.

2) Isolation: Enteric precautions for known and suspected cases.

3) Concurrent disinfection: Of all fecal discharges and soiled articles. In communities with a modern and adequate sewage disposal system, feces can be discharged directly into sewers without preliminary disinfection. Thorough terminal cleaning.

4) Quarantine: Use enteric precautions and cohort methods (see 9A3, above).

5) Immunization of contacts: None.

6) Investigation of contacts and source of infection: Families of discharged babies should be contacted for diarrheal status of the baby (see 9C2, below).

7) Specific treatment: Electrolyte/fluid therapy (oral or IV) is the most important measure (see Cholera, 9B7). Most cases do not require any other therapy. For severe enteropathogenic infant diarrhea, oral co-trimoxazole

(10-50 mg/kg/day) has been shown to ameliorate the severity and duration of diarrheal illness. It should be administered in 3 to 4 divided doses for 5 days. Feeding, including breast feeding, should be continued.

C. *Epidemic measures:* For nursery epidemics (see 9B1, above) the following—

1) All babies with diarrhea should be placed in one nursery under enteric precautions. Admit no more babies to the contaminated nursery. Suspend maternity service unless a clean nursery is available with separate personnel and facilities; promptly discharge infected infants when medically possible. For the babies exposed in the contaminated nursery, provide separate medical and nursing personnel skilled in the care of infants with communicable diseases. Observe contacts for at least 2 weeks after the last case leaves the nursery; promptly remove each new case to one nursery ward used for these infants. Maternity service may be resumed after discharge of all contact babies and mothers, and thorough cleaning and terminal disinfection. Put into practice recommendations of 9A, above, so far as feasible in the emergency.

2) Carry out a thorough epidemiologic investigation into the distribution of cases by time, place, person and exposure to risk factors to determine how transmission is occurring.

D. *Disaster implications:* None.

E. *International measures:* WHO Collaborating Centres (see Preface).

IV. DIARRHEA CAUSED BY ENTEROHEMORRHAGIC STRAINS (EHEC)

1. **Identification**—This category of diarrheagenic *E. coli* has been recognized since 1982 when a multistate epidemic of hemorrhagic colitis occurred in the USA and was shown to be due to a specific serotype. Watery stools contain gross blood but no fecal leukocytes. EHEC strains can also cause the hemolytic-uremic syndrome. EHEC elaborate potent cytotoxins called Shiga-like toxins 1 and 2 (because of their close resemblance to Shiga toxin of *S. dysenteriae* 1); they are also called Vero toxins I and II. Elaboration of these toxins depends on the presence of certain phages carried by the bacteria. In addition, EHEC strains have a plasmid that codes for a novel type of fimbria that is involved in

attachment of the bacteria to intestinal mucosa.

EHEC can be diagnosed by demonstrating the presence of Shiga-like toxins, by serotyping (e.g., identifying characteristic serotypes) or by DNA probes that identify the toxin genes or the presence of the EHEC plasmid. Absence of fecal leukocytes differentiates this from shigellosis and dysentery caused by EIEC.

2. **Infectious agent**—While the main EHEC serotype is O157:H7, other serotypes such as O26:H11 and O111:H8 have been implicated.

3. **Occurrence**—These infections are now recognized to be an important problem in N America, Europe and the cone of S America. Their relative importance in the rest of the world is not yet established.

4. **Reservoir**—Cattle are believed to be the reservoir of EHEC; man may also serve as a reservoir for transmission within custodial institutions. Both calves and humans can develop hemorrhagic colitis due to EHEC.

5. **Mode of transmission**—Transmission occurs by means of contaminated food, most often poorly cooked beef (especially ground beef) and also raw milk. Sustained outbreaks in custodial institutions have been observed, suggesting that transmission by direct contact may occur in high-risk populations.

6. **Incubation period**—Estimated to range from 12 to 60 hours, with a median of 48 hours.

7. **Period of communicability**—The duration of excretion of the pathogen, which is notably short.

8. **Susceptibility and resistance**—Little is known about susceptibility and immunity. Old age appears to be a risk factor, so hypochlorhydria may be a factor contributing to susceptibility.

9. **Methods of control**—Same as for ETEC diarrhea, above.

DIARRHEA CAUSED BY ENTEROAGGREGATIVE E. COLI (EAggEC)

This is a less well-defined category of diarrheagenic *E. coli;* it causes infant diarrhea in less-developed countries, and preliminary evidence suggests that, at least in some areas, some strains may cause persistent diarrhea in infants. In animal models, these *E. coli* evoke a characteristic histopathology. At present, the most widely available method to identify EAggEC is by the HEp-2 assay, wherein these strains cause a characteristic aggregative pattern as they attach to one another and to the HEp-2 cells; this is a plasmid-dependent characteristic. A DNA probe has been described.

EAggEC is an important cause of infant diarrhea in some parts of the world, as well as a cause of persistent diarrhea in infants.The incubation period is estimated to be 20-48 hours.

DIPHTHERIA   ICD-9 032

1. **Identification**—An acute bacterial disease of tonsils, pharynx, larynx, nose, occasionally of other mucous membranes or skin, and sometimes the conjunctivae or genitalia. The characteristic lesion, caused by liberation of a specific cytotoxin, is marked by a patch or patches of an adherent grayish membrane with a surrounding inflammation. The throat is moderately sore in faucial or pharyngotonsillar diphtheria, with cervical lymph nodes somewhat enlarged and tender; in severe cases, there is marked swelling and edema of the neck. Laryngeal diphtheria is serious in infants and young children, while nasal diphtheria is mild, often chronic, and marked by one-sided nasal discharge and excoriations. Inapparent infections outnumber clinical cases. The lesions of cutaneous diphtheria are variable and may be indistinguishable from, or a component of, impetigo. Late effects of absorption of toxin, appearing after 2-6 weeks, include cranial and peripheral motor and sensory nerve palsies and myocarditis (which may occur early), and are often severe. Case fatality rates of 5-10% for noncutaneous diphtheria have changed little in 50 years.

Diphtheria should be suspected in the differential diagnosis of bacterial and viral pharyngitis, Vincent's angina, infectious mononucleosis, oral syphilis and candidiasis.

Administration of antibiotics for sore throats before obtaining a culture, on the assumption that most are streptococcal, may delay diagnosis and appropriate treatment of diphtheria, with a fatal result.

Presumptive diagnosis is based on observation of a whitish membrane, especially if extending to the uvula and soft palate, in association with tonsillitis, pharyngitis or cervical lymphadenopathy, or a serosanguinous nasal discharge. The diagnosis is confirmed by bacteriologic examination of lesions. If diphtheria is strongly suspected, specific treatment with antibiotics and antitoxin should be initiated while studies are pending, and should be continued even in the face of a negative laboratory report.

2. **Infectious agent**—*Corynebacterium diphtheriae* of gravis, mitis or intermedius biotype. Toxin production results when the bacteria are infected by corynebacteriophage containing the gene *tox*. Non-toxigenic strains rarely produce local lesions.

3. **Occurrence**—A disease of colder months in temperate zones,

involving primarily unimmunized children under 15 years of age; often found among adults in population groups whose immunization was neglected. Formerly a prevalent disease, it has largely disappeared in those areas where effective immunization programs have been carried out. In the USA, from 1980 to 1987, an average of fewer than 3 cases was reported annually; two-thirds of the affected persons were ≥20 years of age. In the tropics, seasonal trends are less distinct; inapparent, cutaneous and wound diphtheria cases are much more common.

4. **Reservoir**—Man.

5. **Mode of transmission**—Contact with a patient or carrier; more rarely, contact with articles soiled with discharges from lesions of infected persons. Raw milk has served as a vehicle.

6. **Incubation period**—Usually 2-5 days, occasionally longer.

7. **Period of communicability**—Variable, until virulent bacilli have disappeared from discharges and lesions; usually 2 weeks or less and seldom more than 4 weeks. Effective antibiotic therapy promptly terminates shedding. The rare chronic carrier may shed organisms for 6 months or more.

8. **Susceptibility and resistance**—Infants born of immune mothers are relatively immune; protection is passive and usually lost before the sixth month. Recovery from a clinical attack is not always followed by lasting immunity; immunity is often acquired through inapparent infection. Prolonged active immunity can be induced by toxoid. Serosurveys in the USA indicate that more than 40% of adults lack protective levels of circulating antitoxin; decreasing immunity levels have also been found in Canada, Australia and several European countries. Antitoxic immunity protects against systemic disease but not against local infection in the nasopharynx.

9. **Methods of control**—

A. *Preventive measures:*

1) Educational measures are important to inform the public, and particularly the parents of young children, of the hazards of diphtheria and the necessity for active immunization.

2) The only effective control is widespread active immunization with diphtheria toxoid, including an adequate program to maintain immunity. Immunization should be initiated in infancy with a triple antigen containing diphtheria toxoid, tetanus toxoid and pertussis vaccine (DTP).

3) The following schedules are recommended for use in the USA. (Some countries may recommend different ages for specific doses or fewer than 4 doses in the primary series.)

Some, as Australia, use DTP up to 8 years of age.

a) For children less than 7 years of age—

A primary series of four doses of diphtheria toxoid with tetanus toxoid and pertussis vaccine as DTP. The first three doses are given at 4- to 8-week intervals beginning when the infant is 6-8 weeks old. While these elicit good antitoxic responses which are maintained by exposure to organisms in areas of high prevalence, the fourth dose given 6 months to 1 year after the third dose (usually administered at 15-18 months of age) assures greater and longer protection in developed areas with low prevalence of diphtheria. This schedule does not need to be restarted because of any delay in administering the scheduled doses. A fifth dose is usually given prior to school entry; this dose is not necessary if the fourth dose is given after the fourth birthday. If the pertussis component of DTP is contraindicated, diphtheria and tetanus toxoids for children (DT) should be substituted, with two doses 4 to 8 weeks apart followed by a third dose 6-12 months later. A fourth dose is indicated between 4 and 6 years of age unless the third dose was given after the fourth birthday.

b) For persons 7 years of age and older—

Because adverse reactions may increase with age, a preparation with a reduced concentration of diphtheria toxoid (adult Td) is used after the 7th birthday. For a previously unimmunized individual, a primary series of 3 doses of adsorbed tetanus and diphtheria toxoids, adult type (Td) is given. The first 2 doses are given at 4- to 8-week intervals and the third dose 6 months to 1 year after the second dose.

c) Active protection should be maintained by administering a dose of Td every 10 years thereafter. This is not the practice in the UK.

4) Special efforts should be made to ensure that persons who are at higher risk of patient exposure, such as health workers, are fully immunized and receive a booster dose of Td every 10 years.

B. *Control of patient, contacts and the immediate environment:*

1) Report to local health authority: Case report is obligatory in most states (USA) and countries, Class 2A (see Preface).

2) Isolation: Strict isolation for pharyngeal diphtheria, contact isolation for cutaneous diphtheria, until two cultures

from both throat and nose (and skin lesions in cutaneous diphtheria) taken not less than 24 hours apart, and not less than 24 hours after cessation of antimicrobial therapy, fail to show diphtheria bacilli. Where culture is impractical, isolation may be ended after 14 days of appropriate antibiotic treatment (see 9B7, below).

3) Concurrent disinfection: Of all articles in contact with patient, and all articles soiled by discharges of patient. Terminal cleaning.

4) Quarantine: Adult contacts whose occupations involve handling food, especially milk, or close association with unimmunized children, should be excluded from that work until bacteriologic examination proves them not to be carriers.

5) Management of contacts: All close contacts should have cultures taken and should be kept under surveillance for 7 days. If cultures are positive, they should be treated with antibiotics (see 9B7, below), and those who handle food or work with school children should be excluded from work or school until bacteriologic examination proves them not to be carriers. Previously immunized contacts should receive a booster dose of a diphtheria toxoid vaccine, and a primary series should be initiated in unimmunized contacts, using Td, DT or DTP vaccine depending on age. Contacts who are unimmunized or inadequately immunized should also be given an appropriate antibiotic (oral erythromycin or IM penicillin).

6) Investigation of contacts and source of infection: The search for carriers by use of nose and throat cultures is not ordinarily useful or indicated if provisions of 9B5, above, are carried out.

7) Specific treatment: If diphtheria is strongly suspected, antitoxin (only antitoxin of equine origin is available) should be given immediately after bacteriologic specimens are taken, without waiting for results. After completion of tests to rule out hypersensitivity, a single dose of 20,000 to 100,000 units is given IM, depending upon the duration of symptoms, area of involvement and severity of the disease. Intramuscular administration usually suffices; in severe infections, both intravenous and intramuscular administration may be indicated. Both erythromycin and penicillin are effective against the organism, and one of these should be administered after cultures have been obtained, in conjunction with, but not as a substitute for, antitoxin.

If a carrier state is demonstrated: For adults, give

erythromycin 1.0 g/day orally for 7 days; or aqueous procaine penicillin, 600,000 to 2 million units IM daily for 10 days. For children, erythromycin, 40 mg/kg/day for 7 days; or procaine penicillin—for those ≤10 kg (or 20 pounds), give 300,000 units, for >10 kg (or 20 pounds), give 600,000 units; or benzathine penicillin, 1.2 million units (600,000 units for children <27 kg or 60 pounds).

C. *Epidemic measures:*

1) Immunize the largest possible proportion of the population group involved, with emphasis on protection of infants and preschool children. Repeat immunization efforts 1 month later to provide at least 2 doses to the recipients.

2) In areas with appropriate facilities, carry out a prompt field investigation of reported cases to verify diagnosis, determine biotype and toxigenicity of *C. diphtheriae*, identify contacts, and define population groups at special risk.

D. *Disaster implications:* Outbreaks can occur when social or natural conditions lead to crowding of susceptible groups, especially infants and children.

E. *International measures:* Give primary immunization to susceptible persons traveling to or through countries where either faucial or cutaneous diphtheria is common, or a booster dose of Td for those previously immunized.

DIPHYLLOBOTHRIASIS ICD-9 123.4
(Dibothriocephaliasis, Broad or Fish tapeworm infection)

1. **Identification**—An intestinal tapeworm infection of long duration; symptoms commonly are trivial or absent. A few patients in whom the worms are attached to the jejunum develop vitamin B_{12} deficiency anemia. Massive infections may be associated with diarrhea, obstruction of the bile duct or intestine, and toxic symptoms.

Diagnosis is confirmed by identification of eggs or segments (proglottids) of the worm in feces.

2. **Infectious agents**—*Diphyllobothrium latum (Dibothriocephalus latus), Diphyllobothrium pacificum* and other species; cestodes.

3. Occurrence—The disease occurs in lake regions in subarctic, temperate and tropical zones, where eating raw or partly cooked freshwater fish is popular. Prevalence increases with age. In N America, endemic foci have been found among Eskimos in Alaska and Canada. Infections in the USA are sporadic and usually come from eating uncooked fish from Alaska or, less commonly, from midwestern or Canadian lakes.

4. Reservoir—People. Mainly infected hosts discharging eggs in feces; reservoir hosts other than people include dogs, bears and other fish-eating mammals.

5. Mode of transmission—People acquire the infection by eating raw or inadequately cooked fish. Eggs in mature segments of the worm are discharged in feces into bodies of fresh water, where they mature, hatch, and infect the first intermediate host (copepods of the genera *Cyclops* and *Diaptomus*) and become procercoid larvae. Susceptible species of freshwater fish (pike, perch, turbots) ingest infected copepods and become second intermediate hosts in which the worms transform into the plerocercoid (larval) stage, which is infective for people and fish-eating mammals, such as the fox, mink, bear, cat, dog, pig, walrus and seal. The egg-to-egg cycle takes at least 11 weeks.

6. Incubation period—Three to six weeks from ingestion to passage of eggs in the stool.

7. Period of communicability—Not directly transmitted from person to person. People and other definitive hosts continue to disseminate eggs into the environment as long as worms remain in the intestine, sometimes for many years.

8. Susceptibility and resistance—People are universally susceptible. No apparent resistance follows infection.

9. Methods of control—

A. *Preventive measures:* Thorough heating (56°C/133°F for 5 minutes) of freshwater fish, or freezing for 24 hours at -18°C (0°F) insures protection.

B. *Control of patient, contacts and the immediate environment:*

1) Report to local health authority: Official report not ordinarily justifiable, Class 5 (see Preface). Report is indicated if a commercial source is implicated.
2) Isolation: None.
3) Concurrent disinfection: None; sanitary disposal of feces.
4) Quarantine: None.
5) Immunization of contacts: None.

6) Investigation of contacts and source of infection: Not usually justified.

7) Specific treatment: Praziquantel (Biltricide®) or niclosamide (Niclocide®) is the drug of choice.

C. *Epidemic measures:* None.

D. *Disaster implications:* None.

E. *International measures:* None.

DRACUNCULIASIS   ICD-9 125.7
(Guinea-worm infection, Dracontiasis)

1. **Identification**—An infection of the subcutaneous and deeper tissues by a large nematode. A blister appears, usually on a lower extremity (especially the foot) when the gravid, 60-100 cm long, adult female worm is ready to discharge its larvae. Burning and itching of the skin in the area of the lesion, and frequently fever, nausea, vomiting, diarrhea, dyspnea, generalized urticaria and eosinophilia may accompany or precede vesicle formation. After the vesicle ruptures, the worm discharges larvae whenever the infected part is immersed in water. The prognosis is good unless there are multiple worms or unless a bacterial infection occurs which may produce severe crippling sequelae.

Diagnosis is made by microscopic identification of larvae or recognition of the adult worm.

2. **Infectious agent**—*Dracunculus medinensis,* a nematode.

3. **Occurrence**—In India, Pakistan and Africa, especially in regions with dry climates. Local prevalence varies greatly: In some localities, nearly all inhabitants are infected, in others, few; mainly young adults.

4. **Reservoir**—Man; there are no significant animal reservoirs.

5. **Mode of transmission**—Larvae discharged by the parent worm into fresh water are ingested by minute crustacean copepods and, in about 2 weeks, develop into the infective stage. People swallow the infected copepods in drinking water from infested step-wells and ponds; larvae are liberated in the stomach or duodenum, migrate through the viscera and become adults. The female, after mating, migrates to the subcutaneous tissues (most frequently of the legs) where she grows and develops to full maturity.

6. **Incubation period**—About 12 months.

7. Period of communicability—From rupture of vesicle until larvae have been completely evacuated from the uterus of the gravid worm, usually 2 to 3 weeks. In water, the larvae are infective for the copepods for about 5 days; after ingestion by copepods, the larvae become infective for people after 12-14 days at temperatures $>25°C$ ($>77°F$), and remain infective in the copepods for over one month. Not directly transmitted from person to person.

8. Susceptibility and resistance—Susceptibility is universal. No acquired immunity; multiple and repeated infections may occur in the same person.

9. Methods of control—The provision of safe drinking water to the populations at risk could lead to eradication of the disease. Foci of disease formerly present in some parts of the Middle East have been eliminated in this manner.

A. Preventive measures:

    1)   Provide health education programs in endemic communities to convey three messages: (1) that guinea-worm comes from their drinking water; (2) that villagers with blisters or ulcers should not enter any source of drinking water; and (3) that water should be boiled, or filtered through fine mesh cloth (such as nylon gauze with a mesh size of 100 μm) to remove copepods.

    2)   Provide potable water. Abolish step-wells or convert them to draw wells. Construction of wells or rainwater catchments can provide non-infected water.

    3)   Control copepod populations in ponds, tanks, reservoirs and step-wells by use of the insecticide temephos (Abate®), which is effective and safe. Treat drinking water chemically with chlorine or iodine to kill the larvae and copepods.

B. Control of patient, contacts and the immediate environment:

    1)   Report to local health authority: Case report required wherever the disease occurs, as part of the WHO elimination program, Class 2B (see Preface).

    2)   Isolation: None.

    3)   Concurrent disinfection: None.

    4)   Quarantine: None.

    5)   Immunization of contacts: None.

    6)   Investigation of contacts and source of infection: Obtain information as to source of drinking water at probable time of infection (about 1 year previously). Search for other cases.

7) Specific treatment: Thiabendazole (Mintezol®), niridazole (Ambilar®), metronidazole (Flagyl®) and mebendazole (Vermox®) have been used; they help to reduce inflammation and hasten expulsion of the worm, but their efficacy is undetermined.

C. *Epidemic measures:* In hyperendemic situations, field survey to determine prevalence, discover sources of infection and guide control measures as described in 9A, above.

D. *Disaster implications:* None.

E. *International measures:* The World Health Assembly has adopted a resolution (WHA 42.29, 19 May 1989) to eliminate dracunculiasis as a public health problem from the world in the 1990s.

EBOLA-MARBURG VIRUS DISEASES   ICD-9 078.89
(African hemorrhagic fever, Marburg virus disease, Ebola virus hemorrhagic fever)

1. Identification—Systemic viral febrile illnesses, usually characterized by sudden onset with malaise, fever, myalgia, headache and pharyngitis, followed by vomiting, diarrhea, a maculopapular rash, limited renal and hepatic involvement and a hemorrhagic diathesis. Laboratory findings indicate multiple system involvement, primarily of liver, spleen and kidney; to a lesser degree, pancreas, CNS and heart. Lymphopenia, severe thrombocytopenia and transaminase (SGOT) elevation are characteristic. Approximately 25% of reported primary cases of Marburg virus infection have been fatal; case fatality rates of Ebola infections in Africa have ranged from 50% to nearly 90%.

Diagnosis is made by IFA, ELISA or Western blot detection of specific IgG antibody (presence of IgM antibody suggests recent infection); by visualization of the virus antigen in liver cells by use of monoclonal antibody in IFA test; or by virus isolation in cell culture or guinea pigs. Virus may sometimes be seen in liver sections by EM . Laboratory studies represent an extreme biohazard, and should be carried out only where protection against infection of the staff and community is available (BSL4 containment).

2. Infectious agents—Virions are 80 nm in diameter and 790 (Marburg) or 970 (Ebola) nm in length, and are members of the Filoviridae. Longer, bizarre virion-related structures may be branched or coiled and reach 10 microns in length. The two viruses, Ebola and Marburg, are antigenically distinct, and are not related to other known infectious agents. Ebola strains from Zaire and from Sudan differ in their antigenic and biologic properties.

3. **Occurrence**—Marburg disease has been recognized on four occasions: In 1967, 31 persons (7 fatalities) in the Federal Republic of Germany and Yugoslavia were infected following exposure to African green monkeys *(Cercopithecus aethiops)* from Uganda; in 1975, the index fatal case of 3 diagnosed in South Africa had originated in Zimbabwe; in 1980, there were two confirmed cases in Kenya, one fatal; and in 1987, a fatal case occurred in Kenya.

Ebola disease was first recognized in the western equatorial province of the Sudan and the nearby region of Zaire in 1976; a second outbreak occurred in the same area in Sudan in 1979. A serologic survey disclosed antibodies in 7% of asymptomatic individuals in the epidemic area. Antibodies have been found in residents of several other areas of sub-Saharan Africa, but their relation to the highly virulent Ebola virus is unknown.

Ebola-related filoviruses have been isolated from cynomolgus monkeys *(Macacca fascicularis)* imported since November 1989 into the USA from the Philippines; many of these monkeys have died. Antibodies to these viruses are also seen in monkeys from Indonesia and East Africa. The pathogenicity and frequency of infection in humans by these new viruses have not yet been determined. Four of five animal handlers with daily exposure to these monkeys have developed specific antibodies with no antecedant fevers or other illness.

4. **Reservoir**—Unknown despite extensive studies. African green monkeys have not been incriminated as a natural reservoir of Marburg virus.

5. **Mode of transmission**—Person-to-person transmission occurs by direct contact with infected blood, secretions, organs or semen. Nosocomial infections have been frequent; all Ebola (Zaire) cases acquired from contaminated syringes and needles died. Transmission through semen has occurred 7 weeks after clinical recovery.

6. **Incubation period**—Three to 9 days in Marburg and 2-21 days in Ebola virus disease.

7. **Period of communicability**—As long as blood and secretions contain virus. Secondary infections with Ebola virus occurred in about 5% of case contacts in Zaire and in 10-15% in Sudan, among those with greatest direct contact. Ebola virus was isolated from the seminal fluid on the 61st, but not on the 76th day after onset of illness, in a laboratory-acquired case.

8. **Susceptibility and resistance**—All ages are susceptible.

9. **Methods of control**—Control measures in Lassa fever, 9B, C, D and E apply; plus restriction of sexual intercourse until semen can be assumed to be free of virus.

ECHINOCOCCOSIS   ICD-9 122

This disease of man is produced by cysts of varying sizes, which are the larval stages of the tapeworm, *Echinococcus*. The adult worms are found in dogs and other carnivores. Three closely related species cause different clinical manifestations: (1) unilocular echinococcosis or cystic hydatid disease, (2) multilocular or alveolar hydatid disease, and (3) polycystic hydatid disease.

Signs and symptoms consistent with space-occupying lesions and a history of travel to endemic areas warrant inclusion of echinococcosis in the differential diagnosis. The lesions can be defined by x-ray, CT scanning and sonography. The diagnosis is supported by positive results in serologic tests; since most tests are not specific, positive results should be confirmed with tests that detect antibody against genus-specific antigens. Definitive diagnosis is made by microscopic identification of parasitic tissue from cyst fluid obtained surgically, at necropsy, or from sputum after the rupture of pulmonary cysts.

I. ECHINOCOCCOSIS DUE TO   ICD-9 122.4
ECHINOCOCCUS GRANULOSUS
(Unilocular echinococcosis, Cystic hydatid disease)

1. **Identification**—Signs and symptoms vary according to the size, number and location of the cysts. These grow slowly and eventually may exceed 10 cm in diameter in middle and older age groups. Cysts of *E. granulosus* are unilocular, have a laminated noncellular wall, are usually surrounded by a fibrous pericyst of host origin and are found frequently in the liver and lungs and less commonly in the kidney, spleen, bone, CNS and elsewhere; no organ of the body is exempt. Infection may be asymptomatic and cysts are frequently found on routine chest x-rays or at autopsy. However, cysts in vital organs may cause severe symptoms and death. Species identification is based on the thick laminated cyst walls, brood capsules, and the structure and measurements of the protoscolex hooks.

2. **Infectious agent**—*Echinococcus granulosus,* a small tapeworm of the dog.

3. **Occurrence**—This parasite is common where dogs are used to herd grazing animals and also have intimate contact with people. The Middle East, Greece, Sardinia, North Africa, Kenya, Asia including China, western Canada and Alaska, Argentina, Uruguay, southern Brazil, Peru and Chile are enzootic areas. Human cases have been completely eliminated in Iceland and greatly reduced in Cyprus, Australia and New Zealand. Most infections acquired within mainland USA have been found in rural areas in northern Arizona and southern Utah involving ethnic populations.

4. **Reservoir**—Definitive hosts are the dog, wolf, dingo and other Canidae infected with adult worms; the usual intermediate hosts are herbivores. In domestic life cycles, the dog is the definitive host and sheep, goats, pigs, cattle and horses are intermediate hosts.

5. **Mode of transmission**—By hand-to-mouth transfer of tapeworm eggs from dog feces. Exposure occurs in handling dogs and objects soiled with dog feces and through contaminated food and water. Eggs may survive for several months in pastures, gardens and around households. Ingested eggs hatch in the intestine; the larvae migrate through the mucosa and are carried by the blood to various organs where they produce cysts, in which many infectious protoscolices develop. This stage may occur in a variety of herbivores as well as people. Carnivores become infected by eating viscera containing hydatid cysts. The dog-sheep cycle is important in most areas where *E. granulosus* is endemic. In other regions, the dog-cattle, dog-horse, dog-camel, dog-kangaroo, or dog-pig cycle predominates. In northwest Canada and Alaska, the disease is maintained in a wolf-moose cycle, from which dogs may bring the parasite to people.

6. **Incubation period**—Variable, from months to years, depending upon the number and location of cysts and how rapidly they grow.

7. **Period of communicability**—Not directly transmitted from person to person or from one intermediate host to another. Dogs begin to pass eggs of the parasite approximately 7 weeks after infection. Most infections in dogs are lost spontaneously by 6 months, but adult worms may survive as long as 2-3 years. Dogs may be infected repeatedly.

8. **Susceptibility and resistance**—Children are more likely to be exposed to infection through contact with infected dogs; there is no evidence that they are more susceptible to infection than are adults. People do not harbor the adult worm.

9. **Methods of control**—

A. *Preventive measures:*

1) Educate the general public in endemic areas to control environmental contamination by dog feces, of the dangers

       of close association with dogs and of the need for controlled slaughter of animals.

2)   Adequately inspect the carcasses and rigidly control the slaughter of herbivorous animals so that dogs have no access to uncooked viscera.

3)   Incinerate or deep-bury infected organs from dead intermediate hosts.

4)   Periodically treat high-risk dogs; reduce their numbers in endemic areas to a level compatible with occupational requirements for dogs.

5)   Field and laboratory personnel exposed to infection should observe strict safety precautions to avoid ingestion of tapeworm eggs.

B.   *Control of patient, contacts and the immediate environment:*

1)   Report to local health authority: In selected endemic areas; not a reportable disease in most states (USA) and countries, Class 3B (see Preface).

2)   Isolation: None.

3)   Concurrent disinfection: None.

4)   Quarantine: None.

5)   Immunization of contacts: None.

6)   Investigation of contacts and source of infection: Examine families and associates for suspicious tumors. Check dogs kept in and about houses for infection in an attempt to determine source and practices leading to infection.

7)   Specific treatment: Surgical resection of isolated cysts is the treatment of choice. Treatment with mebendazole (Vermox®) and albendazole (Zentel®) has given good results in some cases. Chemotherapy at this time should be restricted to complicated cases in whom surgery is not feasible or has failed. Praziquantel (Biltricide®) reduces the probability of secondary cyst recurrence if administered when spillage of cyst contents occurs; while it does not kill cysts, it is protoscolicidal.

C.   *Epidemic measures:* In highly endemic areas, destroy wild and stray dogs. For mass antihelminthic treatment of dogs, praziquantel (Biltricide®) is drug of choice. Serodiagnostic and ultrasonographic studies of the human population would facilitate early diagnosis and treatment.

D.   *Disaster implications:* None.

E.   *International measures:* Coordinate programs in neighboring countries where the disease is enzootic to control infection in animals and to control the movement of dogs from known enzootic areas.

II. ECHINOCOCCOSIS DUE TO ECHINOCOCCUS MULTILOCULARIS
ICD-9 122.7

(Alveolar hydatid disease, Multilocular echinococcosis)

1. **Identification**—This disease is caused by the poorly circumscribed alveolar larval cysts of *Echinococcus multilocularis*, usually found in the liver and rarely metastatic to the lungs and brain. Because growth of the cysts is not restricted by a thick laminated cyst wall, they continuously grow by external proliferation throughout the liver and contiguous organs to produce chronic space-occupying lesions. The clinical effects of the infection depend upon the size and location of the larval masses; the prognosis is grave because of the invasive and metastatic potentials.

Diagnosis is often based on histopathology, i.e., evidence of the thin host pericyst and multiple microvesicles formed by external proliferation. Man is an abnormal host and the cysts rarely produce brood capsules, protoscolices or calcareous corpuscles. Serodiagnosis using purified *E. multilocularis* antigen is highly sensitive and specific.

2. **Infectious agent**—*Echinococcus multilocularis.*

3. **Occurrence**—Distribution is limited to areas of the Northern Hemisphere: central Europe, the USSR, Siberia, northern Japan, Alaska, Canada and north-central USA. The disease is usually diagnosed in adults.

4. **Reservoir**—The adult tapeworms are found in foxes, wolves, dogs, coyotes and cats; the intermediate hosts are voles, lemmings, shrews and mice. *E. multilocularis* is commonly maintained in nature in fox-rodent cycles.

5. **Mode of transmission**—By ingestion of infective eggs passed in the feces of infected Canidae and Felidae. Fecally soiled dog hair, harnesses and environmental fomites serve as vehicles of infection.

6., 7., 8., and 9. **Incubation period, Period of communicability, Susceptibility and resistance, and Methods of control**—As in Section I., *Echinococcus granulosus,* above, except that surgical removal is less often successful. For nonresectable cases, continuous treatment with mebendazole, and possibly albendazole, may prevent progression of the disease.

ECHINOCOCCOSIS DUE TO ECHINOCOCCUS VOGELI
ICD-9 122.9

(Polycystic hydatid disease)

This disease is caused by the cysts of *Echinococcus vogeli,* which occur in the liver, lungs and other organs. Symptoms are variable according to cyst size and location. The species is distinguishable on the basis of its rostellar hooks. The polycystic hydatid is unique in that the germinal membrane proliferates externally to form new cysts and internally to form septae that divide the cavity into numerous microcysts. Brood capsules containing many protoscolices develop in the microcysts.

Cases have been reported in Colombia, Ecuador, Panamá, Brazil and Venezuela. The principal definitive host is the bush dog, *Speothos venaticus;* the main intermediate hosts are the paca *(Cuniculus paca)* and the spiny rat. Domestic hunting dogs are also definitive hosts, and serve as an important source of human infection.

EHRLICHIOSIS   ICD-9 083.8
(Sennetsu fever, Human ehrlichiosis found in USA)

1. **Identification**—Ehrlichiosis is an acute febrile bacterial illness caused by a group of small, pleomorphic organisms that survive in the phagosomes of mononuclear or polymorphonuclear leukocytes of the infected host. The organisms are sometimes observed within these cells.

Sennetsu fever, so far convincingly documented only in Japan, is characterized by sudden onset, with fever, chills, general malaise, headache, muscle and joint pain, sore throat and sleeplessness. Generalized lymphadenopathy, with tenderness of the enlarged nodes, is common. Lymphocytosis, with postauricular and posterior cervical lymphadenopathy, is similar to that seen in infectious mononucleosis. The disease is usually benign; fatal cases have not been reported.

Human ehrlichiosis in the USA is a newly-recognized disease of man. The spectrum of disease ranges from an illness so mild that no medical care is sought, to a severe, life-threatening or fatal disease. Symptoms are usually nonspecific; most common complaints are fever, headache, anorexia, nausea, vomiting and myalgia. The disease may be confused clinically with Rocky Mountain spotted fever (RMSF) but differs by rarity of a prominent rash. Laboratory findings include leukopenia and thrombocytopenia, and elevation of one or more liver function tests. In hospitalized cases, the laboratory findings may be only slightly abnormal on admission, and become more abnormal during hospitalization.

Differential diagnosis includes RMSF, Lyme disease and other febrile illnesses. The clinical diagnosis of sennetsu fever is confirmed by IFA tests, using the etiologic organisms isolated in macrophage cultures. Diagnosis of ehrlichiosis in the USA is based on clinical and laboratory findings and the development of antibody to *Ehrlichia canis* in the IFA test, using an antigen derived from a canine isolate. On rare occasions, inclusions typical of *Ehrlichia* may be observed in the cytoplasm of circulating leukocytes.

2. **Infectious agents**—*Ehrlichia sennetsu* is the etiologic agent of sennetsu fever. The organisms are members of the genus *Ehrlichia*, tribe Ehrlichiae and family Rickettsiaceae; until 1984, they were classified as members of the genus *Rickettsia*. The causative agent of the type of ehrlichiosis found in the USA has not been isolated; convalescent sera of patients react serologically with *Ehrlichia canis*, the cause of canine ehrlichiosis. However, there is a possibility that the disease is caused by a different species of *Ehrlichia*.

3. **Occurrence**—Sennetsu fever appears to be confined to western Japan. The distribution of ehrlichiosis in N America is not known. The disease has been found primarily in the southeastern and southcentral areas of the USA; 38 cases were reported in 1989.

4. **Reservoir**—Not known for either sennetsu fever or American ehrlichiosis.

5. **Mode of transmission**—Not known for sennetsu fever, although patients with the disease are frequently reported to have visited rivers or swampy areas near the rivers 3-4 weeks prior to onset. Ticks are suspected to be the source of infection for American ehrlichiosis; most patients report a tick bite or an association with wooded, tick-infested areas several weeks prior to onset of illness. Although *E. canis* is transmitted to dogs by the brown dog tick, *Rhipicephalus sanguineus,* dogs have not been found to be reservoirs of human disease.

6. **Incubation period**—Fourteen days for sennetsu fever; not well established for American ehrlichiosis. A majority of patients have reported tick exposure 1-3 weeks prior to onset of illness.

7. **Period of communicability**—No evidence of transmission from person to person.

8. **Susceptibility and resistance**—Susceptibility is believed to be general. No data are available on protective immunity in man from infections caused by these organisms.

9. **Methods of control**—

   A. *Preventive measures:*

   1) None established for sennetsu fever.
   2) Since patients with American ehrlichiosis have a strong association with tick exposure, measures against ticks should be employed (see Lyme disease, 9A).

B. *Control of patient, contacts and the immediate environment:*

1) Report to local health authority: In selected areas (USA), Class 3B (see Preface).
2) Isolation: None.
3) Concurrent disinfection: Remove any ticks.
4), 5), 6) Quarantine, Immunization of contacts, and Investigation of contacts and source of infection: None.
7) Specific treatment: A tetracycline; chloramphenicol for pregnant women and children under 8 years of age.

C. *Epidemic measures:* None.

D. *Disaster implications:* None.

E. *International measures:* None.

ENCEPHALOPATHY, SUBACUTE SPONGIFORM   ICD-9 046
(Slow virus infections of the CNS)

A group of subacute, and usually noninflammatory, degenerative diseases of the brain caused by "unconventional" filterable agents, possibly viruses, with very long incubation periods and no demonstrable immune response. The infectious agents are thought by some to be unique proteins replicating by a yet unknown mechanism; if that proves true, then the recently proposed term "prion" may be an appropriate name for them. Two such diseases are known to occur in humans (Creutzfeldt-Jakob disease and kuru) and four in animals (scrapie of sheep and goats, transmissible mink encephalopathy, chronic wasting disease of American mule deer and elk, and bovine spongiform encephalopathy). Subacute sclerosing panencephalitis (SSPE), progressive multifocal leukoencephalopathy (PML) and AIDS dementia are also subacute infections of the brain associated with conventional viruses—measles, papovavirus and human immunodeficiency virus (HIV), respectively.

CREUTZFELDT-JAKOB DISEASE   ICD-9 046.1
(Jakob-Creutzfeldt syndrome, Subacute spongiform encephalopathy)

1. Identification—An insidious onset with confusion, progressive dementia and variable ataxia in patients age 16 to over 80 years, but almost all are between 40 and 70. Later, myoclonic jerks appear, together with spasticity, wasting and coma. Focal signs sometimes suggest an

intracranial mass. Characteristically, routine laboratory studies of the CSF are normal, and there is no fever. Typical periodic high-voltage complexes are common on electroencephalogram (EEG). The disease progresses rapidly; death usually occurs within 3 to 12 months (median 4 months, mean 7 months). About 10% of cases have a positive family history of presenile dementia. Pathologic changes are limited to the CNS, predominantly the cerebrum and cerebellum. Amorphous amyloid plaques are present in the cerebellum of about 15% of cases.

A familial form of the disease, characterized genetically by the presence of a unique gene mutation encoding a normal amyloid protein, and neuropathologically by many multicentric plaques, is called the Gerstmann-Sträussler syndrome.

Creutzfeldt-Jakob disease must be differentiated from other forms of dementia, especially Alzheimer's disease, from other slow infections, from toxic and metabolic encephalopathies, and occasionally, from tumors and other space-occupying lesions.

Diagnosis is based on clinical signs, EEG and imaging techniques, and can be confirmed by characteristic histopathologic findings and transmission of disease to animals from biopsy specimens. Presence of an abnormal amyloid protein in brain tissue and a pair of different abnormal proteins in CSF can verify the diagnosis; however, the CSF test is not generally available at present.

2. Infectious agent—Caused by a filterable, self-replicating agent transmissible to chimpanzees, monkeys, guinea pigs, mice, hamsters and goats.

3. Occurrence—Creutzfeldt-Jakob disease has been reported from 50 countries. Average annual mortality rates are usually below 1/million, but vary from 0.25 to >30 cases/million in different population groups. Highest reported incidence is found among Libyan Jews in Israel.

4. Reservoir—Human cases constitute the only known reservoir. There is no documentation of human infection acquired from animals, although this has been hypothesized.

5. Mode of transmission—The mode of transmission of most cases is unknown. Iatrogenic cases have been recognized; these include one due to a corneal transplant, two to cortical electrodes that had been used on known Creutzfeldt-Jakob patients, two to grafts of human dura mater, and several to injections of growth hormone prepared from human pituitary glands. Other cases have had a history of brain or eye surgery within 2 years of onset.

6. Incubation period—Fifteen months to possibly more than 20 years in the iatrogenic cases (10 months to 8 years in animals); unknown in most cases, probably as long as in kuru (4 to over 20 years).

7. **Period of communicability**—CNS tissues are infectious throughout symptomatic illness. Other tissues and CSF are sometimes infectious. Infectivity during incubation period is not known, but studies in animals suggest that lymphoid and other organs are probably infectious before signs of illness appear.

8. **Susceptibility and resistance**—Genetic differences in susceptibility resembling those of autosomal dominant traits have been hypothesized to explain patterns of occurrence of the disease in families. Genetic differences in susceptibility to scrapie have been found in animals. Mutations in the "prion protein" gene have been found linked to familial Creutzfeldt-Jakob disease and Gerstmann-Sträussler syndrome.

9. **Methods of control**—

A. *Preventive measures:* Great care must be taken to avoid using tissue from infected patients in transplants and surgical instruments contaminated by tissue from such patients. Instruments must be disinfected before further use.

B. *Control of patient, contacts and the immediate environment:*

1) Report to local health authority: Official case report not ordinarily justifiable, Class 5 (see Preface).
2) Isolation: Universal precautions.
3) Concurrent disinfection: Tissues, surgical instruments and all wound drainage should be considered contaminated and must be inactivated. Steam autoclaving is the surest method of disinfection (2 hours at ≥121°C). Effective disinfectants include 5% sodium hypochlorite and 1N to 2N sodium hydroxide. Aldehydes are ineffective.
4) Quarantine: None.
5) Immunization of contacts: None.
6) Investigation of contacts and source of infection: A complete medical history, including previous surgical or dental procedures and possible exposure to human growth hormone, as well as a family history of dementia should be obtained.
7) Specific treatment: None.

C., D., and E. *Epidemic measures, Disaster implications* and *International measures:* None.

KURU   ICD-9 046.0

A disease of the CNS manifested by cerebellar ataxia, incoordination, tremors, rigidity and progressive wasting in patients ≥4 years of age, which occurred exclusively among women and children of the Fore language group in the Papua New Guinea highlands. It is caused by a filterable, self-replicating agent transmissible to primates and other animals, similar to that in Creutzfeldt-Jakob disease. Kuru was transmitted by traditional burial practices involving intimate contact with infected tissues, including cannibalism. Formerly very common, kuru now occurs in fewer than 10 patients a year.

ENTEROBIASIS   ICD-9 127.4
(Pinworm disease, Oxyuriasis)

1. **Identification**—A common intestinal helminthic infection which is often asymptomatic. There may be perianal itching, disturbed sleep, irritability and sometimes secondary infection of the scratched skin. Other clinical manifestations include vulvovaginitis, salpingitis, and pelvic and liver granulomata. Appendicitis and enuresis have been reported as possible associated conditions, but these are rare events.

Diagnosis is made by applying transparent adhesive tape (scotch-tape swab or pinworm paddle) to the perianal region and examining the tape microscopically for eggs; the material is best obtained in the morning before bathing or defecation. Examination should be repeated 3 or more times before accepting a negative result. Eggs are sometimes found on microscopic stool and urine examination. Female worms may be found in feces, and in the perianal region during rectal or vaginal examinations.

2. **Infectious agent**—*Enterobius vermicularis,* an intestinal nematode.

3. **Occurrence**—Worldwide, affecting all socioeconomic classes, with high rates in some areas. The most common worm infection in the USA; prevalence is highest in school-age children (in some groups near 50%), followed by preschoolers, and is lowest in adults except for mothers of infected children. Infection often occurs in more than one family member. Prevalence is often high in domiciliary institutions.

4. **Reservoir**—Man. Pinworms of animals are not transmissible to people.

5. **Mode of transmission**—Direct transfer of infective eggs by hand from anus to mouth of the same or another person, or indirectly through clothing, bedding, food, or other articles contaminated with eggs of the parasite. Dustborne infection is possible in heavily contaminated households and institutions. Eggs become infective within a few hours after being deposited at the anus by migrating gravid females; eggs survive less than 2 weeks outside the host. Larvae from ingested eggs hatch in the small intestine; young worms mature in the cecum and upper portions of

the colon. Gravid worms usually migrate actively from the rectum and may enter adjacent orifices.

6. **Incubation period**—The life cycle requires 2 to 6 weeks to be completed. Symptomatic disease with high worm burdens results from successive reinfections occurring within months after the initial exposure.

7. **Period of communicability**—As long as gravid females are discharging eggs on perianal skin and eggs remain infective in an indoor environment, usually about 2 weeks.

8. **Susceptibility and resistance**—Susceptibility is universal. Differences in frequency and intensity of infection are due primarily to differences in exposure.

9. **Methods of control**—

A. *Preventive measures:*

1) Educate the public in personal hygiene, particularly the need to wash hands before eating or preparing food. Keep nails short; discourage scratching bare anal area and nail-biting.
2) Remove sources of infection by treatment of cases.
3) Daily morning bathing, with showers (or stand-up baths) preferred to tub baths.
4) Frequent change to clean underclothing, night clothes and bed sheets, preferably after bathing.
5) Clean/vacuum house daily for several days after treatment of cases.
6) Reduce overcrowding in living accommodations.
7) Provide adequate toilets; maintain cleanliness in these facilities.

B. *Control of patient, contacts and the immediate environment:*

1) Report to local health authority: Official report not ordinarily justifiable, Class 5 (see Preface).
2) Isolation: None.
3) Concurrent disinfection: Change bed linen and underwear of infected person daily, with care to avoid dispersing eggs into the air. Use closed sleeping garments. Eggs on discarded linen are killed by exposure to temperatures of 55°C (131°F) for a few seconds; either boil bed clothing or use a properly functioning household washing machine. Clean/vacuum sleeping and living areas daily for several days after treatment.
4) Quarantine: None.
5) Immunization of contacts: None.

6) Investigation of contacts and source of infection: Examine all members of an affected family or institution.

7) Specific treatment: Pyrantel pamoate (Antiminth®, Combantrin®), mebendazole (Vermox®), albendazole (Zentel®), or pyrvinium pamoate (Povanyl®). In intensive infections, treatment should be repeated after 2 weeks; concurrent treatment of the whole family may be advisable if several members are infected.

C. *Epidemic measures:* Multiple cases in schools and institutions can best be controlled by systematic treatment of all infected individuals and their household contacts.

D. *Disaster implications:* None.

E. *International measures:* None.

ERYTHEMA INFECTIOSUM
HUMAN PARVOVIRUS INFECTION
(Fifth disease)

ICD-9 057.0

1. **Identification**—Erythema infectiosum is a mild, usually nonfebrile, viral disease with an erythematous eruption, occurring sporadically or in epidemics, especially among children. Characteristic is a striking erythema of the cheeks (slapped-face appearance) followed in 1 to 4 days by a lace-like rash on the trunk and extremities which fades but may recur for 1 to 3 weeks on exposure to sunlight or heat (e.g., bathing). Mild constitutional symptoms may precede onset of rash. In adults, the rash is often atypical or absent, but arthralgias or arthritis lasting days to months may occur; 25% or more of infections may be asymptomatic. Differentiation from rubella and scarlet fever is often necessary.

Severe complications of infection with the causal virus are unusual, but persons with chronic hemolytic diseases may develop transient aplastic crises, often in the absence of a preceding rash; intrauterine infection does not cause congenital anomalies, but has been demonstrated to result sometimes in fetal anemia with hydrops fetalis and fetal death. Immunosuppressed persons may develop severe, chronic anemia.

Diagnosis is usually made on clinical and epidemiologic grounds; it can be confirmed where testing is available by detection of specific IgM antibodies against parvovirus B19 (B19), or by a fourfold rise in B19 IgG antibodies. IgM titers begin to decline 30-60 days after the onset of symptoms. Parvovirus B19 antigens can be detected in the acute sera of persons with aplastic crises and in autopsy tissues of infected fetuses by nucleic acid hybridization and other techniques.

2. **Infectious agent**—Parvovirus B19, a 20-25-nm DNA virus belonging to the family Parvoviridae, which grows in erythroid precursor cells in bone marrow explant culture systems.

3. **Occurrence**—Worldwide. Common in children; both sporadic and epidemic. In the USA, the prevalence of B19 IgG antibodies ranges from 5-10% in children <5 years old, to ≥50% in adults. In temperate zones, epidemics tend to occur in winter and spring, with a periodicity of 5-7 years in any given community.

4. **Reservoir**—Man.

5. **Mode of transmission**—Primarily through contact with infected respiratory secretions; also, vertically from mother to fetus, and rarely parenterally by transfusion of blood and blood products.

6. **Incubation period**—Variable; 4-20 days to development of rash or symptoms of aplastic crisis.

7. **Period of communicability**—In persons with rash-illness alone, greatest before onset of rash and probably not communicable after onset of rash. Persons with aplastic crisis are communicable up to 1 week after onset of symptoms. Immunosuppressed persons with chronic infection and severe anemia may be communicable for months to years.

8. **Susceptibility and resistance**—Universal susceptibility; protection appears to be conferred with development of B19 antibodies. Attack rates of erythema infectiosum among susceptibles can be high: 50% in household contacts, 10-60% in the day-care or school setting over a 2- to 6-month outbreak period. In the USA, about 50% of adults have serologic evidence of past infection.

9. **Methods of control**—

A. *Preventive measures:*

1) Since the disease is generally benign, prevention should focus on those most likely to develop complications, i.e., those with chronic hemolytic anemias and immunodeficiencies and non-immune pregnant women. These people should avoid exposure to potentially infectious persons in hospital or outbreak settings. Immunoglobulin has not yet had a trial for efficacy.

2) Susceptible women, who are pregnant or who might become pregnant, and have continued close contact to persons with B19 infection (e.g., at school, at home, in health care facilities) should be advised of the potential for acquiring infection and the risk to the fetus. B19 IgG

antibody testing can be used to determine susceptibility. Pregnant women with sick children at home should be advised to wash hands frequently and avoid sharing eating utensils.

3) Health care workers should be advised of the importance of following good infection control measures. Nosocomial outbreaks have been reported.

B. *Control of patient, contacts and the immediate environment:*

1) Report to local health authority: Community-wide outbreaks, Class 4 (see Preface).

2) Isolation: Impractical in the community at large. Cases of transient aplastic crisis in the hospital setting should be placed on respiratory and contact isolation and should be excluded from school contact until 7 days after onset of symptoms.

3) Concurrent disinfection: Strict handwashing after patient contact.

4) Quarantine: None.

5) Immunization of contacts: None.

6) Investigation of contacts and source of infection: Exposed pregnant women should be offered B19 IgG and IgM antibody testing, when available, to determine susceptibility and to assist with management of the fetus should infection occur.

7) Specific treatment: None.

C. *Epidemic measures:* During outbreaks in school or day-care settings, persons with chronic hemolytic anemias, persons with immunodeficiencies and pregnant women should be informed of the possible risk of acquiring and transmitting infection.

D. *Disaster implications:* None.

E. *International measures:* None.

FASCIOLIASIS   ICD-9 121.3

1. **Identification**—A disease of the liver caused by a large trematode that is a natural parasite of sheep, cattle and related animals throughout the world. Flukes measuring up to about 3 cm live in the bile ducts; the young stages live in the liver parenchyma, causing tissue damage and enlargement of the liver. During the early period of parenchymal

invasion, there may be right upper quadrant pain, liver function abnormalities and eosinophilia. After migration to the biliary ducts, the flukes may cause biliary colic or obstructive jaundice. Ectopic infection, especially by *Fasciola gigantica,* may produce transient or migrating areas of inflammation in the skin over the trunk or other areas of the body.

Diagnosis is based on finding eggs in feces or in bile aspirated from the duodenum. Serodiagnostic tests, available in some centers, suggest the diagnosis when positive. Spurious infection may be diagnosed when nonviable eggs appear in the feces after liver from infected animals has been eaten.

2. **Infectious agents**—*Fasciola hepatica* and (less commonly) *F. gigantica.*

3. **Occurrence**—Human infection has been reported in sheep- and cattle-raising areas of S America, the Caribbean, Europe, Australia and the Middle East. Sporadic cases are reported in the USA. *F. gigantica* has a restricted distribution in Africa, the western Pacific and Hawaii.

4. **Reservoir**—Man is an accidental host. The infection in nature is maintained in a cycle between other animal species, mainly sheep and cattle, and snails of the family Lymnaeidae. Cattle, water buffalo, and other large herbivorous mammals harbor *F. gigantica.*

5. **Mode of transmission**—Eggs passed in the feces develop in water, and in about 2 weeks a motile ciliated larva (miracidium) hatches. On entering a snail (lymnaeid), this larva develops to produce large numbers of free-swimming cercariae which attach to aquatic plants and encyst; these encysted forms (metacercariae) are somewhat resistant to drying. Infection is acquired by eating uncooked aquatic plants (such as watercress) bearing metacercariae. On reaching the intestine, the larvae migrate through the wall into the peritoneal cavity, enter the liver and, after development, enter the bile ducts and begin laying eggs 3 to 4 months after initial exposure.

6. **Incubation period**—Variable.

7. **Period of communicability**—Infection is not transmitted directly from person to person.

8. **Susceptibility and resistance**—People of all ages are susceptible; infection persists indefinitely.

9. **Methods of control**—

   A. *Preventive measures:*

      1) Educate the public in endemic areas to abstain from eating watercress or other aquatic plants of wild or unknown origin, especially from areas where sheep or other animals graze.

2) Avoid use of sheep feces for fertilizing water plants.
3) Drain the land or use chemical molluscicides to eliminate the molluscs where it is technically and economically feasible.

B. *Control of patient, contacts and the immediate environment:*

1) Report to local health authority: Official report not ordinarily justifiable, Class 5 (see Preface).
2) Isolation: None.
3) Concurrent disinfection: None.
4) Quarantine: None.
5) Immunization of contacts: None.
6) Investigation of contacts and source of infection: Identification of the source of infection may be useful in preventing additional infections of the patient or others.
7) Specific treatment: Treatment is generally unsatisfactory. Dehydroemetine is the most effective treatment. Cure rates with praziquantel and bithionol (Bitin®; available in the USA from CDC) are inconsistent.

C. *Epidemic measures:* Determine source of infection and identify plants and snails involved in transmission. Prevent eating of aquatic plants from contaminated areas.

D. *Disaster implications:* None.

E. *International measures:* None.

FASCIOLOPSIASIS   ICD-9 121.4

1. **Identification**—A trematode infection of the small intestine, particularly the duodenum. Symptoms result from local inflammation, ulceration of the intestinal wall and systemic toxic effects. Diarrhea usually alternates with constipation; vomiting and anorexia are frequent. Large numbers of flukes may produce acute intestinal obstruction. Patients may show edema of the face, abdominal wall and legs within 20 days after massive infection; ascites is common. Eosinophilia is usual; secondary anemia is occasional. Death is rare; light infections are usually asymptomatic.

Diagnosis is made by finding the large flukes or characteristic eggs in feces; worms are occasionally vomited.

2. **Infectious agent**—*Fasciolopsis buski,* a large trematode or fluke reaching lengths up to 7 cm.

3. **Occurrence**—Widely distributed in rural SE Asia, especially Thailand, central and south China, and parts of India. Prevalence is often high.

4. **Reservoir**—Swine, man and dogs are definitive hosts of adult flukes.

5. **Mode of transmission**—Eggs passed in feces develop in water within 3 to 7 weeks under favorable conditions; miracidia hatch, and penetrate planorbid snails as intermediate hosts; cercariae develop, are liberated and encyst on aquatic plants to become the infective metacercariae. Human infections result from eating these plants uncooked. In China, the chief sources of infection are the nuts of the red water caltrop grown in enclosed ponds, and tubers of the so-called "water chestnut"; infection frequently results when the hull or skin is peeled off with teeth and lips.

6. **Incubation period**—Eggs appear in the feces about 3 months after infection.

7. **Period of communicability**—As long as viable eggs are discharged in feces; without treatment, probably for one year. Not directly transmitted from person to person.

8. **Susceptibility and resistance**—Susceptibility is universal. In malnourished individuals, the ill effects are pronounced; number of worms influences severity of disease.

9. **Methods of control**—

   A. *Preventive measures:*

      1) Educate the public in endemic areas on the mode of transmission and life cycle of the parasite.
      2) Treat nightsoil to destroy eggs.
      3) Bar hogs from contaminating areas where water plants are growing; do not feed water plants to pigs.
      4) Dry suspected plants, or if plants are to be eaten fresh, dip into boiling water for a few seconds; both methods kill metacercariae.

   B. *Control of patient, contacts and the immediate environment:*

      1) Report to local health authority: In selected endemic areas; in most countries not a reportable disease, Class 3C (see Preface).
      2) Isolation: None.
      3) Concurrent disinfection: Sanitary disposal of feces.
      4) Quarantine: None.
      5) Immunization of contacts: None.

6) Investigation of contacts and source of infection: In the individual case, of little value. A community problem (see 9C, below).
7) Specific treatment: Praziquantel (Biltricide®) is the drug of choice.

C. *Epidemic measures:* Identify aquatic plants that harbor encysted metacercariae and are eaten fresh; identify infected snail species living in water with such plants; and prevent contamination of water with human and pig feces.

D. *Disaster implications:* None.

E. *International measures:* None.

FILARIASIS   ICD-9 125

The term "filariasis" can be used to denote infection with any of the several Filarioidea. However, as commonly used, the term refers only to the lymphatic-dwelling filariae listed below. For others, refer to the specific disease.

FILARIASIS DUE TO *WUCHERERIA*   ICD-9 125.0
BANCROFTI
(Bancroftian filariasis)
FILARIASIS DUE TO *BRUGIA MALAYI*   ICD-9 125.1
(Malayan filariasis, Brugian filariasis
FILARIASIS DUE TO *BRUGIA TIMORI*   ICD-9 125.6
(Timorean filariasis, Brugian filariasis)

1. Identification—
A. Bancroftian filariasis is an infection with the nematode *Wuchereria bancrofti*, which normally resides in the lymphatics in infected persons. Female worms produce microfilariae that reach the bloodstream 6 to 12 months after infection. Two biologically different forms occur: In one, the microfilariae circulate in the peripheral blood at night (nocturnal periodicity), with greatest concentrations between 10 pm and 2 am; in the other form, microfilariae circulate continuously in the peripheral blood, but occur in greater concentration in the daytime (diurnal subperiodicity). The latter form is endemic in the S Pacific and in small rural foci in SE Asia where the principal vectors are day-biting *Aedes* mosquitoes.
The spectrum of clinical manifestations in regions of endemic filariasis include: people who are exposed but remain asymptomatic and parasito-

logically negative; those who are asymptomatic with microfilaremia; those with acute recurrent filarial fever, lymphadenitis and retrograde lymphangitis who may or may not have microfilaremia; those with chronic signs including hydrocele, chyluria and elephantiasis of the limbs, breasts and genitalia, who have low-level or undetectable microfilaremia; and those with the tropical pulmonary eosinophilia syndrome, manifested by paroxysmal, nocturnal asthma, chronic interstitial lung disease, recurrent low-grade fever, profound eosinophilia and degenerating microfilariae in tissues but not in the bloodstream (occult filariasis).

B. Brugian filariasis is caused by the nematodes *Brugia malayi* and *B. timori*. The nocturnally-periodic form of *B. malayi* occurs in rural populations living in open rice-growing areas throughout much of SE Asia. The subperiodic form infects man, monkeys and wild and domestic carnivores in the forests of Malaysia and Indonesia. Clinical manifestations are similar to those of Bancroftian filariasis, except that the recurrent acute attacks of filarial fever, adenitis and retrograde lymphangitis are more severe, while chyluria is uncommon and elephantiasis is usually confined to the distal extremities, most frequently to the legs below the knees. Breasts and urogenital tract are rarely, if ever, compromised.

C. *Brugia timori* infections have been described on Timor and other southeastern islands of Indonesia. Clinical manifestations are comparable to those seen in *B. malayi* infections, but abscess formation is more common.

Clinical manifestations of filariasis often occur with no demonstrable circulating microfilariae (occult filariasis). In several thousand cases seen in American military personnel during World War II, microfilariae were found in only 10-15 patients despite repeated blood examinations. In some of these cases, infection was manifested by marked eosinophilia associated with pulmonary infiltrates (tropical eosinophilia syndrome or tropical pulmonary eosinophilia).

Microfilariae are best detected during periods of maximal microfilaremia. Live microfilariae can be seen under low power in a drop of peripheral blood (finger prick) on a slide or in hemolyzed blood in a counting chamber. Giemsa-stained thick and thin smears permit species identification. Microfilariae may be concentrated by filtration through a Nucleopore filter (2-5-μm pore size) in a Swinney adapter and by the Knott technique (centrifugal sedimentation of 2 ml of blood mixed with 10 ml of 2% formalin).

2. **Infectious agents**—*Wuchereria bancrofti, Brugia malayi* and *B. timori;* long threadlike worms.

3. **Occurrence**—*W. bancrofti* is endemic in most of the warm humid regions of the world, including Latin America (scattered foci in Brazil, Surinam, French Guiana, Haiti, the Dominican Republic and Costa Rica), Africa, Asia and the Pacific Islands. It is common in those urban areas

where conditions favor breeding of vector mosquitoes. In general, nocturnal periodicity in *Wuchereria*-infected areas of the Pacific is found west of 140° E longitude and diurnal subperiodicity east of 180° E longitude. *B. malayi* is endemic in rural southwest India, Sri Lanka, SE Asia, central and northern coastal areas of China, and S Korea. *B. timori* occurs on the rural islands of Timor, Flores, Alor and Roti in SE Indonesia. High prevalence depends on a large reservoir of infection and abundant vectors.

4. **Reservoir**—Man with microfilariae in the blood for *W. bancrofti,* periodic *B. malayi* and *B. timori.* In Malaysia, the Philippines and Indonesia, cats, civets and nonhuman primates serve as reservoirs for subperiodic *B. malayi.*

5. **Mode of transmission**—By bite of a mosquito harboring infective larvae. *W. bancrofti* is transmitted by many species, the most important being *Culex quinquefasciatus, Anopheles gambiae, An. funestus, Aedes polynesiensis, Ae. scapularis* and *Ae. pseudoscutellaris. B. malayi* is transmitted by various species of *Mansonia, Anopheles* and *Aedes. B. timori* is transmitted by *An. barbirostris.* In the female mosquito, ingested microfilariae penetrate the stomach wall and develop in the thoracic muscles into elongated, infective filariform larvae that migrate to the proboscis. When the mosquito feeds, the larvae emerge and enter the punctured skin following the mosquito bite. They travel via the lymphatics to the lymph nodes where they molt twice before becoming adults.

6. **Incubation period**—While allergic inflammatory manifestations may appear as early as a month after infection, microfilariae may not appear in the blood until 2-3 months in *B. malayi* or 6-12 months in *W. bancrofti* infections.

7. **Period of communicability**—Not directly transmitted from person to person. Man may infect mosquitoes if microfilariae are present in the peripheral blood; microfilaremia may persist for 5 years or longer after initial infection. The mosquito becomes infective about 12-14 days after an infective blood meal.

8. **Susceptibility and resistance**—Universal susceptibility to infection, but considerable geographic difference in the type and severity of disease. Repeated infections occur in endemic regions and lead to the severe manifestations such as elephantiasis.

9. **Methods of control**—

    A. Preventive measures:

        1) Educate the public on the mode of transmission and methods of mosquito control.

        2) Identify the vectors by detecting infective larvae in mosquitoes caught on human bait; identify times and places of

mosquito biting and locate breeding places. If indoor night-biters are responsible, spray inside walls with a residual insecticide, screen houses, or use bed nets and insect repellents. Eliminate breeding places, such as open latrines, old tires, coconut husks, etc., and treat others with larvicides. Where *Mansonia* species are vectors, clear ponds of vegetation *(Pistia),* or apply herbicides to plants which serve as sources of oxygen for the larvae.

3) Long-term control may involve changes in housing construction to include screening, and environmental control to eliminate mosquito breeding sites.

4) Mass treatment with diethylcarbamazine (DEC, Banocide®, Hetrazan®, Notezine®), especially when followed by monthly treatment with low-dose (25-50 mg/kg body weight) DEC for 1-2 years, has proven efficacious. However, in some instances, adverse reactions have discouraged community participation, especially where onchocerciasis is endemic (see Mazzotti reaction). Ivermectin may ultimately replace DEC.

B. *Control of patient, contacts and the immediate environment:*

1) Report to local health authority: In selected endemic regions; in most countries, not a reportable disease, Class 3C (see Preface). Reporting of cases with demonstrated microfilariae provides information on potential areas of transmission.

2) Isolation: Not practicable. As far as possible, patients with microfilaremia should be protected from mosquitoes to reduce transmission.

3) Concurrent disinfection: None.

4) Quarantine: None.

5) Immunization of contacts: None.

6) Investigation of contacts and source of infection: Only as part of a general community effort (see 9A and 9C).

7) Specific treatment: Diethylcarbamazine (DEC, Banocide®, Hetrazan®, Notezine®) results in rapid disappearance of most or all microfilariae from the blood, but may not destroy the adult worms. Low-level microfilaremia may reappear after treatment. Therefore, treatment must usually be repeated at specified intervals. Low-level microfilaremia can be detected only by concentration techniques. DEC may cause acute generalized reactions during the first 24 days of treatment due to death and degeneration of microfilariae; these reactions are often controlled by aspirin, antihistamines or corticosteroids. Localized lymphadenitis and lymphangitis may

follow the death of the adult worms.

C. **Epidemic measures:** Vector control is the fundamental measure. In areas of high endemicity, it is essential to appraise correctly the bionomics of mosquito vectors, prevalence and incidence of disease, and environmental factors responsible for transmission in each locale. Even partial control by antimosquito measures may reduce incidence and restrict the focus. Measurable results are slow because of the long incubation period.

D. **Disaster implications:** None.

E. **International measures:** None.

DIROFILARIASIS   ICD-9 125.6
(Zoonotic filariasis)

Certain species of filaria commonly seen in wild or domestic animals occasionally infect man, but microfilaremia rarely occurs. The genus *Dirofilaria* causes pulmonary and cutaneous disease in man. *D. immitis*, the dog heartworm, has caused pulmonary disease in the USA (about 50 cases), with a few reported infections in Japan, Asia and Australia. Transmission to man is by mosquito bite. The worm lodges in a pulmonary artery where it may form the nidus of a thrombus, which leads to vascular occlusion, coagulation, necrosis and fibrosis. Common symptoms are chest pain, cough and hemoptysis. Eosinophilia is infrequent. The fibrotic nodule, 1-3 cm in diameter, is recognizable by x-ray as a "coin lesion."

Cutaneous disease is caused by various species, including *D. tenuis*, a parasite of the raccoon in the USA; *D. ursi*, a parasite of bears in Canada; and adult *D. repens*, a parasite of dogs and cats in Europe, Africa and Asia. The worms develop in or migrate to the conjunctivae and the subcutaneous tissues of the scrotum, breasts, arms and legs, but microfilaremia is rare. Others *(Brugia)* localize in lymph nodes. Diagnosis is usually by the finding of worms in tissue sections of surgically excised lesions.

OTHER NEMATODES PRODUCING MICROFILARIAE IN MAN

Several other nematodes may infect man and produce microfilariae. These include *Onchocerca volvulus* and *Loa loa*, causing onchocerciasis and loiasis, respectively (see under each disease listing). Other infections are forms of mansonellosis (ICD-9 125.4 and 125.5): *Mansonella (Dipetalonema, Tetrapetalonema, Acanthocheilonema) perstans* is widely distributed in West Africa and northeastern S America; the adult is found in the body cavities and the unsheathed microfilariae circulate with no regular periodicity. Infection is usually asymptomatic, but eye infections by immature stages have been reported from persons residing in Oregon. In some countries of West and Central Africa infection with *D. streptocerca* (ICD-9 125.6) is common and is suspected of causing cutaneous edema and thickening of the skin, hypopigmented macules, pruritis and papules. The adults and unsheathed microfilariae occur in the skin as in onchocerciasis. *M. ozzardi* (ICD-9 125.5) occurs from the Yucatan Peninsula in Mexico to northern Argentina and in the West Indies; diagnosis is based on the demonstration of the circulating unsheathed nonperiodic microfilaria. Infection is generally asymptomatic but may be associated with allergic manifestations such as articular pain, pruritis, headaches and lymphadenopathy. *Culicoides* midges are the main vectors for the last three parasites; in the Caribbean area, *M. ozzardi* is also transmitted by blackflies. *M. rodhaini,* a parasite of chimpanzees, was found in 1.7% of skin snips taken in Gabon.

DEC is effective against *M. streptocerca* and occasionally against *M. perstans* and *M. ozzardi.* There is evidence that ivermectin may be effective against *M. ozzardi.*

FOODBORNE DISEASE   ICD-9 005
(Food poisoning, Foodborne infections)

Food poisoning, foodborne intoxication and foodborne infections are generic terms applied to illnesses acquired through consumption of contaminated food or water. The terms apply to intoxications caused by chemical contaminants (heavy metals and others), toxins elaborated by bacterial growth (*Staphylococcus aureus, Clostridium perfringens* and others), and a variety of noxious organic substances that may be present in natural foods, such as certain mushrooms, mussels, eels, scombroid fish, and other seafood. This definition also includes acute foodborne infections such as salmonellosis (q.v.), discussed elsewhere, as well as intoxications such as botulism (q.v.).

This chapter will present those conditions with short incubation periods which can be considered as intoxications, i.e., caused by toxins produced by infectious agents present in the ingested food, and infections with short incubation periods in which toxins may be formed within the intestinal tract. Included are diseases caused by *S. aureus, Clostridium perfringens, Vibrio parahaemolyticus* and *Bacillus cereus;* botulism is presented elsewhere (q.v.).

Food "poisoning" outbreaks are usually recognized by the occurrence of illness within a short period of time after consumption, among individuals who have consumed foods in common. Prompt and thorough laboratory evaluation of cases and implicated foods is essential. Single cases of food poisoning are difficult to identify unless, as in botulism, there is a distinctive clinical syndrome. Food poisoning may be one of the most common causes of acute illness; many cases and outbreaks are underrecognized and underreported.

Prevention and control of these diseases, regardless of the specific cause, are based on the same technical principles: avoidance of food contamination, destruction or denaturation of the contaminants, and prevention of further spread or multiplication of contaminants. Specific problems and appropriate modes of intervention may vary from one country to another depending on environmental, economic, political, technological and sociocultural factors. Ultimately, prevention depends on education of foodhandlers in proper practices in cooking and storage of food, and personal hygiene. Toward this end, WHO has developed "Ten Golden Rules for Safe Food Preparation." These are:

1. Choose food processed for safety.
2. Cook food thoroughly.
3. Eat cooked food immediately.
4. Store cooked food carefully.
5. Reheat cooked foods thoroughly.
6. Avoid contact between raw foods and cooked foods.
7. Wash hands repeatedly.
8. Keep all kitchen surfaces meticulously clean.
9. Protect foods from insects, rodents, and other animals.
10. Use pure water.

I. STAPHYLOCOCCAL FOOD POISONING   ICD-9 005.0

1. **Identification**—An intoxication (not an infection) of abrupt and sometimes violent onset, with severe nausea, cramps, vomiting and prostration, often accompanied by diarrhea, and sometimes with subnormal temperature and lowered blood pressure. Deaths are rare; duration of illness is commonly not more than a day or two, but the intensity of symptoms may require hospitalization and may result in surgical exploration in sporadic cases. Diagnosis is easier when a group of cases is seen with the characteristic acute, predominantly upper GI symptoms and the short interval between eating a common food item and the onset of symptoms.

Differential diagnosis includes other recognized forms of food poisoning as well as chemical poisons.

Recovery of large numbers of enterotoxin-producing staphylococci ($\geq 10^5$ organisms/g) on routine culture media from vomitus, feces or a suspected food item supports the diagnosis. Absence of staphylococci on culture of a heated food does not rule out the diagnosis; a Gram stain of the food may disclose the organisms which have been heat-killed. It may be possible to identify enterotoxin or thermonuclease in the food in the absence of viable organisms. Phage typing and enterotoxin tests may help epidemiologic investigations but are not routinely available or indicated.

2. Toxic agent—Several enterotoxins of *Staphylococcus aureus,* stable at boiling temperature. Staphylococci multiply in food and produce the toxins.

3. Occurrence—Widespread and relatively frequent; one of the principal acute food poisonings in the USA.

4. Reservoir—Man in most instances; occasionally cows with infected udders, as well as dogs and fowl.

5. Mode of transmission—By ingestion of a food product containing staphylococcal enterotoxin. Foods involved are particularly those which come in contact with foodhandlers' hands, either without subsequent cooking or with inadequate heating or refrigeration, such as pastries, custards, salad dressings, sandwiches, sliced meats and meat products. Toxin has also developed in inadequately cured hams and salami, and in non-processed and inadequately processed cheese. When these foods remain at room temperature for several hours before being eaten, toxin-producing staphylococci multiply and elaborate the toxin. The organisms may be of human origin from purulent discharges of an infected finger, infected eyes, abscesses, acneiform facial eruptions, nasopharyngeal secretions, or apparently normal skin; or of bovine origin, such as contaminated milk or milk products.

6. Incubation period—Interval between eating food and onset of symptoms is 30 minutes to 7 hours, usually 2-4 hours.

7. Period of communicability—Not applicable.

8. Susceptibility and resistance—Most persons are susceptible.

9. Methods of control—

    A. Preventive measures:

        1)   Reduce food handling time (initial preparation to service) to an absolute minimum, with no more than 4-5 hours at ambient temperature. Keep perishable foods **hot** (>60°C/140°F) or **cold** (below 10°C /50°F; best ≤4°C/ 39°F) in shallow containers and covered, if they are to be stored for more than 2 hours.

        2)   Temporarily exclude from food handling persons with boils, abscesses and other purulent lesions of hands, face or nose.

3) Educate foodhandlers in strict food hygiene, sanitation and cleanliness of kitchens, proper temperature control, handwashing, cleaning of fingernails; and to the danger of working with skin, nose and eye infections.

B. *Control of patient, contacts and the immediate environment:*

1) Report to local health authority: Report promptly. Obligatory report of outbreaks of suspected or confirmed cases, Class 4 (see Preface)

2), 3), 4), 5), and 6) Isolation, Concurrent disinfection, Quarantine, Immunization of contacts, and Investigation of contacts and source of infection: Not pertinent. Control is of outbreaks; single cases are rarely identified.

7) Specific treatment: Fluid replacement when indicated.

C. *Epidemic measures:*

1) By quick review of reported cases, determine time and place of exposure and the population at risk; obtain a complete listing of the foods served and embargo, under refrigeration, all foods still available. The prominent clinical features, coupled with an estimate of the incubation period, provide useful leads to the most probable etiologic agent. Collect specimens of feces and vomitus for laboratory examination. Alert the laboratory to suspected etiologic agents. Interview a random sample of those exposed. Compare the attack rates for specific food items eaten and not eaten; the implicated food item(s) will usually have the greatest difference in attack rates. Most of the sick will have eaten the contaminated food.

2) Inquire about the origin of the incriminated food and the manner of its preparation and storage before serving. Look for possible sources of contamination and periods of inadequate refrigeration and heating that would permit growth of staphylococci. Submit any leftover suspected foods promptly for laboratory examination; failure to isolate staphylococci does not exclude the presence of the heat-resistant enterotoxin if the food had been heated.

3) Search for foodhandlers with skin infections, particularly of the hands. Culture all purulent lesions and collect nasal swabs from all foodhandlers. Antibiograms and/or phage-typing of representative strains of enterotoxin-producing staphylococci isolated from foods and foodhandlers and from vomitus or feces of patients may be helpful.

D. *Disaster implications:* A potential hazard in situations involving mass feeding and lack of refrigeration facilities. A particular problem of air travel.

E. *International measures:* WHO Collaborating Centres (see Preface).

II. CLOSTRIDIUM PERFRINGENS FOOD POISONING ICD-9 005.2
(*C. welchii* food poisoning, Enteritis necroticans, Pigbel)

1. **Identification**—An intestinal disorder characterized by sudden onset of colic followed by diarrhea; nausea is common, but vomiting and fever are usually absent. Generally it is a mild disease of short duration, one day or less, and rarely fatal in healthy persons. Outbreaks of severe disease with high case fatality rates associated with a necrotizing enteritis have been documented in post-war Germany and Papua New Guinea.

Diagnosis is supported by demonstration of *C. perfringens* in semiquantitative anaerobic cultures of food ($\geq 10^5$/g) and patients' stools ($\geq 10^6$/g) in addition to clinical and epidemiologic evidence. When serotyping can be performed, the same serotype is usually demonstrated in different specimens; serotyping is done routinely only in Japan and the UK.

2. **Infectious agent**—Type A strains of *C. perfringens* (*C. welchii*) cause typical food poisoning outbreaks (they also cause gas gangrene); type C strains cause necrotizing enteritis. Disease is produced by toxins elaborated by the organisms.

3. **Occurrence**—Widespread and relatively frequent in countries with cooking practices that favor multiplication of *Clostridia* to high levels.

4. **Reservoir**—Soil; also the GI tract of healthy persons and animals (cattle, pigs, poultry and fish).

5. **Mode of transmission**—Ingestion of food which was contaminated by soil or feces and then held under conditions which permit multiplication of the organism. Almost all outbreaks are associated with inadequately heated or reheated meats, usually stews, meat pies, and gravies made of beef, turkey or chicken. Spores survive normal cooking temperatures, germinate and multiply during slow cooling, storage at ambient temperature, and/or inadequate rewarming. Outbreaks are usually traced to food-catering firms, restaurants, cafeterias and schools which have inadequate cooking and refrigeration facilities for large-scale service. Heavy bacterial contamination ($>10^5$ organisms/g of food) is usually required for clinical disease.

6. **Incubation period**—From 6 to 24 hours, usually 10-12 hours.

7. **Period of communicability**—Not applicable.

8. **Susceptibility and resistance**—Most persons are probably susceptible. In volunteer studies, no resistance was observed after repeated exposures.

9. **Methods of control**—

    A.   *Preventive measures:*

        1)   Educate foodhandlers on the risks inherent in large-scale cooking, especially of meat dishes. Where possible, encourage serving hot dishes while still hot from initial cooking.

        2)   Serve meat dishes hot, as soon as they are cooked, or cool them rapidly in a properly designed chiller and refrigerate until serving time; reheating, if necessary, should be thorough (internal temperature of at least 70° C/158°F, preferrably ≥75°C/167°F), and rapid. Do not partially cook meat and poultry one day and reheat the next, unless it can be stored at a safe temperature. Large cuts of meat should be thoroughly cooked; for more rapid cooling of cooked foods, divide stews and similar dishes prepared in bulk into many shallow containers and place in a rapid chiller.

    B., C., and *D. Control of patient, contacts and the immediate environment; Epidemic measures;* and *Disaster implications:* See Staphylococcal food poisoning (I9B, C and D, above).

    E.   *International measures:* None.

III. *VIBRIO PARAHAEMOLYTICUS* FOOD POISONING   ICD-9 005.4
(*Vibrio parahaemolyticus* infection)

1. **Identification**—An intestinal disorder characterized by watery diarrhea and abdominal cramps in the majority of cases, and sometimes with nausea, vomiting, fever and headache. Occasionally, a dysentery-like illness is observed with bloody or mucoid stools, high fever and high WBC count. Typically, it is a disease of moderate severity lasting 1-7 days; systemic infection and death rarely occur.

Diagnosis is confirmed by isolating the Kanagawa-positive vibrios from the patient's stool on appropriate media; or ≥10^5 organisms from an epidemiologically incriminated food (usually seafood).

2. **Infectious agent**—*Vibrio parahaemolyticus,* a halophilic vibrio. Twelve different "O" antigen groups and approximately 60 different "K" antigen types have been identified. Pathogenic strains are generally

capable of producing a characteristic hemolytic reaction (the "Kanagawa phenomenon").

3. Occurrence—Sporadic cases and common-source outbreaks have been reported from many parts of the world, particularly Japan, SE Asia and the USA. Cases occur primarily in warm months.

4. Reservoir—Marine coastal environs are the natural habitat. During the cold season, organisms are found in marine silt; during the warm season, they are found free in coastal waters and in fish and shellfish.

5. Mode of transmission—Ingestion of raw or inadequately cooked seafood, or any food cross-contaminated by handling raw seafood, or by rinsing with contaminated seawater. A period of time at room temperature is generally necessary to allow multiplication of organisms to the usual infective level ($\geq 10^6$).

6. Incubation period—Usually between 12-24 hours, but can range from 4 to 96 hours.

7. Period of communicability—Noncommunicable from person to person.

8. Susceptibility and resistance—Most persons are probably susceptible.

9. Methods of control—

A. *Preventive measures:*

1) Educate consumers of the risks associated with eating raw seafood.
2) Educate seafood handlers and processors on the following preventive measures.
3) Ensure that cooked seafood reaches temperatures adequate to kill the organism by heating for 15 minutes at 70°C/158°F (organisms may survive at 60°C/140°F for up to 15 minutes and at 80°C/176°F for several minutes).
4) Handle cooked seafood in a manner that precludes contamination from raw seafood or contaminated seawater.
5) Keep all seafood, raw and cooked, adequately refrigerated before eating.
6) Avoid use of seawater in foodhandling areas, e.g., on cruise ships.

B., C., and D. *Control of patient, contacts and immediate environment; Epidemic measures;* and *Disaster implications:* See Staphylococcal food poisoning (I9B, C and D, above) except for 9B2, Isolation: Enteric precautions.

E. *International measures:* None.

IV. *BACILLUS CEREUS* FOOD POISONING ICD-9 005.8

1. **Identification**—An intoxication characterized in some cases by sudden onset of nausea and vomiting, and in others by colic and diarrhea. Illness generally persists no longer than 24 hours and is rarely fatal.

Diagnosis is supported by identifying the causative organism in the suspected food and in feces of patients, and by performing quantitative cultures with selective media to estimate the number of organisms present (generally $>10^5$ organisms/g of the incriminated food are required). Enterotoxin testing is valuable but may not be widely available.

2. **Toxic agent**—*Bacillus cereus,* an aerobic spore former. Two enterotoxins have been identified, one (heat stable) causing vomiting, and one (heat labile) causing diarrhea.

3. **Occurrence**—A well-recognized cause of foodborne disease in Europe; rarely reported in the USA.

4. **Reservoir**—A ubiquitous organism of soil and commonly found at low levels in raw, dried and processed foods.

5. **Mode of transmission**—Ingestion of food that has been kept at ambient temperatures after cooking, permitting multiplication of the organisms. Outbreaks associated with vomiting have been most commonly associated with cooked rice that had subsequently been held at ambient room temperatures before reheating. A variety of mishandled foods has been implicated in outbreaks associated with diarrhea.

6. **Incubation period**—From 1 to 6 hours in cases where vomiting is the predominant symptom, from 6 to 24 hours where diarrhea is predominant.

7. **Period of communicability**—Not communicable from person to person.

8. **Susceptibility and resistance**—Unknown.

9. **Methods of control**—

   A. *Preventive measures:* Foods should not remain at ambient temperature after cooking, since the ubiquitous *B. cereus* spores can survive boiling, germinate, and multiply rapidly at room temperature. Refrigerate leftover food promptly; reheat thoroughly and rapidly to avoid multiplication of microorganisms.

B., C., and **D.** *Control of patient, contacts and the immediate environment; Epidemic measures;* and *Disaster implications:* See Staphylococcal food poisoning (I9B, C and D, above).

E. *International measures:* None.

GASTROENTERITIS, ACUTE VIRAL   ICD-9 078

Viral gastroenteritis presents as a sporadic or epidemic illness in infants, children and adults. Several enteropathogenic viruses (rotaviruses and, less commonly, enteric adenoviruses, caliciviruses and astroviruses) affect mainly infants and young children as a diarrheal illness which may be severe enough to produce dehydration requiring hospitalization. Other non-cultivable enteric viruses (Norwalk agent and Norwalk-like viruses) affect primarily older children and adults and cause self-limited sporadic gastroenteritis or outbreaks in families, institutions and communities. The epidemiology, natural history and clinical expression of enteric viral infections are best understood for group A rotavirus in infants and Norwalk agent in adults.

I. ROTAVIRAL ENTERITIS   ICD-9 008.8
(Sporadic viral gastroenteritis, Severe viral gastroenteritis of infants and children, Non-bacterial gastroenteritis of infancy)

1. Identification—A sporadic or seasonal, often severe gastroenteritis of infants and young children characterized by fever and vomiting, followed by a watery diarrhea occasionally associated with severe dehydration and death in the young age group. Secondary symptomatic cases among adult family contacts are infrequent, although subclinical infections occur frequently. Rotavirus infection has occasionally been found in pediatric patients with a variety of clinical manifestations, but the virus is probably coincidental rather than causative in these conditions. Rotavirus is a major cause of nosocomial diarrhea of newborns and infants. In any single patient, illness caused by rotavirus is not distinguishable from that caused by other enteric viruses, although rotavirus diarrhea may be more severe, and is more frequently associated with fever and vomiting than is acute diarrhea due to other agents.

Rotavirus is identified in stool or rectal swab by EM, ELISA, LA and other immunologic techniques for which commercial kits are available. Evidence of rotavirus infection can be demonstrated by serologic techniques but diagnosis is usually based on the demonstration of rotavirus antigen in stools.

2. **Infectious agent**—The 70-nm rotavirus belongs to the Reoviridae family. Group A is common, group B is uncommon in infants but has caused large epidemics in adults in China, while group C is rare in humans; groups B, C and D occur in animals. There are 4 major serotypes of group A human rotavirus, based on antigenic differences in the VP7 surface protein, the major neutralization antigen. Another surface protein, designated VP4, is associated with virulence and also plays a role in virus neutralization.

3. **Occurrence**—In both developed and developing countries, rotavirus is associated with about one-third of the hospitalized cases of diarrheal illness in infants and young children less than 5 years of age. All children are infected in their first 3-4 years of life, and most first infections after the first month of life are associated with diarrhea. Rotavirus is more frequently associated with severe diarrhea than are other enteric pathogens. In developing countries, it is responsible for an estimated 870,000 diarrheal deaths each year.

In temperate climates, it occurs almost exclusively in the cooler months; in tropical climates, throughout the year and with less pronounced peaks. Neonatal infections are frequent in certain settings but are usually asymptomatic. Infection of adults is usually subclinical; outbreaks of clinical disease occur in geriatric units. Rotavirus has caused travelers' diarrhea in adults, diarrhea in immunocompromised (and AIDS) patients, among parents of children with rotavirus diarrhea, in the elderly and among children in day-care settings.

4. **Reservoir**—Probably man. The pathogenicity of animal viruses for man has not been found when searched for, except for group B and group C rotaviruses which may be primarily animal rotaviruses.

5. **Mode of transmission**—Probably fecal-oral and possibly fecal-respiratory. Although rotaviruses do not effectively multiply in the respiratory tract, they may be swallowed with respiratory secretions.

6. **Incubation period**—Approximately 24 to 72 hours.

7. **Period of communicability**—During acute stage of disease, and later while virus shedding continues. Rotavirus is not usually detectable after about the eighth day of illness, although excretion of virus for ≥ 30 days has been reported in immunocompromised patients. Symptoms last for an average of 4-6 days.

8. **Susceptibility and resistance**—Susceptibility is greatest between 6 and 24 months of age. By age 3, most individuals have acquired rotavirus antibody. Immunocompromised infants are at particular risk for prolonged rotavirus diarrhea.

9. **Methods of control—**

A. *Preventive measures:*

1) Undetermined. Hygienic measures applicable to diseases transmitted via fecal-oral route may not be effective in preventing transmission.

2) Prevent exposure of infants and young children to individuals with acute gastroenteritis in family and institutional (day-care or hospital) settings.

3) Passive immunization by oral administration of IG has been shown to protect low-birth-weight neonates. Breast feeding does not affect infection rates, but may reduce the severity of the gastroenteritis. Studies are under way on the efficacy of attenuated rotavirus as an orally administered vaccine.

B. *Control of patient, contacts and the immediate environment:*

1) Report to local health authority: Obligatory report of epidemics; no individual case report, Class 4 (see Preface).

2) Isolation: Enteric precautions, with frequent handwashing by caretakers of infants.

3) Concurrent disinfection: Sanitary disposal of diapers.

4) Quarantine: None.

5) Immunization of contacts: None.

6) Investigation of contacts and source of infection: Sources of infection should be sought, especially in the home and institutions.

7) Specific treatment: None. Oral rehydration therapy with oral glucose-electrolyte solution is adequate in most cases. Parenteral fluids are needed in cases with vascular collapse or uncontrolled vomiting (see Cholera, 9B7).

C. *Epidemic measures:* Search for vehicles of transmission and source on epidemiologic bases.

D. *Disaster implications:* A potential problem.

E. *International measures:* WHO Collaborating Centres (see Preface).

II. EPIDEMIC VIRAL GASTROENTEROPATHY

ICD-9 078.8, 078.82

(Viral gastroenteritis in adults, Epidemic viral gastroenteritis, Norwalk type disease, Acute infectious nonbacterial gastroenteritis, Viral diarrhea, Epidemic diarrhea and vomiting, Winter vomiting disease, Epidemic nausea and vomiting)

1. **Identification**—Usually a self-limited, mild to moderate disease

that often occurs in outbreaks, with clinical symptoms of nausea, vomiting, diarrhea, abdominal pain, myalgia, headache, malaise, low-grade fever, or a combination of these symptoms. Gastrointestinal symptoms characteristically last 24-48 hours.

The virus may be identified in stools of ill individuals by IEM or, for the Norwalk virus, also by RIA. Serologic evidence of infection may be demonstrated by IEM or, for the Norwalk virus, by RIA. Diagnosis requires collection of a large volume of stool, with aliquots stored at 4°C (39°F) for EM, and at -20°C (-4°F) for antigen assays. Acute and convalescent sera (3-4 week interval) are essential to link particles observed by IEM with disease etiology.

2. **Infectious agents**—The small, 27-32-nm Norwalk virus, an atypical calicivirus, has been implicated as the etiologic agent in about one-third of the nonbacterial gastroenteritis outbreaks. Other agents that are morphologically similar, but antigenically distinct, have been associated with gastroenteritis outbreaks. These include Hawaii, Ditchling or W, Cockle, Parramatta, Snow Mountain agents and the Marin County agent (an astrovirus). Outbreaks have also been associated with adenoviruses (types 40, 41 and probably 31), several types of astroviruses and 20-35-nm caliciviruses, the 33-39-nm Sapporo agent, the similar Otofuke agent, parvoviruses and coronaviruses. With the exception of the enteric adenoviruses, some astroviruses and caliciviruses, the role of these agents as a cause of severe diarrhea of infants and young children is unclear.

3. **Occurrence**—Worldwide and common; most often in outbreaks but also sporadically affecting all age groups. In a study in the USA, antibodies to Norwalk agent were acquired slowly; by the fifth decade of life, >60% of the population had antibodies. In most developing countries studied, antibodies are acquired much earlier. Seroresponse to Norwalk virus was detected in infants and young children in Bangladesh; this agent was associated with 1-2% of diarrhea episodes.

4. **Reservoir**—Man is the only known reservoir.

5. **Mode of transmission**—Unknown; probably by fecal-oral route principally, although airborne transmission from fomites has been suggested to explain the rapid spread in hospital settings. Several recent outbreaks have strongly suggested primary community foodborne and waterborne transmission, with secondary transmission to family members.

6. **Incubation period**—Twenty-four to 48 hours; in volunteer studies with Norwalk agent, the range was 10-50 hours.

7. **Period of communicability**—During acute stage of disease and up to 48 hours after Norwalk diarrhea stops.

8. **Susceptibility and resistance**—Susceptibility is widespread. Short-term immunity lasting up to 14 weeks has been demonstrated in volunteers after induced Norwalk illness but long-term immunity was variable; some individuals became ill on rechallenge 27-42 months later. Levels of pre-existing serum antibody to Norwalk virus did not correlate with susceptibility or resistance.

9. **Methods of control**—

A. *Preventive measures:* Undetermined. Use hygienic measures applicable to diseases transmitted via fecal-oral route (see Typhoid fever, 9A).

B. *Control of patient, contacts and the immediate environment:*

1) Report to local health authority: Obligatory report of epidemics; no individual case report, Class 4 (see Preface).
2) Isolation: Enteric precautions.
3) Concurrent disinfection: None.
4) Quarantine: None.
5) Immunization of contacts: None.
6) Investigation of contacts and source of infection: Search for means of spread of infection in outbreak situations.
7) Specific treatment: Fluid and electrolyte replacement in severe cases.

C. *Epidemic measures:* Search for vehicles of transmission and source; determine course of outbreak to define the epidemiology.

D. *Disaster implications:* A potential problem.

E. *International measures:* None.

GIARDIASIS   ICD-9 007.1
(Giardia enteritis, Lambliasis)

1. **Identification**—A protozoan infection principally of the upper small intestine; while usually asymptomatic, it may occasionally be associated with a variety of intestinal symptoms, such as chronic diarrhea, steatorrhea, abdominal cramps, bloating, frequent loose and pale greasy stools, fatigue and weight loss. Malabsorption of fats or of fat-soluble vitamins may occur. There is usually no extra-intestinal invasion, but occasionally trophozoites may migrate into the bile or pancreatic ducts

producing inflammatory processes; damage to duodenal and jejunal mucosal cells may occur in severe giardiasis.

Diagnosis is made by the identification of cysts or trophozoites in feces (repeated at least 3 times before considered negative) or of trophozoites in duodenal fluid (by aspiration or string test) or in mucosa obtained by small intestine biopsy; the latter may be more reliable when results of stool examination are questionable, but is rarely necessary. Because *Giardia* infection is usually asymptomatic, the presence of *G. lamblia* (either in stools or duodenum) does not necessarily indicate that *Giardia* is the cause of illness. Tests for improved detection of antigen in the stool and humoral antibodies are under development.

2. **Infectious agent**—*Giardia lamblia (G. intestinalis)*, a flagellate protozoan.

3. **Occurrence**—Worldwide. Children are infected more frequently than adults. Prevalence is higher in areas of poor sanitation and in institutions with children not toilet trained, including day-care centers. The prevalence of stool positivity in different areas may range between 1% and 30%, depending on the community and age group surveyed. Waterborne outbreaks in the USA occur most often in mountain communities and those that derive drinking water from streams or rivers without a water filtration system. It is prevalent in certain temperate as well as tropical countries, with frequent infection of tour groups related epidemiologically to drinking inadequately treated water.

4. **Reservoir**—Man; possibly beaver and other wild and domestic animals. Cysts from human sources are more infectious to man than those from animal sources.

5. **Mode of transmission**—Person-to-person transmission occurs by hand-to-mouth transfer of cysts from the feces of an infected individual, especially in institutions and day-care centers; this is the principal mode of spread. Asymptomatic infected individuals (being very common) are probably more responsible for transmission than those with diarrhea. Localized outbreaks may occur from ingestion of cysts in fecally contaminated water and less often from fecally contaminated food. Concentrations of chlorine used in routine water treatment do not kill *Giardia* cysts, especially when the water is cold; unfiltered stream and lake waters that are open to contamination by human and animal feces are a frequent source of infection.

6. **Incubation period**—Five to 25 days or longer; median 7-10 days.

7. **Period of communicability**—Entire period of infection.

8. **Susceptibility and resistance**—Asymptomatic carrier rate is high; infection is frequently self-limited. Pathogenicity of *G. lamblia* for humans has been established by clinical studies. Host factors associated

with resistance have not been defined.

9. **Methods of control—**

A. *Preventive measures:*

1) Educate families, personnel and inmates of institutions, and especially adult personnel of day-care centers, in personal hygiene and the need for handwashing before eating and after toilet use.

2) Filter public water supplies that are at risk of human or animal fecal contamination.

3) Protect public water supplies against contamination with human and animal feces.

4) Dispose of feces in a sanitary manner.

5) Emergency water supplies are best boiled. Less reliable is chemical treatment with hypochlorite or iodine, using 0.1 to 0.2 ml (2 to 4 drops) of household bleach or 0.5 ml of 2% tincture of iodine per liter for 20 minutes (longer if the water is cold or turbid). See Amebiasis, 9A5, for more detailed treatment of water.

B. *Control of patient, contacts and the immediate environment:*

1) Report to local health authority: Case report in selected areas, Class 3B (see Preface).

2) Isolation: Enteric precautions.

3) Concurrent disinfection: Of feces and articles soiled therewith. In communities with a modern and adequate sewage disposal system, feces can be discharged directly into sewers without preliminary disinfection. Terminal cleaning.

4) Quarantine: None.

5) Immunization of contacts: None.

6) Investigation of contacts and source of infection: Microscopic examination of feces of household members and other suspected contacts, especially those who are symptomatic, supplemented by search for environmental contamination.

7) Specific treatment: Metronidazole (Flagyl®) and tinidazole (not licensed in the USA) are the drugs of choice. Quinacrine is an alternative; furazolidone is available in pediatric suspension for young children and infants. Relapses may occur with any drug.

C. *Epidemic measures:* Epidemiologic investigation of clustered cases in an area or institution to determine source of infection and mode of transmission; a common vehicle, such as water or association with a day-care center, should be sought; institute applicable preventive or control measures. Control of person-to-person transmission requires special emphasis on personal cleanliness and sanitary disposal of feces.

D.   Disaster implications: None.

E.   International measures: None.

GONOCOCCAL INFECTIONS   ICD-9 098

Urethritis, epididymitis, proctitis, cervicitis, Bartholinitis, salpingitis (pelvic inflammatory disease), and pharyngitis of adults; vulvovaginitis of children and conjunctivitis of the newborn and adults are localized inflammatory conditions caused by *Neisseria gonorrhoeae*. Gonococcal bacteremia results in the arthritis-dermatitis syndrome, occasionally associated with endocarditis or meningitis. Other complications include perihepatitis and the neonatal amniotic infection syndrome.

Clinically similar infections of the same genital structures may be caused by *Chlamydia trachomatis* and other infectious agents.

I. GONOCOCCAL INFECTION OF   ICD-9 098.0-098.3 THE GENITOURINARY TRACT
(Gonorrhea, Gonococcal urethritis, Gonococcal vulvovaginitis, Gonococcal cervicitis, Gonococcal Bartholinitis, Clap, Strain, Gleet, Dose, GC)

1. **Identification**—A sexually transmitted bacterial disease limited to columnar and transitional epithelium, which differs in males and females in course, severity and ease of recognition.

In males, a purulent discharge from the anterior urethra with dysuria appears 2-7 days after an infecting exposure. The infection may be self-limited, or may occasionally result in a chronic carrier state. Asymptomatic anterior urethral carriage also may occur. Rectal infection, common among homosexual males, is usually asymptomatic but may cause pruritis, tenesmus and discharge.

In females, a few days after exposure, an initial urethritis or cervicitis occurs, frequently so mild as to pass unnoticed. In about 20% there is uterine invasion at the first, second or later menstrual period, with symptoms of endometritis, salpingitis or pelvic peritonitis, and subsequent risk of infertility. Chronic endocervical infection is common. Prepubescent girls may develop gonococcal vulvovaginitis subsequent to direct genital contact with exudate from infected persons.

In both sexes, pharyngeal and anorectal infections are common. Conjunctivitis occurs rarely in adults but may cause blindness if not rapidly and adequately treated. Septicemia may occur in 0.5-1% of all gonococcal infections, with arthritis, skin lesions, and (rarely) endocarditis and meningitis. Arthritis can produce permanent joint damage if appropriate antibiotic treatment is delayed. Death is rare except among persons with endocarditis.

Nongonococcal urethritis (NGU) and nongonococcal mucopurulent cervicitis are usually caused by sexually transmitted agents and seriously complicate the clinical diagnosis of gonorrhea; frequently these coexist with gonococcal infections. In many populations, the incidence of NGU exceeds that of gonorrhea. About 30% of NGU in the USA and the UK is caused by *Chlamydia trachomatis* (see Chlamydial infections).

Diagnosis is made by bacteriologic culture on selective media (e.g., modified Thayer-Martin). Typical Gram-negative intracellular diplococci can be considered diagnostic in male urethral smears; they are highly suggestive when seen in smears from the cervix. In females, repeated cervical and anorectal cultures may be necessary to detect infection. Because of the frequent presence of commensal *Neisseriaceae*, positive cultures from cervix, pharynx or anorectum should be confirmed as *N. gonorrhoeae* by biochemical or serologic methods. Presently available serologic tests for diagnosis of gonorrhea can not distinguish current from prior infection.

2. **Infectious agent**—*Neisseria gonorrhoeae*, the gonococcus. The presence of plasmids coding for beta-lactamases render some strains resistant to penicillin (penicillinase-producing *Neisseria gonorrhoeae* or PPNG strains). Plasmid-mediated tetracycline resistance (TRNG) also occurs. Chromosomally mediated resistance to penicillin, tetracycline and cefoxitin is seen with increasing frequency. High-level resistance to spectinomycin is endemic in the Far East.

3. **Occurrence**—Common worldwide, affecting both sexes and practically all ages, especially younger adult groups. Incidence is highest in inner-city areas. In the last two decades, incidence has increased worldwide; in the USA, the number of reported cases has decreased by at least 22% since 1985. Incidence of all types of resistant strains (PPNG, TRNG, and chromosomally mediated) is increasing worldwide.

4. **Reservoir**—Man; strictly a human disease.

5. **Mode of transmission**—By contact with exudates from mucous membranes of infected persons, almost always as a result of sexual activity. In children older than 1 year, it is most frequently a result of sexual contact or molestation.

6. **Incubation period**—Usually 2-7 days, sometimes longer.

7. **Period of communicability**—May extend for months in un-treated, asymptomatic individuals. Effective therapy usually ends commu-nicability within hours.

8. **Susceptibility and resistance**—Susceptibility is general. Humoral and secretory antibodies have been demonstrated, but gonococcal strains are antigenically heterogeneous and reinfection is common. Women using an intrauterine contraceptive device have higher risks of salpingitis; some persons deficient in complement components are uniquely suscep tible to bacteremia. Since only columnar and transitional epithelium can be infected by the gonococcus, the vaginal epithelium of adult women (which is covered by stratified squamous epithelium) is resistant to infection, whereas the prepubertal columnar or transitional vaginal epi-thelium is susceptible.

9. **Methods of control**—

A. *Preventive measures:* Same as for syphilis (see Syphilis, 9A), except for measures which apply specifically to gonorrhea, i.e., the use of prophylactic agents in the eyes of the newborn (II, 9A2, below) and special attention (prophylactic treatment) to contacts of infectious patients (I, 9B6, below).

B. *Control of patient, contacts and the immediate environment:*

1) Report to local health authority: Case report is required in all states (USA) and many countries, Class 2B (see Preface).

2) Isolation: None. Effective antibiotics in adequate dosage promptly render discharges noninfectious. Patients should refrain from sexual intercourse until antimicrobial therapy is completed, and, to avoid reinfection, abstain from sex with previous sexual partners until they have been treated.

3) Concurrent disinfection: Care in disposal of discharges from lesions and contaminated articles.

4) Quarantine: None.

5) Immunization of contacts: Not available.

6) Investigation of contacts and source of infection: Inter-view patients and notify sex partners. Trained interview-ers obtain the best results with uncooperative patients, but clinicians can motivate most patients to help arrange for treatment of their partners. Sexual contacts within the preceding 30 days should be examined, cultured and treated presumptively. Urethral, vaginal, orogastric and rectal cultures should be made on all infants born to infected mothers.

7) Specific treatment: On clinical, laboratory or epidemiologic grounds (contacts of a diagnosed case), adequate treatment must be given as follows:

For uncomplicated gonorrhea in adults (both antibiotic resistant and susceptible infections) ceftriaxone, 125-250 mg IM in a single dose, plus doxycycline, 100 mg orally twice daily for 7 days (to cure any concurrent chlamydial infection), is the recommended treatment. For patients who cannot take ceftriaxone, spectinomycin, 2.0 g IM in a single dose, followed by doxycycline is an alternate regimen. Spectinomycin is not effective for pharyngeal gonorrhea; ceftriaxone, 250 mg IM, or oral ciprofloxacin, 500 mg as a single dose, is effective; repeat throat culture 4-7 days after treatment.

If the infecting gonococci are known to be penicillin-susceptible, a penicillin such as amoxicillin, 3.0 g orally as a single dose, with probenecid, 1 g orally, may be used, followed by doxycycline as above. Tetracycline may be substituted for doxycycline for chlamydia control; neither tetracycline nor doxycycline alone is considered adequate therapy for GC.

Pregnant women should be cultured at the first prenatal visit; recommended treatment for infection is ceftriaxone, 125-250 mg IM once, plus erythromycin base for chlamydial coverage, 500 mg orally four times daily for seven days. Follow-up culture 4-7 days after treatment. Quinolones are contraindicated during pregnancy.

Treatment failure following combined ceftriaxone and doxycycline therapy is rare and culture as test of cure is not essential except for pregnant women. Rescreen after 1-2 months to pick up reinfections. If ceftriaxone is not available and alternative therapeutic regimes were used, culture as test of cure is indicated 4-7 days after completion of treatment. Examine serologically for syphilis. Patients should be offered confidential counseling and testing for HIV infection. Because up to 45% of gonorrhea patients have also been infected with chlamydia, gonorrhea treatment should be followed by tetracycline/doxycycline (or erythromycin in pregnant women) as therapy for chlamydia (q.v.).

C. *Epidemic measures:* Intensification of routine procedures, especially therapy of contacts on epidemiologic grounds.

D. *Disaster implications:* None.

E. *International measures:* See Syphilis, 9E.

II. GONOCOCCAL CONJUNCTIVITIS   ICD-9 098.40 (NEONATORUM)
(Gonorrheal ophthalmia neonatorum)

1. **Identification**—Acute redness and swelling of the conjunctiva of one or both eyes, with mucopurulent or purulent discharge in which gonococci are identifiable by microscopic and culture methods. Corneal ulcer, perforation and blindness may occur if specific treatment is not given promptly.

Gonococcal ophthalmia neonatorum is only one of a number of acute inflammatory conditions of the eye or the conjunctiva occurring within the first three weeks of life, collectively known as ophthalmia neonatorum. The gonococcus is the most serious, but not the most frequent, infectious agent. The most common cause is *Chlamydia trachomatis,* producing inclusion conjunctivitis which tends to be less acute than gonococcal conjunctivitis and usually appears 5-14 days after birth (see Conjunctivitis, Chlamydial). All purulent neonatal conjunctivitides should be considered gonococcal until proven otherwise.

2. **Infectious agent**—*Neisseria gonorrhoeae,* the gonococcus.

3. **Occurrence**—Varies widely according to the prevalence of maternal infection and the measures for prevention of eye infections in the newborn at delivery; infrequent where infant eye prophylaxis is adequate. Globally, the disease continues to be an important cause of blindness.

4. **Reservoir**—Infection of the cervix.

5. **Mode of transmission**—Contact with the infected birth canal during childbirth.

6. **Incubation period**—Usually 1-5 days.

7. **Period of communicability**—While discharge persists if untreated; for 24 hours following initiation of specific treatment.

8. **Susceptibility and resistance**—Susceptibility is general.

9. **Methods of control**—

   A. *Preventive measures:*

   1) The best prevention of gonococcal conjunctivitis in the neonate is diagnosis and treatment of GC in pregnant women. Routine cervical and rectal culturing for gonococci during the prenatal period, especially in the third trimester, should be considered.

   2) Use an established effective preparation for protection of babies' eyes at birth; instillation of 1% silver nitrate aqueous solution stored in individual wax capsules re-

mains the prophylactic agent most widely used. Erythromycin (0.5%) and tetracycline (1%) ophthalmic ointments are also effective.

B. *Control of patient, contacts and the immediate environment:*

1) Report to local health authority: Case report is required in all states (USA) and many countries, Class 2B (see Preface).

2) Isolation: Contact isolation for the first 24 hours after administration of effective therapy. Patients should be hospitalized if possible. Bacterial cure after therapy should be confirmed by culture.

3) Concurrent disinfection: Care in disposal of conjunctival discharges and contaminated articles.

4) Quarantine: None.

5) Immunization of contacts: Not applicable; prompt treatment on diagnosis or clinical suspicion of infection.

6) Investigation of contacts and source of infection: Examination and treatment of mothers and their sexual partners.

7) Specific treatment: For gonococcal infections when antibiotic susceptibility is not known, or for penicillin-resistant organisms, ceftriaxone, 25-50 mg/kg/day (IV or IM) once daily for 7 days; or cefotaxime, 25 mg/kg (IV or IM) every 12 hours for 7 days, is recommended. For organisms known to be penicillin-sensitive, crystalline penicillin G, 100,000 units/kg/day (IV) in 2 equal doses (4 equal doses/day for infants older than 1 week) for 7 days. Mother and infant should also be treated for chlamydia.

C. *Epidemic measures:* None.

D. *Disaster implications:* None.

E. *International measures:* None.

GRANULOMA INGUINALE　　　　　ICD-9 099.2
(Donovanosis)

1. **Identification**—A nonfatal, chronic and progressive bacterial disease of the skin and mucous membranes of the external genitalia, inguinal and anal region with low communicability. A small beefy-red nodule, vesicle or papule becomes a slowly spreading, exuberant, granulomatous,

ulcerative, or cicatricial process, which is frequently painless and extends peripherally with characteristic rolled edges and formation of fibrous tissue. In many cases the lesion is predominantly granulomatous. Lesions have a predilection for warm and moist surfaces such as the folds between scrotum and thighs or labia and vagina. If neglected, the process may result in extensive destruction of genital organs and spread by autoinoculation to other parts of the body.

Laboratory diagnosis is based on demonstration of intracytoplasmic rod-shaped organisms (Donovan bodies) in Giemsa-stained smears of granulation tissue or by histologic examination of biopsy specimens. Culture is difficult and unreliable. *Haemophilus ducreyi* should be excluded by culture on appropriate selective media.

2. Infectious agent—*Calymmatobacterium granulomatis (Donovania granulomatis)*, a Gram-negative bacillus, is the presumed etiologic agent; this is not certain.

3. Occurrence—Rare in industrialized countries; endemic in tropical and subtropical areas, such as southern India, Papua New Guinea, central, eastern and southern Africa, West Indies and S America. It is more frequent among males than females and among persons of lower socioeconomic status; predominant in ages 20 to 40. In the USA, more common among homosexuals; relatively rare in heterosexual partners of cases.

4. Reservoir—Man.

5. Mode of transmission—Presumably by direct contact with lesions during sexual activity.

6. Incubation period—Unknown; probably between 1 week and 3 months.

7. Period of communicability—Unknown; probably for the duration of open lesions on the skin or mucous membranes.

8. Susceptibility and resistance—Susceptibility is variable; immunity apparently does not follow attack.

9. Methods of control—

    A. *Preventive measures:* Except for those measures applicable only to syphilis, preventive measures are those described in Syphilis, 9A.

    B. *Control of patient, contacts and the immediate environment:*

        1) Report to local health authority: A reportable disease in most states (USA) and countries, Class 3B (see Preface).

        2) Isolation: None; avoid close personal contact until lesions are healed.

3) Concurrent disinfection: Care in disposal of discharges from lesions and articles soiled therewith.
4) Quarantine: None.
5) Immunization of contacts: Not applicable; prompt treatment upon recognition or clinical suspicion of infection.
6) Investigation of contacts and source of infection: Examination of sexual contacts.
7) Specific treatment: Tetracyclines, co-trimoxazole, and chloramphenicol have been reported to be effective. Therapy is continued for 3 weeks or until the lesions have resolved; recurrence is not rare but usually responds to a second course of therapy unless malignancy is present.

C. **Epidemic measures:** Not applicable.

D. **Disaster implications:** None.

E. **International measures:** See Syphilis, 9E.

HEMORRHAGIC FEVER, ARGENTINE   ICD-9 078.7 & BOLIVIAN
(Junin h.f., Machupo h.f., Arenaviral h.f.)

1. **Identification**—Acute febrile viral illnesses; duration is 7-15 days. Onset is gradual, with malaise, headache, retro-orbital pain, conjunctival injection, and sustained fever and sweats, followed by prostration. There may be petechiae and ecchymoses, accompanied by erythema of the face, neck and upper thorax. An enanthem with petechiae on the soft palate is frequent. Severe infections result in epistaxis, hematemesis, melena, hematuria and gingival hemorrhage; encephalopathies, intention tremors and depressed deep tendon reflexes are frequent. Bradycardia and hypotension with clinical shock are common findings, and leukopenia and thrombocytopenia are characteristic. Moderate albuminuria is present, with many cellular and granular casts and vacuolated epithelial cells in the urine. Relapses may occur. Case fatality rates range from 5 to 30%.

Diagnosis is made by isolation of virus from blood, and serologically by titer rises of ELISA, IFA or neutralizing antibodies. Laboratory studies require BSL 4.

2. **Infectious agents**—The Junin virus of the Tacaribe group of arenaviruses for the Argentine disease, and the closely related Machupo virus for the Bolivian disease. (These viruses are related to the viruses of Lassa fever and lymphocytic choriomeningitis.)

3. **Occurrence**—Argentine hemorrhagic fever was first described among corn harvesters in Argentina in 1955. About 300-600 cases are reported from endemic areas of the Argentine pampas each year. Disease occurs primarily from March to October (autumn and winter), with a peak in May or June. It occurs mainly between ages 15-44 years and is five times more frequent in males than females. A similar disease, Bolivian hemorrhagic fever, caused by the related virus, was subsequently described in a series of epidemics in small villages of northeastern Bolivia; no cases have been reported since 1975.

4. **Reservoir**—In Argentina, wild rodents of corn fields (especially *Akodon azarae* and *Calomys musculinus*) are principal vertebrate hosts but *Mus musculus*, the house mouse, may also be involved; in Bolivia, *C. callosus* is the reservoir animal.

5. **Mode of transmission**—Airborne transmission may occur via dust contaminated with infected rodent excreta; both saliva and excreta of infected rodents contain the virus. Abraded skin may also be a protal of entry for infection. Laboratory infections occur. There is no confirmed evidence of arthropod transmission, but mites have been found infected with the Junin virus.

6. **Incubation period**—Commonly seven to 16 days.

7. **Period of communicability**—Not often directly transmitted from person to person, although this has occurred in both Argentine and Bolivian diseases.

8. **Susceptibility and resistance**—All ages appear to be susceptible but protective immunity of unknown duration follows infection. Subclinical infections occur.

9. **Methods of control**—

    A. ***Preventive measures:*** Specific rodent control in houses has been successful in Bolivia. In Argentina, human contact most commonly occurs in the fields, and rodent dispersion makes control impractical. A live-attenuated vaccine is currently in field trials.

    B. ***Control of patient, contacts and the immediate environment:***

        1) Report to local health authority: In selected endemic areas; in most countries not a reportable disease, Class 3A (see Preface).

        2) Isolation: Strict isolation during the acute febrile period.

        3) Concurrent disinfection: Of sputum and respiratory secretions, and blood-contaminated materials.

        4) Quarantine: None.

        5) Immunization of contacts: None.

6) Investigation of contacts and source of infection: None.
7) Specific treatment: Specific immune plasma given within 8 days of onset is effective in the treatment of Argentine disease. Ribavirin may be a useful adjunct.

C. *Epidemic measures:* Rodent control.

D. *Disaster implications:* None.

E. *International measures:* None.

HEMORRHAGIC FEVER WITH RENAL SYNDROME   ICD-9 078.6

(Epidemic hemorrhagic fever, Korean hemorrhagic fever, Nephropathia epidemica, Hemorrhagic nephrosonephritis)

1. **Identification**—An acute zoonotic viral disease characterized by an abrupt onset of fever lasting 3-8 days, conjunctival injection, prostration, backache, headache, abdominal pain, anorexia and vomiting. Hemorrhagic manifestations may appear from the third to the sixth day, followed by proteinuria, hypotension and sometimes shock. Renal abnormalities may be mild, or progress to acute renal failure and continue for several weeks. The majority of deaths (case fatality rate is about 7% in China and Korea) occur during the hypotensive and anuric phases. Convalescence frequently takes weeks. A milder form of the disease, caused by the Puumala virus, is referred to as nephropathia epidemica, and occurs throughout the Far East; it is the predominant form of disease seen in Scandinavia and Europe. Infections caused by the Seoul virus, carried by the roof rat, are also clinically milder.

Leptospirosis must be considered in the differential diagnosis.

Diagnosis is made by demonstration of specific antibodies using IFA or ELISA; most patients have IgM antibodies at the time of hospitalization. Presence of proteinuria, leukocytosis, thrombocytopenia and elevated blood urea nitrogen assist in supporting the diagnosis.

2. **Infectious agent**—Hantaviruses (a genus of the Bunyaviridae family) are 3-segmented RNA viruses, with spherical to oval particles, 95-110 nm in diameter. Several antigenic subtypes exist, each associated with a single rodent species: the Hantaan virus with *Apodemus* spp. of field mice, the Seoul virus with rats, and the Puumala virus with *Clethrionomys* spp. of bank voles. Laboratory-adapted strains can be propagated in cell cultures and laboratory rats and mice.

3. **Occurrence**—Prior to World War II, Japanese and Soviets reported its presence in Manchuria along the Amur River. Later, it was recognized in Korea among United Nations troops in 1951 and among military personnel and civilians since then. Epidemic hemorrhagic fever is considered a major public health problem in central and southern China, with about 100,000-200,000 cases/year, cases also occur in Japan. Disease occurs throughout the year, but in Korea and China there are two seasonal peaks, one in May-June and one in October-November. The majority of cases are isolated events, but outbreaks have involved 5-20 persons within a small area, apparently acquired at the same time and place. In rural areas of Korea, 100-800 patients are hospitalized per year.

Disease in medical research personnel and animal handlers in Japan was traced to naturally infected laboratory rats. It occurs as a milder (but still sometimes fatal) disease in European USSR, Scandinavia (nephropathia epidemica) and other countries of eastern and southern Europe; in Greece and Yugoslavia, a severe form of disease has been reported. Serologic mapping indicates that Hantaviruses have infected large numbers of people in the region from Japan across central and north Asia to the Scandinavian Peninsula, and southward in Europe to the Balkans. There has been increasing recognition of human illness in most European countries. Other Hantaviruses have been identified in urban rats captured in major Asian and Western cities, including the USA and Brazil. With availability of diagnostic techniques, there is increasing recognition of this infection globally.

4. **Reservoir**—Field rodents (*Apodemus* spp. in Korea, China and the Balkan nations; *Clethrionomys* voles in Scandinavia, USSR, China and the Balkans; *Peromyscus* and *Microtus* rodents in the USA); *Rattus* spp. worldwide. Man is an accidental host.

5. **Mode of transmission**—Aerosol transmission from rodent excreta is presumed. Virus is present in urine, feces and saliva of persistently infected asymptomatic rodents; highest virus concentration is found in the lungs.

6. **Incubation period**—Usually 12-16 days, but varying from 5 to 42 days.

7. **Period of communicability**—Not transmitted directly from person to person.

8. **Susceptibility and resistance**—Persons without serologic evidence of past infection appear to be uniformly susceptible. Inapparent infections occur; second attacks have not been observed.

9. Methods of control—

A. *Preventive measures:*

1) Exclude rodents from houses and other buildings in endemic areas.
2) While details of transmission are unknown, specific rodent control is indicated where the reservoir host has been identified; in endemic areas, minimize personal and environmental exposure to wild rodents.
3) Laboratory rat and mouse colonies should be checked to assure freedom from asymptomatic Hantavirus infection.

B. *Control of patient, contacts and the immediate environment:*

1) Report to local health authority: In selected endemic areas; in most countries not a reportable disease, Class 3A (see Preface).
2) Isolation: None.
3) Concurrent disinfection: None.
4) Quarantine: None.
5) Immunization of contacts: None.
6) Investigation of contacts and source of infection: None.
7) Specific treatment: Ribavirin IV as early as possible during the first few days of illness has shown benefit; appropriate and careful treatment for shock and renal failure to avoid trauma and fluid overload.

C. *Epidemic measures:* Rodent control. Laboratory-associated outbreaks call for evaluation of the associated rodents and, if positive, elimination of the rodents and thorough disinfection with sodium hypochlorite or phenolics.

D. *Disaster implications:* None.

E. *International measures:* None.

HEPATITIS, VIRAL   ICD-9 070

Several distinct infections are grouped as the viral hepatitides; they are similar in many ways, but differ in etiology and in some epidemiologic, immunologic, clinical and pathologic characteristics. Their prevention and control vary greatly. Each will therefore be presented in a separate section.

I. VIRAL HEPATITIS A ICD-9 070.1
(Infectious hepatitis, Epidemic hepatitis, Epidemic jaundice, Catarrhal jaundice, Type A hepatitis, HA)

1. **Identification**—Onset is usually abrupt with fever, malaise, anorexia, nausea and abdominal discomfort, followed within a few days by jaundice. The disease varies in clinical severity from a mild illness lasting 1-2 weeks, to a severely disabling disease lasting several months (rare). Convalescence often is prolonged. In general, severity increases with age, but complete recovery without sequelae or recurrences is the rule. Many infections are asymptomatic; many are mild and without jaundice, especially in children, and recognizable only by liver function tests. The case fatality rate is low (about 0.6%); the rare death usually occurs in an older patient in whom the disease has a fulminant course.

Diagnosis is established by the demonstration of IgM antibodies against hepatitis A virus in the serum of acutely or recently ill patients; IgM may remain detectable for 4-6 months after onset. Diagnosis may also be made by a fourfold or greater rise in specific antibodies in paired sera; virus and antibody can be detected by RIA or ELISA. (Assay kits for the detection of IgM and total antibodies to the virus are available commercially.) If laboratory tests are not available, epidemiologic evidence can provide support for the diagnosis. However, HA cannot be distinguished epidemiologically from hepatitis E, in areas where the latter is endemic.

2. **Infectious agent**—Hepatitis A virus (HAV), a 27-nm picornavirus (i.e., a positive-strand RNA virus). It has been classified as *Enterovirus* type 72, a member of the family Picornaviridae.

3. **Occurrence**—Worldwide, sporadic and epidemic, with a tendency in the past to cyclic recurrences. In developing countries, adults are usually immune and epidemics of HA are uncommon. However, improved sanitation in many parts of the world is leaving many young adults susceptible, and outbreaks are increasing. In developed countries, disease transmission is frequent in day-care centers enrolling diapered children, in household and sexual contacts of acute cases, intravenous drug abusers and travelers to countries where the disease is endemic. Where environmental sanitation is poor, infection is common and occurs at an early age. Epidemics often evolve slowly in developed countries, involve wide geographic areas and last many months; common-source epidemics may evolve explosively. In the USA, nationwide epidemic cycles, with peaks in 1961 and 1971, disappeared in the 1980s. However, since 1983, HA rates have gradually increased. The disease is most common among school-age children and young adults. In recent years, communitywide outbreaks have accounted for most disease transmission, although common-source outbreaks due to food contaminated by foodhandlers, contaminated produce and contaminated water continue to occur.

4. **Reservoir**—Man, and rarely captive chimpanzees; less frequently, certain other nonhuman primates. An enzootic focus has been identified in Malaysia, but there is no suggestion of transmission to man.

5. **Mode of transmission**—Person-to-person by the fecal-oral route. The infectious agent is found in feces, reaching peak levels the week or two before onset of symptoms, and diminishing rapidly after liver dysfunction or symptoms appear, which is concurrent with the appearance of circulating antibodies to HAV. Direct transmission occurs among male homosexuals. Common-source outbreaks have been related to contaminated water; food contaminated by infected foodhandlers, including sandwiches and salads which are not cooked or are handled after cooking; and raw or undercooked molluscs harvested from contaminated waters. Although rare, instances have been reported of transmission by transfusion of blood from a donor during the incubation period.

6. **Incubation period**—Fifteen to 50 days, depending on dose; average 28-30 days.

7. **Period of communicability**—Studies of transmission in humans and epidemiologic evidence indicate maximum infectivity during the latter half of the incubation period, continuing for a few days after onset of jaundice (or during peak aminotransferase activity in anicteric cases). Most cases are probably noninfectious after the first week of jaundice.

8. **Susceptibility and resistance**—Susceptibility is general. Low incidence of manifest disease in infants and preschool children suggests that mild and anicteric infections are common. Homologous immunity after attack probably lasts for life.

9. **Methods of control**—

A. *Preventive measures:*

1) Educate the public about good sanitation and personal hygiene, with special emphasis on careful handwashing and sanitary disposal of feces.

2) Provide proper water treatment and distribution systems, and sewage disposal.

3) Management of day-care centers should stress measures to minimize the possibility of fecal-oral transmission, including thorough handwashing after every diaper change and before eating. If one or more HA cases are associated with a center, IG should be administered to the staff and attendees. IG administration should be considered for family contacts of children ≤2 years of age attending centers where outbreaks are occurring and

cases are recognized in 3 or more families, or where recognition of the outbreak occurs more than 3 weeks after onset of the first case.

4) Travelers to highly endemic areas, including Africa, the Middle East, Asia, and Central and S America, should be given prophylactic doses of IG. For expected exposures up to 3 months, a single dose of 0.02 ml/kg or 2 ml for adults is recommended; for more prolonged exposures, 0.06 ml/kg or 5 ml should be given and repeated every 4-6 months if exposure continues.

5) Use disposable units and properly sterilize syringes, needles and other equipment used for parenteral injections (although the virus is rarely transmitted by this route).

6) Oysters, clams and other shellfish from contaminated areas should be heated to a temperature of 85-90°C (185-194°F) for 4 minutes before eating; steaming for 90 seconds will achieve this.

7) Vaccines for active immunization, both killed and attenuated, are being developed but are not yet available for general use.

B. *Control of patient, contacts and the immediate environment:*

1) Report to local health authority: Obligatory in all states of the USA and in Canada, although not now required in many countries; Class 2A (see Preface).

2) Isolation: For proven hepatitis A, enteric precautions during the first 2 weeks of illness, but no more than 1 week after onset of jaundice.

3) Concurrent disinfection: Sanitary disposal of feces, urine, and blood.

4) Quarantine: None.

5) Immunization of contacts: Passive immunization with IG (IM) 0.02 ml/kg of body weight, should be given as soon as possible after exposure, but within 2 weeks, to all household and sexual contacts. In a day-care center, IG should be given to all classroom contacts. If the center admits children in diapers, IG should be given to all potentially exposed children and staff in the center. IG is not indicated for contacts in the usual office, school or factory situation.

6) Investigation of contacts and source of infection: Search for missed cases and maintain surveillance of contacts in the patient's household or, in a common-source outbreak, persons exposed to the same risk.

7) Specific treatment: None.

C. *Epidemic measures:*

1) Determine mode of transmission by epidemiologic investigation, whether person to person or by common vehicle, and identify the population exposed to increased risk of infection. Eliminate any common sources of infection. If HA occurs in a foodhandler, IG should be given to other foodhandlers in the establishment. IG is usually not offered to patrons; it may be considered if the foodhandlers were involved in the preparation of foods which were not heated and deficiencies in personal hygiene are noted, and if the IG can be given within 2 weeks after last exposure.

2) Make special efforts to improve sanitary and hygienic practices to eliminate fecal contamination of foods and water.

3) Focal outbreaks in institutions may warrant mass prophylaxis with IG.

D. *Disaster implications:* A potential problem in a large collection of people with crowding, inadequate sanitation and water supplies; if cases occur, increased efforts should be exerted to improve sanitation and safety of water supplies. Mass administration of IG is not a substitute for environmental measures.

E. *International measures:* None.

II. VIRAL HEPATITIS B   ICD-9 070.3
(Type B hepatitis, Serum hepatitis, Homologous serum jaundice, Australia antigen hepatitis, HB)

1. Identification—Onset is usually insidious with anorexia, vague abdominal discomfort, nausea and vomiting, sometimes arthralgias and rash, often progressing to jaundice. Fever may be absent or mild. Severity ranges from inapparent cases detectable only by liver function tests, to fulminating, fatal cases of acute hepatic necrosis. The case fatality rate in hospitalized patients is about 1%; higher in those over 40 years of age. Prolonged hepatitis B antigenemia (the HBV carrier state), without overt signs of disease, is found in 0.2-0.9% of adults in N America and in 0.1-20% of persons from other parts of the world; it occurs in 70-90% of children infected very early in life. HBV carriers may or may not have a history of clinical hepatitis. About one-third have an elevated aminotransferase; biopsy findings range from normal to chronic active hepatitis, with or without cirrhosis. The prognosis of the liver disease in such individuals is variable. About 10% of patients with histologic findings of chronic hepatitis or cryptogenic cirrhosis have hepatitis B surface antigen detectable in their sera. HBV may be the cause of up to 80% of all cases of

hepatocellular carcinoma worldwide, second only to tobacco among known human carcinogens. Perinatal infection has a high likelihood of resulting in chronic antigenemia, culminating in chronic hepatitis, cirrhosis, or primary hepatocellular carcinoma.

Diagnosis is usually confirmed by demonstration of hepatitis B surface antigen (HBsAg), less commonly by detection of viral DNA in the blood using nucleic acid hybridization that indicates active viral replication, or demonstration of recent development of antibody to core and/or surface antigens (anti-HBc, anti-HBs, respectively). Three antigen-antibody systems have been identified for HB: HBsAg and anti-HBs, core antigen and antibody (HBcAg and anti-HBc), and e antigen and antibody (HBeAg and anti-HBe). Commercial kits (RIA or ELISA) are available for all markers except HBcAg. HBsAg can be detected in the serum from several weeks before onset of symptoms to days, weeks or months after onset; it persists in chronic infections. Anti-HBc appears at the onset of illness and persists indefinitely. IgM anti-HBc is present in high titer during acute infection and usually disappears within 6 months; this test may reliably diagnose acute HBV infection.

2. **Infectious agent**—The hepatitis B virus (HBV), a hepadnavirus, is a 42-nm partially double-stranded DNA virus, composed of a 27-nm nucleocapsid core (HBcAg), surrounded by an outer lipoprotein coat containing the surface antigen (HBsAg). HBsAg is antigenically heterogeneous, with a common antigen designated a, and two pairs of mutually exclusive antigens, d and y, and w (including several subdeterminants) and r, resulting in 4 major subtypes: adw, ayw, adr, and ayr. The distribution of subtypes varies geographically; protection against one subtype appears to confer protection against the other subtypes, and no differences in clinical features have been related to subtype.

The third hepatitis B antigen, the e antigen (HBeAg), has been identified as a soluble antigen, whose sequences are a subset of those in the core antigen but without cross-reactivity. The hepatitis B virion also contains DNA-dependent DNA polymerase and reverse transcriptase activities. In common usage, antigens are identified as indicated, and the respective antibodies as anti-HBc, anti-HBs, and anti-HBe. In combination with HBsAg, the detection of e antigen (HBeAg) is associated with relatively high infectivity; conversely, presence of anti-HBe correlates with a relative (but not absolute) lack of infectivity. Another correlate of infectivity is the presence of HBV viral DNA in serum; conversely, the absence of HBV viral DNA indicates a relative (but not absolute) lack of infectivity. The presence of e antigen at the time of delivery indicates a very high risk of infection in the newborn infant.

3. **Occurrence**—Worldwide; endemic with little seasonal variation. In areas of Africa and Asia, widespread infection may occur in infancy and childhood; in N America infection is most common in young adults. In the USA and Canada, serologic evidence of previous infection varies

depending on age and socioeconomic class. Overall, 5% of the adult USA population has anti-HBs, and 0.2-0.9% are HBsAg positive; among those from some areas of Asia, overall antigen carrier rates may be 10-15%. In developed countries, HBV infection is common in certain high-risk groups. These include parenteral drug abusers, heterosexuals with multiple partners, homosexual men, clients and staff in institutions for the retarded, patients and employees in hemodialysis centers and persons in certain health care and public safety occupations. Frequent and routine exposure to blood or serous fluids is the common denominator of health care occupational exposure; surgeons, dentists, oral surgeons, pathologists, operating room and emergency room staff, and clinical laboratory workers who handle blood are at highest risk.

In the past, recipients of blood products were at high risk. In the many countries in which pretransfusion screening of blood for HBsAg has been required, and where pooled blood-clotting factors (especially antihemophilic factor) are processed to destroy the virus, this risk has been virtually eliminated. In the past, contaminated and inadequately sterilized syringes and needles have resulted in outbreaks of hepatitis B among patients in clinics and physicians' offices. Occasionally, outbreaks have been traced to tattoo parlors and acupuncturists. Rarely, transmission to patients from HBV-carrier dentists, oral surgeons and obstetric-gynecologic surgeons has been documented.

4. **Reservoir**—Man. Chimpanzees are susceptible but an animal reservoir in nature has not been recognized.

5. **Mode of transmission**—HBsAg has been found in virtually all body secretions and excretions; however, only blood (and serum-derived fluids), saliva, semen and vaginal fluids have been shown to be infectious. The presence of e antigen or viral DNA indicates high virus titer and higher infectivity of these fluids. Transmission occurs by percutaneous (IV, IM, subcutaneous or intradermal) and permucosal exposure to infective body fluids, as may occur in needle stick accidents, perinatal exposure, or sexual exposure. Human blood, plasma, serum, thrombin, fibrinogen, packed RBCs, cryoprecipitate and other blood products may transmit infection if not screened for HBsAg. IG, heat-treated plasma protein fraction, albumin and fibrinolysin are considered safe. Contaminated needles, syringes and other intravenous equipment are important vehicles of spread, especially among drug addicts. The infection may be spread through contamination of skin lesions, or by exposure of mucous membranes to infective blood; this is probably an important source of transmission in health care occupations, institutions for the retarded, and in less developed countries where HBV is endemic. Perinatal transmission is common in hyperendemic areas of SE Asia and the Far East, especially when HBsAg carrier mothers are also HBeAg positive. Infection may also be transmitted between household contacts and between sexual partners, either homosexual or heterosexual, and in toddler-age

children in ethnic groups with high carrier rates. Percutaneous and mucosal inoculations by communally used razors and toothbrushes have been implicated as occasional transmitters of HB. Fecal-oral transmission has not been demonstrated.

6. **Incubation period**—Usually 45-180 days, average 60-90 days. As short as 2 weeks to the appearance of HBsAg, and rarely as long as 6-9 months; the variation is related in part to the amount of virus in the inoculum, the mode of transmission, and host factors.

7. **Period of communicability**—Blood from experimentally inoculated volunteers has been shown to be infective many weeks before the onset of first symptoms and to remain infective through the acute clinical course of the disease and during the chronic carrier state, which may persist for life. Most, if not all, carriers have demonstrable HBsAg and anti-HBc. Chronic antigenemia may follow asymptomatic infections and is common in individuals infected in infancy and in those with immunodeficiency, such as patients with Down syndrome, lymphoproliferative disease, human immunodeficiency virus (HIV) infection, and patients on hemodialysis. The infectivity of chronically infected individuals varies from highly infectious (HBeAg positive) to sparingly infectious (anti-HBe positive); the former may progress to the latter but the reverse rarely occurs.

8. **Susceptibility and resistance**—Susceptibility is general. Usually, the disease is milder and often anicteric in children; in infants it is usually asymptomatic. Protective immunity follows infection if antibody to HBsAg (anti-HBs) develops and HBsAg is negative.

9. **Methods of control—**

   A. *Preventive measures:*

      1) Two types of inactivated vaccines against HB have been licensed and are commercially available. Both have been shown to be safe and highly protective against all subtypes of HBV. The first is a plasma-derived vaccine; it is prepared from plasma from HBsAg-positive carriers. Laboratory studies confirm that each of the 3 inactivating processes used in the production of plasma-derived vaccines licensed in the USA is sufficient to inactivate all human retroviruses including HIV-1, HIV-2, HTLV-I and HTLV-II. The second type is subunit HBsAg-containing vaccine made by recombinant DNA (rDNA) technology. Combined passive-active immunoprophylaxis with hepatitis B immunoglobin (HBIG) and vaccine has been shown to stimulate anti-HBs comparable to vaccine alone.

         a) In hyperendemic areas of the world and in areas of

moderate endemicity as well, only widescale immunization of infants and children can be expected to produce significant disease control; strategies for control differ from those in areas of low endemicity. Currently, the high cost of HB vaccine precludes its widespread use, but many countries are exploring the feasibility of local production of vaccines at lower cost. In addition, newer technologies hold the promise of significantly less costly vaccines in the future.

b) For areas with overall low endemicity of infection, where risk is limited to a few high-risk groups, vaccination is recommended for those at increased and continuing risk of infection. These include users of parenteral drugs, the sexually active (both heterosexuals and male homosexuals), health-care and public-safety personnel (especially those who come into contact with blood and secretions), staff and clients in institutions for the developmentally disabled, hemodialysis patients, patients who receive clotting factor concentrates, and household and sexual contacts of carriers.

c) Tests to exclude persons with pre-existing anti-HBs or anti-HBc are not required prior to vaccination, but may be desirable as a cost-saving method where there is a high level of pre-existing immunity.

d) Vaccines licensed in different parts of the world may have varying dosages and schedules; the vaccines currently licensed in the USA should be administered in 3 IM doses: initially and 1 and 6 months later; or in 4 doses given 1, 2, and 12 months after the first. Recommended doses are 0.5 ml (10 µg of plasma-derived; 5 µg of recombinant vaccine) for children from birth to 10 years; and 1.0 ml (20 µg or 10 µg) for older children and adults. For dialysis and immuno-compromised patients, plasma- derived vaccine is preferred at a dose of 2.0 ml (40 µg) (two-1.0 ml doses at different sites). Studies under way may result in changes in recommendations; the package insert should be consulted for dosage. Pregnancy is not a definitive contraindication for receiving this inactivated vaccine.

2) The current USA recommendation is to test all pregnant women for the presence of HBsAg; if positive, their infants should be managed as outlined in 9B5, below. Universal vaccination of infants is recommended for certain US populations in whom HBV infection is highly

endemic, including refugees from HBV endemic areas (particularly Africa and eastern Asia), Native Alaskans, and Pacific Islanders.

3) Enforce strict discipline in blood banks. All donated blood should be tested for HBsAg by sensitive tests (RIA or EIA); reject as donors all individuals who have a history of viral hepatitis, show evidence of drug addiction, or have received a blood transfusion or tattoo within the preceding 6 months. Use paid donors only in emergencies.

4) Limit administration of unscreened whole blood or potentially hazardous blood products to those patients in clear and immediate need of such therapeutic measures.

5) Maintain surveillance for all cases of post-transfusion hepatitis, including a register of all persons who donated blood for each case. Notify blood banks of these potential carriers so that future donations may be identified promptly.

6) Adequately sterilize all syringes and needles (including acupuncture needles) and stylets for finger puncture or preferably use disposable equipment whenever possible. A sterile syringe and needle are essential for each individual receiving skin tests, other parenteral inoculations, or venipuncture. Discourage tattooing; enforce aseptic sanitary practices in tattoo parlors.

7) Persons with e antigen should exert great care to avoid transmission, especially medical and dental personnel who routinely perform invasive procedures, and sexually active persons. Children in special education classes will require close supervision by the staff; immunization of the uninfected children should be considered.

B. *Control of patient, contacts and the immediate environment:*

1) Report to local health authority: Official report is obligatory in the USA, although not now required in many countries; Class 2A (see Preface).

2) Isolation: Universal precautions; especially blood and body fluid precautions until disappearance of HBsAg and appearance of anti-HBs.

3) Concurrent disinfection: Of equipment contaminated with blood, saliva, or semen.

4) Quarantine: None.

5) Immunization of contacts: Products available for postexposure prophylaxis include hepatitis B immunoglobulin (HBIG) and hepatitis B vaccine. HBIG has high titers of anti-HBs (>1:100,000). When indicated, it is important

to administer HBIG as soon after exposure as possible.

a) Infants born to HBsAg-positive mothers should be given a single dose of HBIG (0.5 ml IM) within 12 hours of birth to provide immediate passive protection, and a complete series of 3 doses of vaccine should be initiated as soon after birth as possible, to provide long-lasting active immunity. The first dose (0.5 ml; 10 μg or 5 μg; see 9A1d, above) should be given concurrently with HBIG at birth but in a separate site. If vaccine is not immediately available, the first dose should be given as soon as possible. The second and third doses of vaccine (without HBIG) are given 1 and 6 months later. If vaccine is delayed until 3 months of age, a second dose of HBIG is needed at that time. It is recommended to test the infant for HBsAg and anti-HBs at 12-15 months to monitor the success or failure of therapy.

b) After percutaneous (e.g., needle-stick) or mucous membrane exposures to HBsAg-positive material (unless a rapid test indicates the presence of anti-HBs in the exposed person) a single dose of HBIG (0.06 ml/kg or 5 ml for adults) should be given as soon as possible, but at least within 24 hours after high-risk needle-stick exposure, and the HB vaccine series should be started. If active immunization is not accepted, a second dose of HBIG should be given 1 month after the first. HBIG is not usually given for needle-stick exposure to blood which is not known or highly suspected to be positive for HBsAg since the risk of infection in these instances is small; however, initiation of HB vaccination is recommended if the person had not previously been immunized.

c) After sexual exposure to an HBsAg-positive contact, a similar dose of HBIG is recommended if it can be given within 14 days of the last sexual contact. For all exposed sexual contacts of acute HBV cases and HBV carriers, vaccine is the treatment of choice.

6) Investigation of contacts and source of infection: See 9C, below.

7) Specific treatment: None. Anti-inflammatory drugs such as steroids are not indicated in acute or chronic hepatitis B. Studies with a variety of antiviral agents are under way; controlled studies have indicated that adenine arabinoside is not helpful.

C. *Epidemic measures:* When two or more cases occur in association with some common exposure, conduct a search for additional cases. Institute strict aseptic techniques. If a plasma derivative such as antihemophilic factor, fibrinogen, pooled plasma or thrombin is implicated, withdraw the lot from use and trace all recipients of the same lot in a search for additional cases.

D. *Disaster implications:* Relaxation of sterilization precautions and emergency use of unscreened blood for transfusions may result in an increased number of cases.

E. *International measures:* None.

III. VIRAL HEPATITIS C ICD-9 070.5
(Parenterally transmitted Non-A Non-B hepatitis [PT-NANB], Non-B transfusion-associated hepatitis, Post-transfusion non-A non-B hepatitis, HC)

1. **Identification**—Onset is usually insidious, with anorexia, vague abdominal discomfort, nausea and vomiting, progressing to jaundice less frequently than hepatitis B. Severity ranges from inapparent cases to fulminating, fatal cases (rare). It is usually less severe in the acute stage, but chronicity is common, occurring more frequently than with hepatitis B in adults. Chronic infection may be symptomatic or asymptomatic. Chronic hepatitis C may progress to cirrhosis, but more often improves clinically after 2-3 years.

Diagnosis currently depends on the exclusion of hepatitis A, B and delta viruses and other causes of liver injury. A serologic test for antibody to the agent mentioned below has been developed and is being established as a screening test for blood donors. This test for antibody to hepatitis C virus (anti-HCV) is positive in the majority of patients with chronic hepatitis C; in patients with acute disease, there may be a prolonged interval between exposure to the virus or the onset of illness and detection of anti-HCV.

2. **Infectious agent**—There is evidence for more than one type of agent from epidemiologic and transmission studies in primates. A putative agent has been identified: The lipid-enveloped agent is between 30 and 50 nm in diameter; it is a positive-strand, RNA virus whose genome is about 10-12 kb with one long open reading frame. These findings suggest a flavivirus, proposed as hepatitis C virus.

3. **Occurrence**—Hepatitis C is parenterally transmitted and has been found in every part of the world where it has been sought. It is the most common post-transfusion hepatitis in the USA, accounting for approximately 90% of this disease, and is more common when paid donors are used. Most cases are not associated with blood transfusion and hepatitis C accounts for 15-40% of community-acquired hepatitis cases. Antibodies

to the hepatitis C virus are found in samples from around the world. Preliminary evidence links antibody positivity to development of liver cancer in Japan.

4. **Reservoir**—Man; has been transmitted experimentally to chimpanzees.

5. **Mode of transmission**—Transmission occurs by percutaneous exposure to contaminated blood and plasma derivatives. Like HB, contaminated needles and syringes are important vehicles of spread, especially among parenteral drug users. Groups at highest risk include transfusion recipients, parenteral drug users, and dialysis patients. Health-care work that entails frequent contact with blood, and household or sexual contact with persons who have had hepatitis in the past have also been documented in some studies as risk factors for acquiring hepatitis C. The importance of person-to-person contact and sexual activity in the transmission of this disease have not been well defined.

6. **Incubation period**—Ranges from 2 weeks to 6 months; most commonly, within 6-9 weeks.

7. **Period of communicability**—From one or more weeks before onset of the first symptoms through the acute clinical course of the disease, and indefinitely in the chronic carrier stages. Based on infectivity studies in chimpanzees, the titer of hepatitis C virus in the blood appears to be relatively low.

8. **Susceptibility and resistance**—Susceptibility is general. The degree of immunity following infection is not known; repeated bouts of acute hepatitis C have been reported, but it is not known whether these represent infection by different agents or recrudescence of the original infection.

9. **Methods of control**—

A. *Preventive measures:* General control measures against HBV infection apply (see Hepatitis B, above). The value of prophylactic IG is not clear. In blood bank operations, discarding donor units with elevated liver enzyme levels and those which are positive for anti-HBc has been widely implemented in the USA and is advisable even after the test for hepatitis C has been established.

B. *Control of patient, contacts and the immediate environment:* Control measures against HBV infection apply. The value of prophylactic IG for contacts has not been established. Corticosteroids and acyclovir have not been effective in treatment. Interferon may be useful for the treatment of chronic carriers.

C. *Epidemic measures:* Same as for hepatitis B, above.

D. *Disaster implications:* Same as for hepatitis B, above.

E. *International measures:* None.

IV. DELTA HEPATITIS   ICD-9 070.5
(Viral hepatitis D, Hepatitis delta virus, Δ hepatitis, Delta agent hepatitis, Delta-associated hepatitis)

1. **Identification**—Onset is usually abrupt, with signs and symptoms resembling those of hepatitis B. Hepatitis may be severe and is always associated with a coexistent hepatitis B virus infection. Delta hepatitis may be self-limiting or it may progress to chronic hepatitis. Hepatitis delta virus (HDV) and hepatitis B virus (HBV) may coinfect, or delta virus infection may be superimposed upon the HBV carrier state. In the latter case, delta hepatitis can be misdiagnosed as an exacerbation of chronic hepatitis B. In several studies throughout Europe and the USA, 25-50% of fulminant hepatitis thought to be caused by HBV was associated with concurrent infection with HDV. The most fulminant disease occurs in superinfections rather than co-infections; a chronic outcome is most commonly associated with superinfection.

Diagnosis is made by demonstration of the viral antigen in the serum or liver, or more commonly, by detection of total or IgM antibody. RIA or ELISA is the method of choice. Viral RNA can be detected by nucleic acid hybridization.

2. **Infectious agent**—HDV is a 35-37-nm virus-like particle consisting of a coat of HBsAg and a unique internal antigen, delta antigen. Encapsulated with the delta antigen is the genome, a single-stranded RNA which can have a linear or circular conformation. The RNA does not hybridize with HBV DNA. HDV is unable to infect a cell by itself and requires coinfection with the HBV to undergo a complete replication cycle. Synthesis of HDV, in turn, results in temporary suppression of synthesis of HBV components.

3. **Occurrence**—Worldwide, but its prevalence varies widely. Occurs epidemically or endemically in populations at high risk of HBV infection, including populations in which HB is endemic (in southern Italy, Africa and S America); in hemophiliacs, drug addicts, and others who come in frequent contact with blood; in institutions for the developmentally disabled; and, to a lesser extent, male homosexuals. Severe epidemics have been observed in tropical S America (Brazil, Venezuela, Colombia), in the Central African Republic, and among drug addicts in Worcester, Massachusetts.

4. **Reservoir**—Man. Can be transmitted experimentally to chimpan-

zees and woodchucks that are infected with HBV and woodchuck hepatitis virus, respectively.

5. **Mode of transmission**—Thought to be similar to that of HBV, including exposure to blood and serous body fluids, contaminated needles, syringes and plasma derivatives such as antihemophilic factor, and sexual transmission.

6. **Incubation period**—Approximately 2-10 weeks for experimental infections in chimpanzees; not firmly established in man.

7. **Period of communicability**—Blood is potentially infectious during all phases of active delta hepatitis infection. Peak infectivity probably occurs just prior to onset of acute illness, when particles containing the delta antigen are readily detected in the blood. Following onset, viremia probably falls rapidly to low or undetectable levels. HDV has been transmitted to chimpanzees from the blood of chronically infected patients in which delta antigen-containing particles could not be detected.

8. **Susceptibility and resistance**—All persons susceptible to HB or who are HBV carriers can be infected with HDV. Severe disease can occur even in children.

9. **Methods of control**—

   A. *Preventive measures:* For persons susceptible to HB, as for Hepatitis B, above. Prevention of HBV infection prevents infection with HDV. Among HBV carriers, avoidance of exposure to any potential source of HDV is the only effective measure. HBIG, IG and HB vaccine do not protect HBV carriers from infection by HDV.

   B., C., D., and E. *Control of patient, contacts and the immediate environment, Epidemic measures, Disaster implications,* and *International measures:* Same as for Hepatitis B, above.

V. VIRAL HEPATITIS E   ICD-9 070.5
(Enterically transmitted non-A non-B hepatitis [ET-NANB], Epidemic non-A non-B hepatitis, Fecal-oral non-A non-B hepatitis)

1. **Identification**—The epidemiology and clinical course are similar to that of hepatitis A; there is no evidence of a chronic form. The case fatality rate is similar to that of hepatitis A, except in pregnant women where the rate may reach 20% during the third trimester of pregnancy. Epidemic and sporadic cases have been described.

Diagnosis depends on exclusion of other etiologies of hepatitis, especially hepatitis A, by serologic means. At present, a serologic test is being developed for one characterized agent of hepatitis E.

2. Infectious agent—There is evidence that one virus or virus family is responsible for hepatitis E. A 32-nm virus-like particle has been found in stools during the early acute phase of infection with a sedimentation coefficient of 183 S (compared to 157 S for HAV), which reacts by IEM with acute phase sera from several areas around the world.

3. Occurrence—Epidemics consistent with a hepatitis E virus etiology have been identified in India, Myanmar (Burma), Nepal, Pakistan, the USSR, Algeria, Libya, Somalia, Mexico and China. Often these have occurred as waterborne epidemics, but sporadic cases and epidemics not clearly related to water have been reported. The attack rate is highest in young adults, often with a male predominance. Cases are uncommon in children and the elderly.

4. Reservoir—Man; transmissible to chimpanzees, cynomolgus macaques and tamarins.

5. Mode of transmission—Contaminated water and probably from person to person by the fecal-oral route.

6. Incubation period—Fifteen to 64 days; mean incubation period has varied from 26 to 42 days in different epidemics.

7. Period of communicability—Not known, but may be similar to HA.

8. Susceptibility and resistance—Susceptibility unknown. Estimates for secondary transmission in households are low. Unexplained is the occurrence of major epidemics among young adults in geographic regions where other enteric viruses are highly endemic and infection of most of the population is in infancy.

9. Methods of control—

    A.   *Preventive measures:* Provide educational programs to stress sanitary disposal of feces and careful handwashing after defecation and before handling food. Basic measures to prevent fecal-oral transmission, as listed under Typhoid fever, 9A. It is unlikely that IG prepared from the serum of donors in the USA or Europe will protect against hepatitis E.

    B.   *Control of patient, contacts and the immediate environment:*

        1), 2), 3) Report to local health authority, Isolation, and Concurrent disinfection: Same as for hepatitis A, above.

        4)   Quarantine: None.

        5)   Immunization of contacts: None. The efficacy of IG has not been established.

        6)   Investigation of contacts and source of infection: Same as for hepatitis A, above.

        7)   Specific treatment: None.

C. *Epidemic measures:* Same as for hepatitis A, except that administration of IG is not indicated; however, administration of IG to prevent possible concurrent hepatitis A infections should be considered.

D. *Disaster implications:* Same as for hepatitis A, above.

E. *International measures:* None.

HERPES SIMPLEX   ICD-9 054
(Alphaherpesviral disease, Herpesvirus hominis, Human herpesviruses 1 and 2)

1. **Identification**—Herpes simplex is a viral infection characterized by a localized primary lesion, latency and a tendency to localized recurrence. The two etiologic agents—designated herpes simplex virus (HSV) types 1 and 2—generally produce distinct clinical syndromes, depending on the portal of entry. Either may infect the genital tract and the term "genital herpes" is now being used.

The primary infection with HSV type 1 may be mild and inapparent and occur in early childhood. In approximately 10% of primary infections, overt disease may appear as an illness of varying severity, marked by fever and malaise lasting a week or more; it may be associated with gingivostomatitis accompanied by vesicular lesions in the oropharynx, severe keratoconjunctivitis, a generalized cutaneous eruption complicating chronic eczema, meningoencephalitis, or some of the fatal generalized infections in newborn infants (congenital herpes simplex, ICD-9 771.2). It causes about 2% of acute pharyngotonsillitis, usually as a primary infection.

Reactivation of latent infection commonly results in herpes labialis (fever blisters or cold sores) manifested by superficial clear vesicles on an erythematous base, usually on the face and lips, which crust and heal within a few days. Reactivation is precipitated by various forms of trauma, fever, physiologic changes, or intercurrent disease, and may also involve other body tissues; it occurs in the presence of circulating antibodies which are seldom elevated by reactivation. Severe and extensive disease may occur in immunosuppressed individuals.

CNS involvement usually occurs in association with a primary infection but may appear following a recrudescence. HSV type 1 is a common cause of meningoencephalitis. Fever, headache, leukocytosis, meningeal irritation, drowsiness, confusion, stupor, coma and focal neurologic signs frequently referable to one or the other temporal region, may occur. The condition may be confused with a variety of other intracranial lesions including brain abscess and tuberculous meningitis. Because antiviral therapy may reduce the high mortality, biopsy of cerebral tissue should be performed early in clinically suspected cases to establish the diagnosis.

HSV type 2 usually produces genital herpes, although it can also be caused by type 1 virus. Genital herpes occurs mainly in adults and is sexually transmitted. Primary and recurrent infections occur, with or without symptoms. In women, the principal sites of primary disease are the cervix and the vulva; recurrent disease generally involves the vulva, perineal skin, legs and buttocks. In men, lesions appear on the glans penis or prepuce, and in the anus and rectum of receptive homosexuals. Other genital or perineal sites, as well as the mouth, may be involved in either sex, depending on sexual practices. This virus has been associated with aseptic meningitis and radiculitis rather than meningoencephalitis. Vaginal delivery in pregnant women with active genital infections (particularly if primary) carries a high risk of infection to the fetus or newborn, causing disseminated visceral infection, encephalitis and death. Genital infection with HSV type 2 in adult women may be a risk factor in cancer of the cervix, especially in conjunction with papillomavirus as the more important oncogen.

Diagnosis is suggested by characteristic cytologic changes (multinucleated giant cells with intranuclear inclusions in tissue scrapings or biopsy), but is confirmed by direct FA tests or isolation of the virus from oral or genital lesions, or from a brain biopsy in cases of encephalitis. Diagnosis of primary infection can be confirmed by testing paired sera by neutralization or other serologic tests; demonstration of herpes-specific IgM is suggestive but not conclusive evidence of primary infection. Reliable techniques to differentiate type 1 from type 2 antibody are now becoming available; virus isolates can be readily distinguished from one another.

2. **Infectious agent**—Herpes simplex virus (HSV) in the virus family Herpesviridae, subfamily Alphaherpesvirinae. HSV types 1 and 2 can be differentiated immunologically (especially when highly specific or monoclonal antibodies are used), and differ with respect to their growth patterns in tissue culture, embryonated eggs and experimental animals.

3. **Occurrence**—Worldwide. Seventy to 90% of adults possess circulating antibodies against HSV type 1. Initial infection with HSV type 1 usually occurs before the fifth year of life, but more primary infections in adults are now being reported. HSV type 2 infection usually begins with sexual activity and is rare before adolescence; type 2 antibody is found in about 20% of adults. The prevalence is greater (up to 60%) in lower socioeconomic groups and sexually promiscuous individuals.

4. **Reservoir**—Man.

5. **Mode of transmission**—Contact with type 1 virus in the saliva of carriers is probably the most important mode of spread. Infection on the hands of health care personnel (e.g., dentists) from patients shedding

HSV results in herpetic whitlow; pre-existing lesions in the recipient may play a significant role. Transmission of HSV type 2 to nonimmune adults is usually by sexual contact. Both types 1 and 2 may be transmitted to various sites during homosexual activity or by oral-genital or oral-anal contact.

6. **Incubation period**—Two to 12 days.

7. **Period of communicability**—Secretion of virus in the saliva has been reported for as long as 7 weeks after recovery from stomatitis. Patients with primary genital lesions are infective for about 7-12 days, with recurrent disease for 4 days to a week. Asymptomatic oral as well as genital infections, with transient viral shedding, are probably common. Reactivation of genital herpes may occur repeatedly in ≥50% of women following either symptomatic or asymptomatic primary infection; reactivation may be asymptomatic with viral shedding only.

8. **Susceptibility and resistance**—Humans are probably universally susceptible.

9. **Methods of control**—

A. *Preventive measures:*

1) Health education and personal hygiene directed toward minimizing the transfer of infectious material.

2) Avoid contaminating the skin of eczematous patients with infectious material.

3) Health personnel should wear gloves when in direct contact with potentially infectious lesions.

4) Cesarean section is advised before the membranes rupture when primary or recurrent genital herpes infections occur in late pregnancy because of the risk of highly fatal neonatal infection.

5) Use of latex condoms in sexual practice may decrease the risk of infection; no antiviral agent has yet been proved to be practical in prophylaxis, although acyclovir may reduce the incidence of recurrences and of herpes infections in immunodeficient patients.

B. *Control of patient, contacts and the immediate environment:*

1) Report to local health authority: Official case report not ordinarily justifiable, Class 5 (see Preface).

2) Isolation: Contact isolation for neonatal and disseminated or severe primary lesions; for recurrent lesions, drainage/secretion precautions. Patients with herpetic lesions should be kept away from newborns, children with eczema or burns, and immunosuppressed patients.

3) Concurrent disinfection: None.

4) Quarantine: None.
5) Immunization of contacts: None.
6) Investigation of contacts and source of infection: Seldom of practical value.
7) Specific treatment: Topical 5-iodo-2'deoxyuridine (Idoxuridine®) may modify the acute manifestations of herpetic keratitis and early dendritic ulcers. Corticosteroids should never be used for ocular involvement unless administered by an ophthalmologist. Adenine arabinoside (vidarabine, Vira-A® or Ara-A®) is effective as an ophthalmic ointment, and is of value in herpes simplex encephalitis, but may not prevent residual neurologic problems. Acyclovir, used orally, intravenous, or topically, has been shown to reduce shedding of virus, diminish pain, and accelerate healing time in primary genital herpes. The oral preparation is most convenient to use and may benefit patients with extensive recurrent infections as well. For CNS disease, acyclovir IV has proven to lower mortality.

C. *Epidemic measures:* Not applicable.

D. *Disaster implications:* None.

E. *International measures:* None.

MENINGOENCEPHALITIS DUE TO CERCOPITHECINE HERPESVIRUS 1

ICD-9 054.3

(B-virus, Simian B disease)

While HSV type 1 (rarely type 2) can cause meningoencephalitis, the picture is distinctly different from B-virus infection, a CNS disease caused by cercopithecine herpesvirus 1, a virus closely related to HSV. This causes an ascending encephalomyelitis occurring in veterinarians, laboratory workers and other individuals having close contact with Old World monkeys or monkey-cell cultures. After an incubation period of 3 days to 3 weeks, there is an acute febrile onset, with headache, often local vesicular lesions, lymphocytic pleocytosis and variable neurologic patterns, usually ending in death in over 70% of cases, 1 day to 3 weeks after onset of symptoms. The occasional recoveries have been associated with considerable residual disability, but a few recent cases, treated with acyclovir, have recovered completely.

The virus causes a natural infection of monkeys analogous to HSV infection in man. Human disease is acquired by the bite of apparently normal monkeys, or by exposure of naked skin or mucous membrane to infected saliva or monkey-tissue cultures. Prevention depends on proper use of protective gauntlets and care to minimize exposure to monkeys.

All bite or scratch wounds incurred from macaques or from cages that might be contaminated with macaque secretions and result in bleeding should be immediately and thoroughly scrubbed and cleansed with soap and water. Prophylactic treatment with an antiviral agent such as acyclovir may be considered when an animal handler sustains a deep, penetrating wound that cannot be adequately cleansed; the B-virus status of the monkey should be determined. The appearance of any skin lesions or neurologic symptoms, such as itching, pain, or numbness, near the site of the wound calls for expert medical consultation for diagnosis and possible treatment.

HISTOPLASMOSIS   ICD-9 115

Two clinically different mycoses have been designated as histoplasmosis because the pathogens that cause them cannot be distinguished morphologically when growing on culture media as molds. Detailed information will be given for the infection caused by *Histoplasma capsulatum* var. *capsulatum,* followed by a brief resumé of histoplasmosis caused by *H. capsulatum* var. *duboisii.*

INFECTION BY *HISTOPLASMA*   ICD-9 115.0
CAPSULATUM
(Histoplasmosis capsulati, Histoplasmosis due to *H. capsulatum* var. *capsulatum,* American histoplasmosis, Classical histoplasmosis)

1. **Identification**—A systemic mycosis of varying severity, with the primary lesion usually in the lungs. While infection is common, overt clinical disease is not. Five clinical forms are recognized:

(1) asymptomatic with only hypersensitivity to histoplasmin;

(2) acute benign respiratory, which varies from a mild respiratory illness to temporary incapacity with general malaise, weakness, fever, chest pains, and dry or productive cough, occasional erythema multiforme and erythema nodosum, and sometimes multiple, small scattered calcifications in the lung, hilar lymph nodes and spleen;

(3) acute disseminated with hepatosplenomegaly, accompanied by septic-type fever, prostration, and a rapid course often resembling miliary tuberculosis, most frequent in infants and young children and patients with AIDS and, without therapy, usually fatal;

(4) chronic disseminated with variable symptoms, such as unexplained fever, anemia, patchy pneumonia, hepatitis, endocarditis, meningitis, mucosal ulcers of mouth, larynx, stomach or bowel, adrenal infection

common but usually asymptomatic (more common in the adult male and may follow cytotoxic or corticosteroid therapy), a subacute course with progression over weeks up to a few years and usually fatal unless treated; and

(5) chronic pulmonary, which clinically and radiologically resembles chronic pulmonary tuberculosis, is more common in males over 40 years old and progresses over months or years, with periods of quiescence and sometimes spontaneous cure.

Clinical diagnosis is confirmed by culture or by visualizing the fungus in Giemsa- or Wright-stained smears of ulcer exudates, bone marrow, sputum or blood; special stains are necessary to demonstrate the fungus in biopsies of ulcers, liver, lymph nodes, or lung. The histoplasmin skin test is helpful in epidemiologic studies but not in diagnosis. Among the available serologic tests, the immunodiffusion test is the most specific and reliable. A rise in CF titers in paired sera may be encountered early in acute infection and is suggestive evidence of active disease; however, recent positive skin tests with histoplasmin can raise the titer against the mycelial form, and the serologic tests can cross-react with other mycoses. False-negative tests are common enough that negative serologic tests do not exclude the diagnosis.

2. **Infectious agent**—*Histoplasma capsulatum* var. *capsulatum (Ajellomyces capsulatus)*, a dimorphic fungus growing as a mold in soil and as a yeast in animal and human hosts.

3. **Occurrence**—Focal infections are common over wide areas of the Americas, Africa, eastern Asia and Australia; rare in Europe. Clinical disease is far less frequent, and severe progressive disease is rare. Histoplasmin hypersensitivity indicating antecedent infection, sometimes in as much as 80% of a population, is prevalent in parts of eastern and central USA. Prevalence increases from childhood to 30 years of age; differences by sex are usually not observed except that the chronic pulmonary form is more common in males. Outbreaks have occurred in families and in groups of workmen with common exposure to bird or bat droppings or recently disturbed contaminated soil. Histoplasmosis also occurs in dogs, cats, cattle, horses, rats, skunks, opossums, foxes and other animals, often with a clinical picture comparable to the disease in man.

4. **Reservoir**—Soil around old chicken houses, in caves harboring bats, and around starling and blackbird roosts; also around houses sheltering the common brown bat, in other soils with high organic content, and in decaying trees.

5. **Mode of transmission**—Growth of the organisms in soil produces spore forms known as conidia; infection results from inhalation of airborne conidia. Person-to-person transmission can occur only if infected tissue is inoculated into a healthy person.

6. **Incubation period**—Symptoms appear within 5-18 days after exposure, commonly 10 days.

7. **Period of communicability**—Not transmitted from person to person.

8. **Susceptibility and resistance**—Susceptibility is general. Inapparent infections are extremely common in endemic areas and usually result in increased resistance to infection.

9. **Methods of control**—

A. *Preventive measures:* Minimize exposure to dust in a contaminated environment, such as chicken coops and their surrounding soil. Spray with water or oil to reduce dust; use protective masks. Infectious foci can be decontaminated with 3% formalin.

B. *Control of patient, contacts and the immediate environment:*

1) Report to local health authority: In selected endemic areas (USA); in many countries not a reportable disease, Class 3B (see Preface).
2) Isolation: None.
3) Concurrent disinfection: Of sputum and articles soiled therewith. Terminal cleaning.
4) Quarantine: None.
5) Immunization of contacts: None.
6) Investigation of contacts and source of infection: Household and occupational contacts for evidence of infection from a common environmental source.
7) Specific treatment: Oral ketoconazole is the drug of choice for patients with chronic fibrocavity pulmonary histoplasmosis and immunocompetent patients with indolent disseminated histoplasmosis outside the CNS. For other patients with disseminated histoplasmosis, amphotericin B (Fungizone®) IV is the drug of choice.

C. *Epidemic measures:* Occurrence of grouped cases of acute pulmonary disease in or outside of an endemic area, particularly with history of exposure to dust within a closed space as within caves or construction sites, should arouse suspicion of histoplasmosis. Suspected sites such as chicken houses, barns, silos, caves, starling and blackbird roosts, attics and basements should be investigated.

D. *Disaster implications:* None. Possible hazard if large groups, especially from nonendemic areas, are forced to move through or live in areas where the mold is prevalent.

E. *International measures:* None.

HISTOPLASMOSIS DUBOISII ICD-9 115.1
(Histoplasmosis due to *H. capsulatum* var. *duboisii*, African histoplasmosis)

This usually presents as a subacute granuloma of the skin or bone. Infection, though usually localized, may be disseminated in the skin, subcutaneous tissue, lymph nodes, bones and joints, lungs and abdominal viscera. Disease is more common in males and may occur at any age, but especially in the second decade of life. Thus far, the disease has been recognized only in Africa and Madagascar. Diagnosis is made by culture and by demonstrating the yeast cells of *H. capsulatum* var. *duboisii* in tissue by smear or biopsy. These cells are much larger than the yeast cells of *H. capsulatum* var. *capsulatum*. The true prevalence of histoplasmosis duboisii, its reservoir, mode of transmission, and incubation period are unknown. It is not communicable from person to person. Amphotericin B (Fungizone®) is an effective therapeutic agent.

HOOKWORM DISEASE ICD-9 126
(Ancylostomiasis, Uncinariasis, Necatoriasis)

1. **Identification**—A common chronic parasitic infection with a variety of symptoms, usually in proportion to the degree of anemia. In heavy infections, the bloodletting activity of the nematode leads to iron deficiency and hypochromic, microcytic anemia, the major cause of disability. Children with heavy, long-term infection may have hypoproteinemia and may be retarded in mental and physical development. Occasionally, severe acute pulmonary and GI reactions follow the exposure to infective larvae. Death is infrequent and usually can be attributed to other infections. Light hookworm infections generally produce few or no clinical effects.

Infection is confirmed by finding hookworm eggs in feces; stool examination may be negative early in the course of the infection until the worms mature. Species differentiation requires microscopic examination of larvae cultured from the feces, or examination of adult worms expelled by purgation following a vermifuge.

2. **Infectious agents**—*Necator americanus, Ancylostoma duodenale* and *A. ceylanicum*.

3. **Occurrence**—Widely endemic in tropical and subtropical countries where sanitary disposal of human feces is not practiced, and the soil, moisture and temperature conditions favor development of infective larvae. May also occur in temperate climates under similar environmental

conditions (e.g., in mines). Both *Necator* and *Ancylostoma* occur in many parts of Asia (particularly in SE Asia), the S Pacific and East Africa. *N. americanus* is the prevailing species throughout SE Asia, most of tropical Africa and America; *A. duodenale* prevails in north Africa, including the Nile Valley, in northern India, northern parts of the Far East and in the Andean areas of S America. *A. ceylanicum* occurs in SE Asia, but is less common than either *N. americanus* or *A. duodenale.*

4. **Reservoir**—Man for *N. americanus* and *A. duodenale;* cats and dogs for *A. ceylanicum.*

5. **Mode of transmission**—Eggs in feces are deposited on the ground and hatch; under favorable conditions of moisture, temperature and soil type, larvae develop to the third stage, becoming infective in 7 to 10 days. Infection of man occurs when the infective larvae penetrate the skin, usually of the foot; in so doing, they produce a characteristic dermatitis (ground itch). The larvae normally enter the skin and pass via lymphatics and bloodstream to the lungs, enter the alveoli, migrate up the trachea to the pharynx, are swallowed, and reach the small intestine where they attach to the intestinal wall, develop to maturity and typically produce eggs in 6 to 7 weeks (3-4 weeks in the case of *A. ceylanicum*). Infection with *Ancylostoma* may also be acquired by ingesting infective larvae.

6. **Incubation period**—Symptoms may develop after a few weeks to many months, depending on intensity of infection and iron intake of the host. Pulmonary infiltration, cough and tracheitis may occur during the lung migration phase of infection, particularly in *Necator* infections. *A. duodenale* may become dormant after entering the body for about 8 months, after which development resumes, with a patent (stools containing eggs) infection a month later.

7. **Period of communicability**—Not transmitted from person to person, but infected persons can contaminate soil for several years in the absence of treatment. Under favorable conditions, larvae remain infective in soil for several weeks.

8. **Susceptibility and resistance**—Universal; some immunity is thought to develop with infection.

9. **Methods of control**—

   A. *Preventive measures:*

   1) Educate the public to the dangers of soil contamination by human, cat or dog feces, and in preventive measures, including wearing shoes in endemic areas.

   2) Prevent soil contamination by installation of sanitary disposal systems for human feces, especially sanitary privies in rural areas. Nightsoil and sewage effluents are hazardous, especially where they are used as fertilizer.

3) Examine and treat people migrating from endemic to receptive nonendemic areas, especially those who work barefooted in mines, constructing dams or in the horticultural sector.

B. *Control of patient, contacts and the immediate environment:*

1) Report to local health authority: Official report not ordinarily justifiable, Class 5 (see Preface).
2) Isolation: None.
3) Concurrent disinfection: Sanitary disposal of feces to prevent contamination of soil.
4) Quarantine: None.
5) Immunization of contacts: None.
6) Investigation of contacts and source of infection: Each infected contact and carrier is a potential or actual indirect spreader of infection.
7) Specific treatment: Mebendazole (Vermox®), albendazole (Zentel®), or pyrantel pamoate (Antiminth®); adverse reactions are infrequent. Bephenium hydroxynaphthoate (Alcopar®) and tetrachloroethylene are effective alternatives. Follow-up stool examination is indicated after 2 weeks, and therapy should be repeated if a heavy worm burden persists. Iron supplementation will correct the anemia without worm eradication. Transfusion may be necessary for severe anemia.

C. *Epidemic measures:* Survey for prevalence in highly endemic areas and provide periodic mass treatment; health education in sanitation of the environment and personal hygiene, and provide facilities for excreta disposal.

D. *Disaster implications:* None.

E. *International measures:* None.

HYMENOLEPIASIS
HYMENOLEPIASIS DUE TO
HYMENOLEPIS NANA
(Dwarf tapeworm infection)

ICD-9 123.6

1. **Identification**—An intestinal infection with tapeworms that are so small that they are often not detected in the feces; light infections are usually asymptomatic. Massive numbers of the worms may cause enteritis

with or without diarrhea, abdominal pain, and other vague symptoms such as pallor, loss of weight, and weakness.

Diagnosis is made by microscopic identification of eggs in feces.

2. **Infectious agent**—*Hymenolepis nana* (dwarf tapeworm), the only human tapeworm without an obligatory intermediate host.

3. **Occurrence**—Cosmopolitan, more common in warm than cold, and in dry than wet, climates. Dwarf tapeworm is the most common human tapeworm in southern USA, and Latin America; it is common in Australia, Mediterranean countries, the Near East and India.

4. **Reservoir**—Man; possibly mice.

5. **Mode of transmission**—Eggs of *H. nana* are infective when passed in the feces. Infection is acquired through ingestion of eggs in contaminated food or water; directly from fecally contaminated fingers (i.e., person-to-person transmission); or by ingestion of insects bearing larvae that have developed from eggs ingested by the insect. When *H. nana* eggs are ingested, they hatch in the intestine, liberating an oncosphere that enters a mucosal villus and develops into a cysticercoid; this ruptures into the lumen and produces the adult tapeworm. Some *H. nana* eggs are immediately infective when released from the proglottids in the human gut, so autoinfections can occur. If *H. nana* eggs are ingested by meal worms, larval fleas or other insects, they may hatch in the insect's intestine liberating an oncosphere that penetrates into the insect's body cavity; this develops into a cysticercoid that is infective to man as well as to rodents when ingested.

6. **Incubation period**—Onset of symptoms is variable; the development of mature worms requires about 2 weeks.

7. **Period of communicability**—As long as eggs are passed in the feces. *H. nana* infections may persist for several years.

8. **Susceptibility and resistance**—Universal; children are more susceptible than adults; infection produces resistance to reinfection. Intensive infection occurs in immunodeficient and malnourished children.

9. **Methods of control**—

    A. Preventive measures:

        1) Educate the public in personal hygiene and sanitary disposal of feces.

        2) Provide and maintain clean toilet facilities.

        3) Protect food and water from contamination with human and rodent feces.

        4) Treat to remove sources of infection.

        5) Eliminate rodents from the home environment.

B. *Control of patient, contacts and the immediate environment:*

1) Report to local health authority: Official report not ordinarily justifiable, Class 5 (see Preface).
2) Isolation: None.
3) Concurrent disinfection: Sanitary disposal of feces.
4) Quarantine: None.
5) Immunization of contacts: Not applicable.
6) Investigation of contacts and source of infection: Fecal examination of family or institution members.
7) Specific treatment: Praziquantel (Biltricide®) or niclosamide (Yomesan®, Niclocide®) is effective.

C. *Epidemic measures:* Outbreaks in schools and institutions can be controlled best by treatment of infected individuals and by special attention to personal and group hygiene.

D. *Disaster implications:* None.

E. *International measures:* None.

HYMENOLEPIASIS DUE TO HYMENOLEPIS DIMINUTA
ICD-9 123.6

(Rat tapeworm infection, Hymenolepiasis diminuta)

Rat tapeworm, caused by *H. diminuta,* occurs accidentally in man, most usually in young children. The eggs passed in rodent feces are ingested by insects such as flea larvae, grain beetles and cockroaches where cysticercoids develop in the hemocele. The mature tapeworm develops in rats, mice or other rodents when the insect is ingested. People are rare accidental hosts, usually of a single or few tapeworms; rarely symptomatic. Definitive diagnosis is based on the characteristic egg in the feces; treatment as for *H. nana.*

DIPYLIDIASIS
ICD-9 123.8

(Dog tapeworm infection)

Toddler-age children are occasionally infected with dog tapeworm *(Dipylidium caninum),* the adult of which is found worldwide in dogs and cats. It rarely if ever produces symptoms in the child but is distressful to the parent who sees motile, seed-like proglottids (tapeworm segments) at the anus or on the surface of the stool. Infection is acquired when the child ingests fleas which, in their larval stage, have eaten eggs from proglottids that have migrated from the anus of the animal or have been passed in the feces. In 3-4 weeks the tapeworm becomes mature. Infection is prevented by keeping dogs and cats free of fleas and worms; niclosamide or praziquantel is effective for treatment.

INFLUENZA ICD-9 487

1. **Identification**—An acute viral disease of the respiratory tract characterized by fever, headache, myalgia, prostration, coryza, sore throat and cough. Cough is often severe and protracted, but other symptoms are usually self-limited with recovery in 2-7 days. Recognition is commonly by epidemiologic characteristics; sporadic cases can be identified only by laboratory procedures. Influenza in children may be indistinguishable from disease caused by other respiratory viruses. The common cold, croup, viral pneumonia, and undifferentiated acute respiratory disease may be caused by influenza virus. Gastrointestinal tract manifestations (nausea, vomiting, diarrhea) may occur, particularly in children, and have been reported in up to 25% of children in school outbreaks of influenza B and A (H1N1).

Influenza derives its importance from the rapidity with which epidemics evolve, the widespread morbidity, and the seriousness of complications, notably viral and bacterial pneumonias. During major epidemics, severe disease and deaths occur primarily among the elderly and those debilitated by chronic cardiac, pulmonary, renal or metabolic disease, anemia or immunosuppression. Most epidemics are associated with a general mortality rate much in excess of nonepidemic expectancy. Current case fatality rates generally are low, and deaths occur mostly among elderly persons. However, in the 1918 epidemic, the highest case fatality rates were among young adults. Reye syndrome, involving the CNS and liver, is a rare complication in children who have ingested salicylates; it occurs mainly in children with influenza B disease and less frequently with influenza A.

During the early febrile stage of disease, laboratory confirmation is made by isolation of influenza viruses from pharyngeal or nasal secretions or washings in cell culture or embryonated eggs, and/or by direct identification of viral antigens in nasopharyngeal cells by FA test or ELISA. Infection may also be confirmed by demonstration of a specific serologic response in acute and convalescent sera.

2. **Infectious agent**—Three types of influenza virus are recognized: A, B and C. Type A includes three subtypes (H1N1, H2N2 and H3N2) that have been associated with recent widespread epidemics and pandemics; type B has been associated with regional or widespread epidemics; type C has been associated with sporadic cases and minor localized outbreaks. Virus type is determined by the antigenic properties of the antigenically stable nucleoprotein. Influenza A subtypes are classified by the antigenic uniqueness of the surface glycoproteins, with the hemag-

glutinin designated as H and the neuraminidase as N. Frequent mutations of the genes encoding the surface glycoproteins of the influenza A subtypes and influenza B result in emergence of variants that are described by the geographic site of isolation, the culture number and the year of isolation. Examples of prototype strains with these designations include A/Japan/ 305/57 (H2N2), A/Hong Kong/1/68 (H3N2), A/USSR/ 90/77 (H1N1) and B/USSR/2/87. Emergence of completely new subtypes (antigenic shift) occurs at irregular intervals and only with type A viruses; they are responsible for pandemics. Minor antigenic changes (antigenic drift) are responsible for the annual epidemics and regional outbreaks.

3. **Occurrence**—In pandemics, epidemics (localized and widespread), and as sporadic cases. During the past 100+ years, pandemics began in 1889, 1918, 1957 and 1968. Clinical attack rates during epidemics range from 10% to 30% in the general community, to >50% in closed populations such as boarding schools or nursing homes. Epidemics of influenza occur in the USA almost every year: Type A viruses cause most epidemics, while those caused by influenza B occur every 2-3 years; mixed A and B epidemics also occur. In temperate zones, epidemics tend to occur in winter; in the tropics, they often occur in the rainy season, but outbreaks or sporadic cases may occur in any month.

Influenza viral infections with different antigenic types also occur naturally in swine, horses, mink and seals, and in many domestic and wild avian species in many parts of the world. Transmission from animals to man has been demonstrated only on very rare occasions.

4. **Reservoir**—Man for human infections, although animal reservoirs are suspected as sources of new human subtypes, perhaps by reassortment with human strains.

5. **Mode of transmission**—Airborne spread among crowded populations in enclosed spaces predominates; transmission also occurs by direct contact through droplet spread. Transmission by direct contact may be important since the influenza virus persists for hours in dried mucus.

6. **Incubation period**—Short, usually 1-5 days.

7. **Period of communicability**—Probably 3-5 days from clinical onset in adults; up to 7 days in young children.

8. **Susceptibility and resistance**—When a new subtype appears, all are susceptible except those who have lived through earlier epidemics caused by a related subtype. Infection produces immunity to the specific infecting virus, but the duration and breadth of immunity depend on the degree of antigenic drift and the number of previous infections. Vaccines produce serologic responses specific for the included viruses and elicit booster responses to related strains with which the individual has had prior experience.

Age-specific attack rates during an epidemic reflect existing immunity from past experience with strains related to the epidemic subtype and the amount of exposure, so that incidence of infection is often highest in school-age children. Thus, with the H1N1 influenza epidemics occurring after 1977, the incidence of disease has been greatest among those born after 1957; most persons born before this time had partial immunity from infection with antigenically related H1N1 viruses that circulated between 1918 and 1957.

9. Methods of control—

   A. *Preventive measures:*

   1) Educate the public and health care personnel in basic personal hygiene, especially the danger of unprotected coughs and sneezes, and hand-to-mucous membrane transmission.

   2) Active immunization with available killed virus vaccines may give 70%-80% protection against infection in healthy young adults when the vaccine antigen closely matches the prevailing wild strain of virus; however, in the elderly, vaccination may not necessarily prevent infection but may reduce complications and severity of disease. A single dose suffices for those with prior exposure to influenza A and B viruses (i.e., persons ≥12 years old); two doses of vaccine are required for younger persons who have no previous vaccination history. Routine immunization programs should be directed primarily at persons at the greatest risk of serious complication or death (see section 1, above), and those who might spread infection to them (health care personnel and household contacts of high-risk persons). Immunization is also recommended for those on long-term aspirin therapy to prevent the development of Reye syndrome.

   Immunization should also be considered for those engaged in essential community services and is recommended for military personnel. However, any individual may benefit from immunization. Immunization should be accomplished each year before influenza is expected in the community. For those living or traveling outside the USA, timing of immunization should be based on the different seasonal patterns of influenza (e.g., in the Southern Hemisphere and tropics). Yearly recommendations for vaccine components are based on the viral strains currently circulating, as determined by international surveillance.

   Contraindications: Allergic hypersensitivity to eggs is a

contraindication; the individual can be skin-tested using the influenza vaccine as antigen. (During the swine influenza vaccine program in 1976, an increased risk of developing Guillain-Barré syndrome (GBS) within 6 weeks following receipt of the vaccine was reported in the USA. Surveillance since then has shown no such association with subsequent influenza vaccinations.)

3) Amantadine hydrochloride or rimantadine (100 mg/day for those ≥20 kg; and 4.4 mg/kg/day in 2 divided doses in those <20 kg) is effective in the chemoprophylaxis of influenza A, but not type B. Amantadine is associated with CNS side effects in 5-10% of recipients; these may be more severe in the elderly or those with impaired kidney function. For this reason, persons with underlying renal disease should have reductions in dosage reflecting the degree of renal impairment. Rimantadine (which is not yet licensed in the USA) has fewer CNS side effects. The use of these drugs should be considered in unimmunized persons or groups at high risk of complications, when an appropriate vaccine is not available, or as a supplement to vaccine when maximal protection is desired.

B. *Control of patient, contacts and the immediate environment:*

1) Report to local health authority: Reporting outbreaks or laboratory-confirmed cases assists disease surveillance. Report identity of the infectious agent as determined by laboratory examination if possible, Class 1A (see Preface).

2) Isolation: Impractical under most circumstances because of the delay in diagnosis, unless rapid direct viral tests are available. In epidemics, due to increased patient load, it would be desirable to isolate patients (especially infants and young children) believed to have influenza, by placing them in the same room (cohorting) during the initial 5 to 7 days of illness.

3) Concurrent disinfection: None.

4) Quarantine: None.

5) Protection of contacts: A specific role has been shown for antiviral chemoprophylaxis with amantadine or rimantadine against type A strains (see 9A3, above).

6) Investigation of contacts and source of infection: Of no practical value.

7) Specific treatment: Amantadine or rimantadine given early in the course of influenza A reduces symptoms and virus titers in respiratory secretions. Dosages are 4.4

mg/kg/day in 2 divided doses for those 1-9 years of age, and 200 mg/day in 2 doses for those >9 years (if weight is less than 45 kg, use 4.4 mg/kg/day in 2 doses) for 2 to 5 days. Doses should be reduced for persons ≥65 years of age and those with decreased renal function.

Drug-resistant mutants may emerge late in the illness and may be transmitted to others; therefore, cohorting persons on therapy should be considered, especially in closed populations with many high-risk individuals. Patients should be watched for development of bacterial complications and only then should antibiotics be administered. Because of the association with Reye syndrome, salicylates should be avoided.

C. *Epidemic measures:*

1) The severe and often disrupting effects of epidemic influenza on community activities may be reduced in part by effective health planning and education, particularly locally organized vaccination programs for high-risk patients and their care providers. Surveillance by health authorities of the extent and progress of outbreaks and the reporting of findings to the community are important.

2) Closing of individual schools has not proven to be an effective control measure; it has generally been done too late and only because of high absenteeism of students and staff.

3) Hospital administrators should anticipate the increased demand for medical care during epidemic periods; there may also be excessive absenteeism of health care personnel as a result of influenza. To prevent this, health care personnel should be immunized annually or use amantadine or rimantadine during influenza A epidemics.

D. *Disaster implications:* Aggregations of people in emergency shelters will favor outbreaks of disease if the virus is introduced.

E. *International measures:* A Disease under Surveillance by WHO. The following are recommended:

1) Report epidemics within a country to WHO.

2) Identify the causative virus in reports, and submit prototype strains to one of the two WHO Centres for Reference and Research on Influenza (Atlanta and London). Throat secretion specimens, nasopharyngeal aspirates and paired blood samples may be sent to any WHO-recognized national influenza center.

3) Epidemiologic studies and prompt identification of viruses by national health agencies.
4) Efforts to ensure enough commercial and/or governmental facilities to provide rapid production of sufficient quantities of vaccine, and programs for vaccine administration to high-risk persons and essential personnel.
5) Maintain adequate supplies of amantadine or rimantadine for use by selected high-risk people and essential personnel, in the event of a new pandemic strain for which no suitable vaccine is available.

KAWASAKI SYNDROME   ICD-9 446.1
(Kawasaki disease, Mucocutaneous lymph node syndrome, Acute febrile mucocutaneous lymph node syndrome)

1. **Identification**—An acute febrile syndrome of early childhood, presumably of infectious or toxic origin, characterized clinically by a high, spiking fever unresponsive to antibiotics (usually of more than five days duration) associated with pronounced irritability and mood change, nonsuppurative cervical adenopathy, bilateral conjunctival injection, and an enanthem consisting of a "strawberry tongue," injected oropharynx or dry fissured or erythematous lips; limb changes consisting of edema, erythema, or periungual or generalized desquamation; and a polymorphous erythematous exanthem which is usually truncal. Typically there are three phases: (1) an acute febrile phase of about 10 days characterized by high, spiking fever, rash, adenopathy, peripheral erythema or edema, conjunctivitis, and enanthem; (2) a subacute phase lasting about two weeks characterized by thrombocytosis, desquamation, and resolution of fever; and (3) a lengthy convalescent phase during which clinical signs fade.

In the later phases of the disease, coronary artery aneurysms due to coronary arteritis occur in 10-20% of patients; the case fatality rate is between 0.3-1.0% with the majority of deaths occuring between the third and sixth weeks of illness. Complications can involve any organ of the body. Long-term prognosis is unknown.

There is no pathognomonic laboratory test for Kawasaki syndrome; diagnosis is based on the presence of fever lasting more than five days, exclusion of other causes, and at least four of the following: (1) bilateral conjunctival injection; (2) injected or fissured lips, or injected pharynx, or "strawberry tongue"; (3) erythema of palms or soles, or edema of the hands or feet, or generalized or periungual desquamation; (4) rash; and/or (5) cervical lymphadenopathy (at least 1 node ≥1.5 cm). The ESR is elevated during the acute phase; the platelet count rises above $500 \times 10^3/$ cu mm during the second and third weeks of the illness and remains elevated for approximately three weeks.

2. **Infectious agent**—Unknown. Antecedent viral respiratory illnesses, infection with a new retrovirus, exposure to mites or freshly shampooed rugs, and association with specific bacterial species have been suggested as causal or possible predisposing risk factors but none has yet been firmly implicated.

3. **Occurrence**—Worldwide, although most cases (>80,000) have been reported in Japan. Most cases are diagnosed in children less than 5 years old, especially those less than 2 years old; more in boys than in girls. In the USA, attack rates are highest in children of Asian ancestry and in black children; cases are more frequent in the winter and spring. Outbreaks have been reported in New York City as well as upstate New York, Los Angeles, Denver, Memphis, Washington DC; and in Hawaii, Illinois, Massachusetts, Maryland, Michigan, Washington and Wisconsin.

4. **Reservoir**—Unknown.

5. **Mode of transmission**—Unknown; no firm evidence of person-to-person transmission. Outbreak occurrence in communities is consistent with infectious etiology.

6. **Incubation period**—Unknown.

7. **Period of communicability**—Unknown.

8. **Susceptibility and resistance**—Children under 5 years, especially those of Asian ancestry, are most likely to develop Kawasaki syndrome. Recurrences are very infrequently reported.

9. **Methods of control**—

   A. *Preventive measures:* Unknown.

   B. *Control of patient, contacts and the immediate environment:*

   1) Report to local health authority: Voluntary in the USA. Clusters and epidemics should be reported immediately, Class 5 (see Preface).
   2) Isolation: None.
   3) Concurrent disinfection: None.
   4) Quarantine: None.
   5) Immunization of contacts: Not applicable.
   6) Investigation of contacts: Not profitable.
   7) Specific treatment: High-dose IG administered intravenously within 10 days of onset of fever may reduce the fever, inflammatory signs and aneurysm formation. High-

dose aspirin is recommended during the acute phase, followed by low doses for several weeks.

C. *Epidemic measures:* Outbreaks and clusters should be investigated to elucidate etiology and risk factors.

D. *Disaster implications:* None.

E. *International measures:* None.

KERATOCONJUNCTIVITIS, ADENOVIRAL
ICD-9 077.1

(Epidemic keratoconjunctivitis [EKC], Shipyard conjunotivitis, Shipyard eye, Infectious punctate keratitis)

1. **Identification**—An acute viral disease of the eye, with unilateral or bilateral inflammation of conjunctivae and edema of the lids and periorbital tissue. Onset is sudden, with pain, photophobia, blurred vision, and occasionally low-grade fever, headache, malaise and tender preauricular lymphadenopathy. Approximately 7 days after onset in about half the cases, the cornea exhibits several small round subepithelial infiltrates, which may eventually form punctate erosions that stain with fluorescein. Duration of acute conjunctivitis is about 2 weeks although the keratitis may continue to evolve, leaving discrete subepithelial opacities which may interfere with vision for a few weeks. In severe cases, conjunctival membranes develop which may be followed by conjunctival scarring.

Diagnosis is confirmed by recovery of virus from appropriate cell cultures inoculated with eye swabs or conjunctival scrapings, and by titer rises in serum neutralization or HAI tests. Virus may be visualized by FA staining of scrapings or by IEM.

2. **Infectious agent**—The "classic" cause is adenovirus type 8; types 3, 7, 19 and 37, and rarely other adenovirus types (e.g., 4, 10, 11 and 14) are involved.

3. **Occurrence**—Presumably worldwide. Both sporadic cases and large outbreaks have occurred in Asia, Hawaii, N America and Europe.

4. **Reservoir**—Man.

5. **Mode of transmission**—Direct contact with eye secretions of an infected person and, indirectly, through contaminated instruments or solutions. In industrial plants, epidemics are centered in first-aid stations and dispensaries where treatment is frequently administered for minor trauma to the eye; transmission then occurs through fingers, instruments

and other contaminated items. Similar outbreaks have originated in eye clinics and medical offices. When dispensary and clinic personnel acquire the disease, they may act as sources of infection. Family spread is common, with children typically introducing the infection.

6. Incubation period—Probably 5-12 days.

7. Period of communicability—From late in the incubation period to 14 days after onset. Prolonged viral shedding has been reported.

8. Susceptibility and resistance—There is usually complete immunity after adenovirus 8 infection. Similar conjunctivitis with minor keratitis may occur with other adenoviruses. Trauma, even minor, and eye manipulation increase the risk of infection.

9. Methods of control—

A. *Preventive measures:*

    1) Avoid communal eye droppers, medicines, eye make-up, instruments, towels, etc.

    2) In ophthalmologic procedures in dispensaries, clinics and offices, asepsis should include vigorous handwashing before examining each patient and systematic sterilization of instruments after use. Medical personnel with overt conjunctivitis should be kept out of contact with patients.

    3) With persistent outbreaks, patients with EKC should be seen in physically separated facilities.

    4) Educate patients about personal cleanliness and the danger of using common towels and toilet articles.

    5) Use safety measures such as goggles in industrial plants.

B. *Control of patient, contacts and the immediate environment:*

    1) Report to local health authority: Obligatory report of epidemics; no individual case report, Class 4 (see Preface).

    2) Isolation: Drainage/secretion precautions; patients should use separate towels and linen during the acute stage. Infected medical personnel should not come in contact with patients.

    3) Concurrent disinfection: Of conjunctival and nasal discharges and articles soiled therewith. Terminal cleaning.

    4) Quarantine: None.

    5) Immunization of contacts: None.

    6) Investigation of contacts and source of infection: In outbreaks, the source of infection should be identified and precautions taken to prevent further transmission.

7) Specific treatment: None during the acute phase. If the residual opacities interfere with the patient's ability to work, topical corticosteroids may be tried.

C. **Epidemic measures:**

1) Educate medical personnel to wash hands and sterilize instruments carefully before and after eye examinations.
2) Organize convenient facilities for prompt diagnosis.

D. **Disaster implications:** None.

E. **International measures:** WHO Collaborating Centres (see Preface).

LASSA FEVER   ICD-9 078.89

1. **Identification**—An acute viral illness of 1-4 weeks duration. Onset is gradual with malaise, fever, headache, sore throat, cough, nausea, vomiting, diarrhea, myalgia, chest and abdominal pain; fever is persistent or intermittent-spiking. Inflammation and exudation of the pharynx and conjunctivitis are commonly observed. In severe cases, hypotension or shock, pleural effusion, hemorrhage, seizures, encephalopathy and edema of the face and neck are frequent. Albuminuria and hemoconcentration are common. Early lymphopenia may be followed by late neutrophilia. Platelet counts are only moderately depressed but platelet function is severely reduced or absent. Disease is more severe in pregnancy, and fetal loss occurs in over 80%. Transient alopecia and ataxia may occur in convalescence, and deafness occurs in 25% of patients with only half recovering some function after 1-3 months. Case fatality rate is about 15% among hospitalized cases; SGOT levels >150 and high viremia indicate poor prognosis. Inapparent infections, diagnosed serologically, are common in endemic areas.

Diagnosis is made by isolation of virus from blood, urine or throat washings, and serologically by ELISA or IFA; half of the patients have specific IgM at the time of admission. Laboratory specimens may be biohazardous and must be handled with extreme care, including BSL4 containment if available.

2. **Infectious agent**—Lassa virus, an arenavirus, serologically related to lymphocytic choriomeningitis, Machupo and Junin viruses.

3. **Occurrence**—Widely distributed over West Africa. Serologically related viruses of lesser virulence for laboratory hosts, from Central African Republic, Mozambique and Zimbabwe, have not yet been associated with human infection or disease.

4. **Reservoir**—Wild rodents; in West Africa, the multimammate mouse, *Mastomys natalensis.*

5. **Mode of transmission**—Primarily through direct or indirect contact with excreta of infected rodents deposited on surfaces such as floors, beds or in food. Person-to-person and laboratory infections occur, especially in the hospital environment, by direct contact with blood (including inoculation with contaminated needles), pharyngeal secretions, and urine of a patient, or by sexual contact. Transmission by droplet exposure has not been clearly demonstrated.

6. **Incubation period**—Commonly 6 to 21 days.

7. **Period of communicability**—Person-to-person spread may occur during the acute febrile phase when virus is present in the throat. Virus may be excreted in urine of patients for 3-9 weeks from onset of illness.

8. **Susceptibility and resistance**—All ages are susceptible; the duration of immunity following infection is unknown.

9. **Methods of control**—

    A. Preventive measures: Specific rodent control.

    B. Control of patient, contacts and the immediate environment:

        1) Report to local health authority: Individual cases should be reported, Class 2A (see Preface).

        2) Isolation: Institute immediate strict barrier isolation in a hospital room away from traffic patterns. Because of the low incidence of nosocomial infections reported from African hospitals, transfer to special isolation units is not considered necessary; however, nosocomial transmission has occurred, and strict procedures for isolation of body fluids and excreta should be maintained.

        3) Concurrent disinfection: Patients' excreta, sputum, blood and all objects with which the patients have had contact, including laboratory equipment used to carry out tests on blood, etc., should be disinfected with 0.5% sodium hypochlorite solution or 0.5% phenol with detergent, and, as far as possible, appropriate heating methods, such as autoclaving, incineration and boiling. Laboratory tests should be carried out in special high-containment facilities; if there is no such facility, tests should be kept to a minimum and specimens handled by experienced technicians using all available precautions such as gloves, hoods, etc. When appropriate, serum may be heat inactivated at 60°C for 30 minutes. In the USA, a portable containment laboratory, together with a qualified laboratory technician, can be obtained from CDC, Atlanta, GA (see

Preface). Thorough terminal disinfection with 0.5% sodium hypochlorite solution or a phenolic compound is adequate; formaldehyde fumigation can be considered.

4) Quarantine: Only surveillance is recommended for close contacts (see 9B6, below).

5) Immunization of contacts: None.

6) Investigation of contacts and source of infection: Identify all close contacts (persons living with, caring for, testing laboratory specimens from, or having non-casual contact with the patient in the 3 weeks preceding the onset of illness). Establish close surveillance of contacts with level of contact as follows: body temperature checks at least 2 times daily for at least 3 weeks after last exposure. In case of temperature >38.3°C (101°F), hospitalize immediately in strict isolation facilities. Determine place of residence of patient during 3 weeks prior to onset, and search for unreported or undiagnosed cases.

In case of a definite exposure, such as a needle stick or similar high-risk incident, oral ribavirin should be administered at a dose of 2 g/day for 10 days.

7) Specific treatment: Ribavirin (Virazole®), most effective within the first six days of illness, should be given intravenously, 30mg/kg initially, followed by 15 mg/kg every 6 hours for 4 days, and 8 mg/kg every 8 hours for 6 additional days.

C. **Epidemic measures:** Not determined.

D. **Disaster implications:** None.

E. **International measures:** Notification of source country and to receiving countries of possible exposures by infected travelers.

LEGIONELLOSIS ICD-9 482.8
(Legionnaires' disease, Legionnaires' pneumonia, Pontiac fever)

1. **Identification**—An acute bacterial disease with two currently recognized, distinct clinicoepidemiologic manifestations: "Legionnaires' disease" and "Pontiac fever." Both are characterized initially by anorexia, malaise, myalgia and headache. Within a day, there is usually a rapidly rising fever associated with chills. A nonproductive cough is common; abdominal pain and diarrhea occur in many patients. Temperatures commonly reach 39°-40.5°C (102°-105°F). In Legionnaires' disease, chest

radiograph may show patchy areas of consolidation which may progress to bilateral involvement and ultimately to respiratory failure; the overall case fatality rate has been as high as 15% in hospitalized cases of Legionnaires' disease; it is generally higher in those with compromised immunity. Pontiac fever is not associated with pneumonia or death; patients recover spontaneously in 2-5 days without treatment; this clinical syndrome may represent reaction to inhaled antigen rather than bacterial invasion.

Diagnosis depends on isolation of the causative organism on special media or its demonstration by direct IF stain of involved tissue or respiratory secretions, or by a fourfold or greater rise in IFA titer between an acute phase serum and one drawn 3-6 weeks later. A single high titer (>256) might be considered diagnostic in patients with a compatible history.

2. Infectious agent—*Legionellae* are poorly staining, Gram-negative bacilli that require cysteine and other nutrients to grow in vitro. Fourteen serogroups of *L. pneumophila* are currently recognized; however, *L. pneumophila* serogroup 1 is most commonly associated with disease. Related organisms, including *L. micdadei, L. bozemanii, L. longbeachae,* and *L. dumoffii* have been isolated, predominantly from immunosuppressed patients with pneumonia. In all, 28 species of *Legionella* with 45 serogroups are currently recognized.

3. Occurrence—Legionellosis is neither new nor localized. The earliest documented case occurred in 1947; the earliest documented outbreak in 1957 in Minnesota. Since then, the disease has been identified in most states as well as in Australia, Africa, Canada, S America and Europe. Although cases occur throughout the year, both sporadic cases and outbreaks are recognized more commonly in summer and autumn. Serologic surveys suggest a prevalence of antibodies to *L. pneumophila* serogroup 1 at a titer of ≥1:128 in 1-20% of the general population in the few locations studied. The proportion of cases with sporadic, previously undiagnosed pneumonias that appear to be Legionnaires' disease ranges from 0.5 to 4%.

Outbreaks of legionellosis usually occur with low attack rates (0.1-5%) in the population at risk. Epidemic Pontiac fever has had a high attack rate (about 95%) in several outbreaks.

4. Reservoir—Probably primarily aqueous. Hot water systems, air-conditioning cooling towers and evaporative condensers have been implicated epidemiologically; the organism has been isolated from water in these, as well as from hot and cold water taps and showers, and from creeks and ponds and the soil from their banks. The organism survives for months in tap and distilled water. An association of Legionnaires' disease with soil disturbances or excavation is not clearly established.

5. Mode of transmission—Epidemiologic evidence supports airborne transmission via aerosol-producing devices; other modes are possible, but none has been proven conclusively.

6. Incubation period—Legionnaires' disease: 2-10 days, most often 5-6 days; Pontiac fever: 5-66 hours, most often 24-48 hours.

7. Period of communicability—Person-to-person transmission has not been documented.

8. Susceptibility and resistance—Susceptibility is general, but the disease is rare in those under 20 years of age, several outbreaks have occurred among hospitalized patients. Unrecognized infections may be common, but prospective studies indicate that at least half of *Legionella* infections are associated with pneumonia. More serious illness tends to occur with increasing age (most cases are at least 50 years of age), especially in smokers; in patients with diabetes mellitus, chronic lung disease, renal disease or malignancy; and in the immunocompromised, particularly those who are receiving corticosteroids or who have had an organ transplant. The male-female ratio is about 2.5/1.

9. Methods of control—

A. *Preventive measures:* Cooling towers should be drained when not in use. They should be mechanically cleaned periodically to remove scale and sediment. Appropriate biocides should be used to limit the growth of slime-forming organisms. Cost-effective preventive guidelines for domestic water systems have not been established.

B. *Control of patient, contacts and the immediate environment:*
   1) Report to local health authority: In selected endemic areas (USA); in many countries, not a reportable disease, Class 3B (see Preface).
   2) Isolation: None.
   3) Concurrent disinfection: None.
   4) Quarantine: None.
   5) Immunization of contacts: None.
   6) Investigation of contacts and source of infection: Search (households, business, etc.) for additional cases due to infection from a common environmental source.
   7) Specific treatment: Erythromycin appears to be the agent of choice. Rifampin may be a valuable adjunct but should not be used alone. Penicillin, the cephalosporins and the aminoglycosides are ineffective.

C. *Epidemic measures:* Search for common exposures among cases and possible environmental sources of infection. Decontamination of implicated sources by chlorination and/or super-heating of water supply has been effective.

D. *Disaster implications:* None known.

E. *International measures:* None.

LEISHMANIASIS   ICD-9 085
I. CUTANEOUS AND   ICD-9 085.1-085.5
MUCOCUTANEOUS LEISHMANIASIS
(Aleppo, Baghdad or Delhi boil, Oriental sore; in the Americas:
Espundia, Uta, Chiclero ulcer)

1. **Identification**—A polymorphic disease of skin and mucous membranes caused by an intracellular protozoan. The disease starts with a papule which enlarges and becomes an indolent ulcer. Lesions may be single or multiple, rarely non-ulcerative and diffuse. Lesions may heal spontaneously within weeks to months, or last for a year or more. In some individuals, certain parasite strains, mainly from the New World, can produce late sequelae of mucocutaneous lesions (espundia) even years after the primary lesion has healed. These sequelae involve nasopharyngeal tissues, are characterized by progressive tissue destruction and often scanty presence of parasites, and can be fatal. Recurrence after apparent cure (recidiva or chronic relapsing form) may occur as ulcers, papules, or nodules at or near the healed original ulcer.

Diagnosis is made by microscopic identification of the intracellular form (amastigotes) in stained smears of material from the edges of lesions, and by culture of the flagellates on suitable media from biopsies or aspirates. An intradermal (Montenegro) test with antigen derived from the flagellated forms (promastigotes) generally is positive in established disease and remains so thereafter; it is not helpful with very early lesions or anergic disease. Serologic (IFA or ELISA) testing can be done, but antibody levels are rather low, so this may not be helpful in diagnosis. Species identification requires testing for biological (development in sandflies, culture media and animals), immunologic (monoclonal antibodies), molecular (DNA techniques) and biochemical (isozyme analysis) criteria.

2. **Infectious agents**—Old World: *Leishmania tropica, L. major, L. aethiopica.* New World: *L. braziliensis* and *L. mexicana* complexes of species, and probably others. Members of the *L. braziliensis* complex are more likely to produce mucocutaneous lesions; *L. tropica* is the usual cause of the "leishmaniasis recidivans" cutaneous lesions. Members of the *L. donovani* complex, which usually cause visceral disease in both the New

and Old World, may cause single cutaneous lesions, as well as post-kala-azar dermal leishmaniasis.

3. **Occurrence**—Pakistan and recently China, the Middle East, including Iran and Afghanistan; southern USSR, the Mediterranean littoral; the sub-Sahara African savanna and Sudan, the highlands of Ethiopia, Kenya and Namibia; southcentral Texas, Mexico (especially Yucatan), all of Central America, and every country of S America except Chile and Uruguay. In some areas, such as the Old World, urban population groups, including children, may be at risk; in the New World, disease is usually restricted to occupational groups, such as those involved in work in forested areas or to those whose homes are in or next to a forest. Generally more common in rural than urban areas.

4. **Reservoir**—Man, wild rodents, edentates (sloths), marsupials, and carnivores (Canidae), often including domestic dogs and, in urban foci, equines; unknown hosts in many areas.

5. **Mode of transmission**—From the zoonotic reservoir host through the bite of infective female phlebotomines (sandflies). After feeding on an infected mammalian host, flagellated forms develop and multiply in the sandfly gut and in 8-20 days, infective parasites develop, which are injected during biting. In man and other mammals, the organisms are taken up by macrophages and transform into amastigote forms, which multiply in macrophages until the cells rupture, enabling spread to other macrophages.

6. **Incubation period**—At least a week, up to many months.

7. **Period of communicability**—As long as parasites remain in lesions; in untreated cases, usually 5 months to 2 years. Eventual spontaneous healing occurs in most cases. A small proportion of patients infected with *L. m. amazonensis* or *L. aethiopica* may develop diffuse cutaneous lesions that are rich in parasites and do not heal spontaneously. Infections with parasites of the *L. braziliensis* complex can heal spontaneously, but a small proportion are followed, months or years later, by metastatic mucocutaneous lesions.

8. **Susceptibility and resistance**—Susceptibility is probably general. Some immunity is present after lesions heal; it is not clear how protective this might be against other species. Factors responsible for late mutilating disease, such as espundia, are unknown; occult infections may be activated years after the primary infection. The most important factor in immunity is the development of an adequate cell-mediated response.

9. **Methods of control**—

   A. *Preventive measures:*

      1) Educate the public concerning modes of transmission and methods of controlling phlebotomines.

2) Control measures vary from area to area, depending on the habits of the mammalian hosts and the vector phlebotomines. Where their habits are known, applicable control measures may be carried out. These include:

a) Systematic case detection and rapid treatment. This applies to all forms as one of the important measures to prevent development of destructive mucocutaneous lesions, particularly in those situations where the reservoir is largely or solely in man.

b) Periodic application of insecticides with residual action. Phlebotomine flies have a relatively short flight range and are highly susceptible to control by systematic spraying with residual insecticides. Spraying should cover exteriors and interiors of doorways and other openings if infection takes place in dwellings; excluding the vectors by screening requires a fine mesh screen (10-12 holes per linear cm or 25-30 holes per linear inch, an aperture size not more than 0.89 mm or 0.035 inches). Possible breeding places of Old World sandflies, such as stone walls, animal houses and rubbish heaps, should be sprayed.

c) Eliminate rubbish heaps and other breeding places for Old World phlebotomines.

d) Destroy animals (and their burrows) implicated as principal reservoirs in local areas.

e) In the New World, avoid sandfly-infested and thickly forested areas, particularly after sundown; use insect repellents and protective clothing if exposure to sandflies is unavoidable.

f) Apply appropriate environmental management and forest clearance (as possible).

B. *Control of patient, contacts and the immediate environment:*

1) Report to local health authority: Official report not ordinarily justifiable, Class 5 (see Preface).

2) Isolation: None. Only of theoretical value.

3) Concurrent disinfection: None.

4) Quarantine: None.

5) Immunization of contacts: None.

6) Investigation of contacts and source of infection: Determine local transmission cycle and interrupt it in most practical fashion.

7) Specific treatment: Mainly pentavalent antimonials. Sodium stibogluconate (Pentostam®), the recommended

drug, is available in the USA from CDC, Atlanta (see Preface). Other compounds, including meglumine antimonate (Glucantime®), are in use in S America and elsewhere. Pentamidine is used as a second-line drug for cutaneous leishmaniasis. Ketoconazole has been reported to be effective in *L. major* infections. Amphotericin B (Fungizone®) may be required in South American mucocutaneous disease when disease does not respond to antimonial therapy. While spontaneous healing of simple cutaneous lesions occurs, infections acquired in geographic regions where mucocutaneous disease is common, should be treated promptly and effectively and on a long-term basis (up to 4 months).

C. *Epidemic measures:* In areas of high incidence, use intensive efforts to control the disease by provision of diagnostic facilities, and appropriate measures directed against phlebotomine flies and the mammalian reservoir hosts.

D. *Disaster implications:* None.

E. *International measures:* WHO Collaborating Centres (see Preface).

II. VISCERAL LEISHMANIASIS   ICD-9 085.0
(Kala-azar)

1. **Identification**—A chronic systemic disease caused by an intracellular protozoan that multiplies in visceral organs. The disease is characterized by fever, hepatosplenomegaly, lymphadenopathy, anemia with leukopenia, and progressive emaciation and weakness. Untreated, it is usually a fatal disease. Fever is of gradual or sudden onset, continued and irregular, often with 2 daily peaks; alternating periods of apyrexia and low-grade fever follow. Post-kala-azar dermal lesions (PKDL) may occur after apparent cure.

Diagnosis is made preferably by culture of the organism from biopsy or aspirated material, or by demonstration of intracellular amastigotes (Leishman-Donovan bodies) in stained smears from bone marrow, spleen, liver, lymph node or blood. (See Leishmaniasis, Cutaneous, above.)

2. **Infectious agents**—*Leishmania donovani, L. infantum* and *L. chagasi.*

3. **Occurrence**—A rural disease of some tropical and subtropical areas, occurring in discrete foci in India, Bangladesh, Pakistan, China, southern USSR, the Middle East including Turkey, the Mediterranean basin, Mexico, Central and S America (mostly in Brazil), and in Sudan, Kenya, Ethiopia and sub-Saharan savanna parts of Africa. In many

affected areas, it occurs commonly as scattered cases among infants, children and adolescents, but occasionally in epidemic waves. Incidence is modified by the use of antimalarial insecticides. Where dog populations have been drastically reduced, human disease also has been reduced.

4. **Reservoir**—Known or presumed reservoirs include man, wild Canidae and domestic dogs, and rodents. Man is the only known reservoir in India, Nepal and Bangladesh.

5. **Mode of transmission**—Through bite of infective phlebotomine sandflies. (See Leishmaniasis, Cutaneous, above.)

6. **Incubation period**—Generally 2-4 months; range is 10 days to 2 years.

7. **Period of communicability**—As long as parasites persist in the circulating blood or skin of the mammalian reservoir host. If man is the reservoir host, infectivity for phlebotomines may persist even after clinical recovery. Transmission from person to person, and by blood transfusion and sexual contact have been reported.

8. **Susceptibility and resistance**—Susceptibility is general. Kala-azar induces apparent lasting homologous immunity; recovery from cutaneous leishmaniasis does not confer immunity against kala-azar. Considerable evidence indicates that inapparent and subclinical infections are common, and that malnutrition predisposes to clinical disease and activation of inapparent infections. Manifest disease occurs among AIDS patients, presumably as reactivation of latent infections.

9. **Methods of control**—

   A. *Preventive measures:* See Leishmaniasis, Cutaneous, 9A, above. Eliminate domestic canine reservoir.

   B. *Control of patient, contacts and the immediate environment:*

   1) Report to local health authority: In selected endemic areas, Class 3B (see Preface).
   2) Isolation: None.
   3) Concurrent disinfection: None.
   4) Quarantine: None.
   5) Immunization of contacts: None.
   6) Investigation of contacts and source of infection: Ordinarily none.
   7) Specific treatment: Sodium stibogluconate (Pentostam®), available from CDC, Atlanta (see Preface) and meglumine antimonate (Glucantime®) are effective. Cases that do not respond to antimony may be treated with amphotericin B or pentamidine; these are not used routinely because of toxicity. In some regions, such as Kenya, the

disease is less responsive to treatment than in Mediterranean countries, requiring much longer antimonial therapy.

C. *Epidemic measures:* Effective control must include an understanding of the local ecology and transmission cycle, followed by adoption of practical measures to stop transmission.

D. *Disaster implications:* None.

E. *International measures:* Institute coordinated programs of control among neighboring countries where the disease is endemic. WHO Collaborating Centres (see Preface).

LEPROSY
(Hansen's Disease)

ICD-9 030

1. **Identification**—A chronic bacterial disease of the skin, peripheral nerves and (in lepromatous patients) the upper airway. The manifestations of the disease vary in a continuous spectrum between the two polar forms, lepromatous and tuberculoid leprosy. In lepromatous leprosy, nodules, papules, macules and diffuse infiltrations are bilaterally symmetrical and usually numerous and extensive; involvement of the nasal mucosa may lead to crusting, obstructed breathing and epistaxis; ocular involvement leads to iritis and keratitis.

In tuberculoid leprosy, skin lesions are single or few, sharply demarcated, anesthetic or hypesthetic, and bilaterally asymmetrical; peripheral nerve involvement tends to be severe. Borderline leprosy has features of both polar forms and is more labile, with a tendency to shift toward the lepromatous form in the untreated patient, and toward the tuberculoid form in the treated patient. An early form of the disease, indeterminate leprosy, is manifested by a hypopigmented macule with ill-defined borders, and, if untreated, may progress to tuberculoid, borderline or lepromatous disease. The clinical manifestations can include "reactions" of leprosy, i.e., acute adverse episodes, which are termed erythema nodosum leprosum (ENL) in lepromatous patients and reversal reactions in borderline leprosy.

Clinical diagnosis is based on complete skin examination; search for signs of peripheral nerve involvement (hypesthesia, anesthesia, paralysis, muscle wasting, trophic ulcers), with bilateral palpation of peripheral nerves (ulnar nerve at the elbow, peroneal nerve at the head of the fibula and the great auricular nerve) for enlargement and tenderness. Skin lesions are tested for sensation (light touch, pin-prick, temperature discrimination).

Differential diagnosis includes many infiltrative skin diseases, including lymphomas, lupus erythematosus, psoriasis, scleroderma and neurofibromatosis. Diffuse cutaneous leishmaniasis, some mycoses, myxedema and pachydermoperiostosis may resemble lepromatous leprosy, but acid-fast bacilli are not present. Several skin conditions, such as vitiligo, tinea versicolor, pityriasis alba, nutritional dyschromia, nevus and scars may resemble tuberculoid leprosy.

The diagnosis in lepromatous leprosy (the multibacillary form) is strongly supported by the demonstration of acid-fast bacilli in skin smears made by the scraped-incision method; in tuberculoid disease (the paucibacillary form), the bacilli may be so few they are not demonstrable. Whenever possible, a skin biopsy confined to the affected area should be sent to a pathologist experienced in leprosy diagnosis. Nerve involvement with acid-fast bacilli is pathognomonic of leprosy.

2. **Infectious agent**—*Mycobacterium leprae*. The organism has not been grown in bacteriologic media or cell cultures. It can be grown in mouse foot pads to 10^6/g of tissue; in disseminated infections of the nine-banded armadillo, it grows to 10^9-10^{10}/g.

3. **Occurrence**—The world prevalence is estimated to be between 10 and 12 million. Prevalence rates of >5/1000 are common in the rural tropics and subtropics; socioeconomic conditions may be more important than climate itself. The chief endemic areas are in South Asia and SE Asia, including the Philippines, Indonesia, some Pacific islands, India, Bangladesh, Myanmar (Burma) and Indonesia; tropical Africa; and some areas of Latin America. Reported rates in the Americas range from <0.1 to 5/1000. Newly recognized cases in the USA are diagnosed principally in California, Hawaii, Texas, Florida, Louisiana and New York City, and in Puerto Rico. Most of these cases are in immigrants and refugees whose disease was acquired in their native countries; however, the disease remains endemic in Hawaii, Texas, California, Louisiana and Puerto Rico.

4. **Reservoir**—Man is the only reservoir of proven significance. Feral armadillos in Louisiana and Texas have been found naturally afflicted with a disease identical to experimental leprosy in this animal, and there have been reports suggesting that disease in armadillos has been naturally transmitted to humans. Naturally acquired leprosy has been observed in a mangabey monkey and in a chimpanzee captured in Nigeria and Sierra Leone, respectively.

5. **Mode of transmission**—Although the exact mode of transmission is not clearly established, household and prolonged close contact appear to be important. Millions of bacilli are liberated daily in the nasal discharges of untreated lepromatous patients, and bacilli have been shown to remain viable for at least 7 days in dried nasal secretions.

Cutaneous ulcers in lepromatous patients may also shed large numbers of bacilli. The organisms probably gain entrance through the upper respiratory tract and possibly through broken skin. In cases in children under 1 year of age, transmission is presumed to be transplacental.

6. **Incubation period**—The incubation period ranges from 9 months to 20 years; the average is probably 4 years for tuberculoid leprosy and twice that for lepromatous leprosy. The disease is rarely seen in children under age 3; however, over 50 cases have been identified in children under 1 year of age, the youngest being 2-1/2 months old.

7. **Period of communicability**—Clinical and laboratory evidence suggests that infectiousness is lost in most instances within 3 months of continuous and regular treatment with dapsone (DDS) or clofazimine, or within 3 days of treatment with rifampin.

8. **Susceptibility and resistance**—The persistence and form of leprosy depend upon the ability to develop effective cell-mediated immunity. The lepromin test is the intradermal injection of autoclaved *M. leprae;* the presence or absence of induration at 28 days is called the Mitsuda reaction. The reaction is negative in lepromatous leprosy and positive in tuberculoid disease and in a proportion of normal adults; thus, the test gives prognostic information but is of no diagnostic value. The rate of positive tests in the general population increases with age. In addition, the high prevalence of *M. leprae*-specific lymphocyte transformation and antibodies specific for *M. leprae* among close contacts of leprosy patients suggests that infection is frequent; clinical disease occurs in only a small proportion.

9. **Methods of control**—The availability of drugs effective in treatment and in rapid elimination of infectiousness, such as rifampin, has changed the management of the patient with leprosy from isolation from society with attendant despair, to one of ambulatory treatment. Hospitalization is reserved only for managing reactions, surgical correction of deformities and the treatment of ulcers resulting from the anesthesia of the extremities.

A. *Preventive measures:*

1) Health education to stress the availability of effective multidrug therapy, the absence of infectivity of patients under continuous treatment, and the prevention of physical and social disabilities.

2) Detect cases, particularly infectious multibacillary cases, early and administer multidrug therapy on a regular outpatient basis whenever possible.

3) In field trials in Uganda and Papua New Guinea, prophylactic BCG apparently effected a considerable reduction in the incidence of tuberculoid leprosy among contacts. A

study in India indicated significant protection against leprosy but not against tuberculosis. A study in Myanmar (Burma) showed less protection. Chemoprophylaxis studies suggest that approximately 50% protection against disease can be achieved with dapsone or acedapsone, but this is not recommended unless closely supervised. A vaccine of live BCG combined with killed *M. leprae* is under study.

B. *Control of patient, contacts and the immediate environment:*

1) Report to local health authority: Case reporting obligatory in many states (USA) and countries and desirable in all, Class 2B (see Preface).

2) Isolation: None for cases of tuberculoid leprosy; contact isolation for cases of lepromatous leprosy. Hospitalization is often indicated during the treatment of reactions. No special procedures are required when cases are hospitalized, but in a general hospital, a separate room may be desirable. No restrictions in employment or attendance at school are indicated for patients whose disease is regarded as noninfectious.

3) Concurrent disinfection: Of nasal discharges of infectious patients. Terminal cleaning.

4) Quarantine: None.

5) Immunization of contacts: Not routinely practiced (see 9A3, above).

6) Investigation of contacts and source of infection: The initial examination is more productive, but periodic examination of household and other close contacts is recommended at 12-month intervals for at least 5 years after last contact with an infectious case.

7) Specific treatment: With the widespread prevalence of dapsone resistance and the emergence of resistance to rifampin, combined chemotherapy regimens are essential. The minimal regimen recommended by WHO for multibacillary leprosy is rifampin, 600 mg once monthly; dapsone (DDS), 100 mg/day; and clofazimine, 300 mg once monthly and 50 mg/day. The monthly rifampin and clofazimine are administered under supervision. The treatment should be continued until skin smears become negative for at least 2 years. For paucibacillary (tuberculoid) leprosy, the recommended regimen is rifampin, 600 mg once a month (supervised), and dapsone, 100 mg/day, both for a period of 6 months. Patients under treatment should be monitored for side effects of drugs, for leprosy reactions, and for the development of trophic ulcers.

Some complications may need to be treated in a referral center.

C. **Epidemic measures:** Not applicable.

D. **Disaster implications:** Any interruption of treatment schedules is serious. During wars, the diagnosis and treatment of leprosy patients has often been neglected.

E. **International measures:** International controls should be limited to untreated infectious cases. WHO Collaborating Centres (see Preface).

LEPTOSPIROSIS
ICD-9 100

(Weil disease, Canicola fever, Hemorrhagic jaundice, Mud fever, Swineherd's disease)

1. **Identification**—A group of zoonotic bacterial diseases with protean manifestations. Common features are fever with sudden onset, headache, chills, severe myalgia (calves and thighs) and conjunctival suffusion. Other manifestations that may be present are diphasic fever, meningitis, rash (palate, exanthem), hemolytic anemia, hemorrhage into skin and mucous membranes, hepato-renal failure, jaundice, mental confusion/depression and pulmonary involvement with or without hemoptysis.

Cases are often misdiagnosed as meningitis or encephalitis; serologic evidence of leptospiral infection is found among 10% of cases with otherwise undiagnosed meningitis and encephalitis. Clinical illness lasts from a few days to 3 weeks or longer. Recovery of untreated cases can take several months. Infections may be asymptomatic; severity varies with the infecting serovar. Case fatality rate is low, but increases with advancing age, and may reach ≥20% in patients with jaundice and kidney damage who have not been treated with renal dialysis; deaths are due predominantly to hepatorenal failure, adult respiratory distress syndrome, or cardiac arrhythmias due to myocardial involvement.

Diagnosis is confirmed by rising titers in serologic tests, such as the microscopic agglutination test (MAT), and by isolation of leptospires from blood (first 7 days) or CSF (days 4-10) during the acute illness, and from urine after the tenth day, in special media or by inoculation of young guinea pigs, hamsters or gerbils. IF and ELISA techniques are also used for detection of leptospires in clinical and autopsy specimens.

2. **Infectious agent**—Leptospires, members of the order Spirochaetales. Pathogenic leptospires belong to the species *Leptospira interrogans*,

which is subdivided into serovars. More than 200 serovars have been identified and these fall into about 23 serogroups based on serologic relatedness. Major changes in leptospiral nomenclature are being made, based on DNA-relatedness. Commonly identified serovars in the USA are *icterohaemorrhagiae, canicola, autumnalis, hebdomadis, australis* and *pomona*. In the UK, New Zealand and Australia, *L. interrogans* serovar *hardjo* infection in man has occurred among those in close contact with infected livestock.

3. **Occurrence**—Worldwide; in urban and rural, developed and primitive areas, except for polar regions. It is an occupational hazard to rice and sugarcane-field workers, farmers, sewer workers, miners, veterinarians, animal husbandrymen, dairymen, abattoir workers, fish workers and military troops; outbreaks occur among those exposed to fresh river, canal and lake water contaminated by urine of domestic and wild animals, and to urine and tissues of infected animals. It is a recreational hazard to bathers, campers and sportsmen in infected areas. Predominantly a disease of males, related to occupation.

4. **Reservoir**—Wild and domestic animals; varies with serovars. Notable are rats *(icterohemorrhagiae)*, swine *(pomona)*, cattle *(hardjo)*, dogs *(canicola)* and raccoons *(autumnalis)*. In the USA, swine appear to be reservoir hosts of *bratislava;* in Europe, also badgers. Alternative animal hosts with usually shorter carrier states abound, including feral rodents, deer, squirrels, foxes, skunks, raccoons, opossums and marine mammals (sea lions). Serovars infecting reptiles and amphibians (frogs) have not been shown to infect man but have been suspected in Barbados and Trinidad. In carrier animals, an asymptomatic infection occurs in the renal tubules, with leptospiruria persisting for long periods of time, especially in reservoir species.

5. **Mode of transmission**—Contact of the skin, especially if abraded, or of mucous membranes, with water, moist soil or vegetation contaminated with urine of infected animals, as in swimming, accidental or occupational immersion; direct contact with urine or tissues of infected animals; occasionally through ingestion of food contaminated with urine of infected rats; and occasionally by inhalation of droplet-aerosols of contaminated fluids.

6. **Incubation period**—Usually 10 days, with a range of 4-19 days.

7. **Period of communicability**—Direct transmission from person to person is rare. Leptospires may be excreted in the urine; usually for one month, but leptospiruria has been observed for as long as 11 months after the acute illness.

8. **Susceptibility and resistance**—Susceptibility of man is general; immunity to the specific serovar follows infection or (sometimes) immu-

nization, but this may not protect against infection with a different serovar.

9. **Methods of control—**

A. *Preventive measures:*

1) Educate the public on modes of transmission, to avoid swimming or wading in potentially contaminated waters, and to use proper protection when work requires such exposure.

2) Protect workers in hazardous occupations by providing boots and gloves.

3) Recognize potentially contaminated waters and soil and drain such waters when possible.

4) Control rodents in human habitations, especially rural and recreational. Burn cane-fields before harvest.

5) Segregate infected domestic animals; prevent contamination of man's living, working and recreational areas by urine of infected animals.

6) Immunization of farm and pet animals prevents disease, but not necessarily infection and renal shedding. The vaccine must contain the dominant local strains.

7) Immunization of man has been carried out against occupational exposures to specific serovars in Japan, China, Italy, Spain, France and Israel.

8) Doxycycline has been shown in Panama to be effective in preventing leptospirosis when administered in an oral dose of 200 mg once weekly during periods of high exposure.

B. *Control of patient, contacts and the immediate environment:*

1) Report to local health authority: Obligatory case report in many states (USA) and countries, Class 2B (see Preface).

2) Isolation: Blood/body fluid precautions.

3) Concurrent disinfection: Articles soiled with urine.

4) Quarantine: None.

5) Immunization of contacts: None.

6) Investigation of contacts and source of infection: Search for exposure to infected animals and potentially contaminated waters.

7) Specific treatment: Penicillins, cephalosporins, lincomycin and erythromycin are inhibitory in vitro. Doxycycline and penicillin G have been shown to be effective in double-blind, placebo-controlled trials; penicillin G and amoxicillin were effective as late as 7 days into an illness.

C. *Epidemic measures:* Search for source of infection, such as a swimming pool; eliminate the contamination or prohibit use. Investigate industrial and occupational sources, including direct animal contact.

D. *Disaster implications:* A potential problem following flooding of certain areas with a high water table.

E. *International measures:* WHO Collaborating Centres (see Preface).

LISTERIOSIS   ICD-9 027.0

1. **Identification**—A bacterial disease usually manifested as meningoencephalitis and/or septicemia. Those at highest risk are neonates, the elderly, immunocompromised individuals including alcoholics, and pregnant women. The onset of meningoencephalitis may be sudden, with fever, intense headache, nausea, vomiting and signs of meningeal irritation, or may be subacute, particularly in an immunocompromised or elderly host. Delirium and coma may appear early; occasionally there is collapse and shock. Endocarditis, granulomatous lesions in the liver and other organs, localized internal or external abscesses, and pustular or papular cutaneous lesions may occur.

The normal host who acquires infection may exhibit only an acute, mild, febrile illness, sometimes with influenza-like symptoms. This may be especially dangerous in pregnant women who transfer the infection to the fetus. Infants may be stillborn, born with septicemia, or develop meningitis in the neonatal period, even though the mother is asymptomatic. The postpartum course of the mother is usually uneventful, but case fatality rate is 30% in newborn infants and approaches 50% when onset occurs in the first 4 days. In a recent epidemic, the case fatality rate among nonpregnant adults was 33%.

Diagnosis is confirmed by isolation of the infectious agent from CSF, blood, meconium, lochia, gastric washings and other sites of infection. *Listeria monocytogenes* can be readily isolated from normally sterile sites on routine media, but care must be taken to distinguish this organism from other Gram-positive rods, particularly "diphtheroids." Isolations from contaminated specimens are more frequent after prolonged incubation at 4°C (39°F); improved selective media are under evaluation. Microscopic examination of CSF or meconium permits presumptive diagnosis; serologic tests are unreliable because of cross reactions with other bacterial species.

2. **Infectious agent**—*Listeria monocytogenes,* a Gram-positive bacte-

rium; types I/2a, I/2b, and 4b are most frequently isolated from man in the USA.

3. **Occurrence**—An uncommonly diagnosed infection with an incidence in the USA of illness requiring hospitalization of about 1:150,000 population. Typically it occurs sporadically; however, several outbreaks have been recognized in recent years, occurring in all seasons. About 30% of clinical cases occur within the first 3 weeks of life; in adults, infection occurs mainly after age 40. Nosocomial acquisition has been reported. Inapparent infections occur at all ages, although these are of importance only during pregnancy. Abortion may occur, sometimes as early as the second month of pregnancy but mainly in the fifth or sixth month; perinatal infection is acquired during the last trimester. European studies have disclosed large numbers of human carriers.

4. **Reservoir**—The principal reservoir of the organism is in forage, water, mud and silage. The seasonal use of silage as fodder is frequently followed by an increased incidence of listeriosis in animals. Other reservoirs include infected domestic and wild mammals, fowl and man; infection of foxes produces an encephalitis simulating rabies. Asymptomatic fecal carriage is common in man (up to 5%) and animals; asymptomatic vaginal carriage occurs in humans. Cheese made from unpasteurized milk may support the growth of listeria during ripening and has caused outbreaks.

5. **Mode of transmission**—Outbreaks of listeriosis have been reported associated with ingestion of unpasteurized milk and cheese and contaminated vegetables; some sporadic cases may also be due to foodborne transmission. Papular lesions on hands and arms may occur from direct contact with infectious material or soil contaminated with infected animal feces.

In neonatal infections, the organism may have been transmitted from mother to fetus in utero or during passage through the infected birth canal. Person-to-person transmission through venereal contact is possible, as is infection from inhalation of the organism. Nursery outbreaks attributed to spread via hands of medical and nursing staff have rarely occurred.

6. **Incubation period**—Variable; outbreak cases have occurred 3 to 70 days following single exposures to an implicated product.

7. **Period of communicability**—Mothers of infected newborn infants may shed the infectious agent in vaginal discharges and urine for 7-10 days after delivery, rarely longer.

8. **Susceptibility and resistance**—Fetuses and newborn infants are highly susceptible. Children and young adults generally are resistant, adults less so after age 40. Disease is frequently superimposed on other debilitating illnesses such as cancer, especially in patients receiving

steroids or other immunosuppressive agents. There is little evidence of acquired immunity, even after prolonged severe infection.

9. **Methods of control—**

A. *Preventive measures:*

   1) Pregnant women and immunocompromised individuals should avoid contact with potentially infective materials such as aborted animal fetuses on farms and known infected persons; they should eat only properly cooked meats and pasteurized dairy products.
   2) Veterinarians and farmers should take proper precautions in handling aborted fetuses.
   3) Ensure safety of foods of animal origin. Pasteurize all dairy products where possible. Monitor non-pasteurized dairy products, such as soft cheeses, by culturing for *Listeria.*

B. *Control of patient, contacts and the immediate environment:*

   1) Report to local health authority: Obligatory case report required in many states (USA) and some countries, Class 2B; in others, report of clusters of cases required, Class 4 (see Preface).
   2) Isolation: Enteric precautions.
   3) Concurrent disinfection: None.
   4) Quarantine: None.
   5) Immunization of contacts: None.
   6) Investigation of contacts and source of infection: Case surveillance data should be analyzed frequently for possible clusters; all suspected clusters should be investigated for common-source exposures.
   7) Specific treatment: Penicillin or ampicillin together with aminoglycosides, ampicillin alone; for penicillin allergic patients, co-trimoxazole, the tetracyclines and chloramphenicol may be effective. Ampicillin is preferred for maternal-fetal listeriosis; the tetracyclines are contraindicated for children less than 8 years.

C. *Epidemic measures:* Investigate outbreaks to identify a common source of infection, and prevent further exposure to that source. A routine Gram-stained smear of meconium from all newborn infants should be examined for short Gram-positive rods resembling *L. monocytogenes.* If positive, prophylactic antibiotics should be administered as a precaution.

D. *Disaster implications:* None.

E. *International measures:* None.

LOIASIS
ICD-9 125.2
(Loa loa infection, Eyeworm disease of Africa)

1. **Identification**—A chronic filarial disease characterized by migration of the adult worm through subcutaneous or deeper tissues of the body, causing transient swellings several centimeters in diameter, located on any part of the body. These swellings may be preceded by localized pain accompanied by pruritus. Pruritis localized on arms, thorax, face and shoulders is a major symptom. Local names include "fugitive swelling" and "Calabar swelling." Migration under the bulbar conjunctivae may be accompanied by pain and edema. Allergic reactions with giant urticaria and fever may occur occasionally, particularly in Caucasians.

Infection with other filariae, such as *Wuchereria bancrofti*, *Onchocerca volvulus*, *Mansonella* (*Dipetalonema*) *perstans* and *M. streptocerca* (which is common in endemic areas of *Loa loa*), requires differentiation in endemic areas.

Larvae (microfilariae) are present in peripheral blood during the daytime, and can be demonstrated in stained thick blood smears, stained sediment of laked blood or by membrane filtration. Eosinophilia is frequent. A travel history is very helpful in diagnosis.

2. **Infectious agent**—*Loa loa,* a filarial nematode.

3. **Occurrence**—Widely distributed in the African rain forest, especially in Central Africa. In the Congo River basin, up to 90% of indigenous inhabitants of some villages are infected.

4. **Reservoir**—Man.

5. **Mode of transmission**—Transmitted by a horsefly or deerfly of the genus *Chrysops*. *Chrysops dimidiata*, *C. silacea* and other species ingest blood containing microfilariae; the larvae develop within 10-12 days in the fat body of the fly. The developed larvae migrate to the proboscis and are transferred to a human host by the bite of the infective fly.

6. **Incubation period**—Symptoms usually do not appear until several years after infection, but may occur as early as 4 months. Microfilariae may appear in the peripheral blood 5-6 months after infection.

7. **Period of communicability**—The adult worm may live in man, and microfilariae may be present in the blood for as long as 17 years; in the fly, communicability is from 10-12 days after its infection and until all infective larvae have migrated, or until the fly dies.

8. **Susceptibility and resistance**—Susceptibility is universal; repeated infections occur and immunity, if present, has not been demonstrated.

9. **Methods of control—**

A. *Preventive measures:*

   1) Measures directed against the fly larvae are effective, but have not proven practical because the moist, muddy breeding areas are usually too extensive.
   2) Diethyltoluamide (Deet®, Autan®) or dimethyl phthalate applied to exposed skin is effective fly repellent.
   3) Wear long trousers; screen houses.
   4) For temporary residents of endemic areas whose risk of exposure is high or prolonged, a weekly dose of diethylcarbamazine (300 mg) will prevent infection.

B. *Control of patient, contacts and the immediate environment:*

   1) Report to local health authority: Official report not ordinarily justifiable, Class 5 (see Preface).
   2) Isolation: As far as possible, patients with microfilaremia should be protected from *Chrysops* bites to reduce transmission.
   3) Concurrent disinfection: None.
   4) Quarantine: None.
   5) Immunization of contacts: None.
   6) Investigation of contacts and source of infection: None; a community problem.
   7) Specific treatment: Diethylcarbamazine (DEC, Banocide®, Hetrazan®, Notezine®) causes disappearance of microfilariae and may kill the adult worm with resulting cure. During therapy, however, hypersensitivity reactions (sometimes severe) are common but controllable with steroids and/or antihistamines; thus, treatment with DEC must be undertaken with medical supervision. Ivermectin seems to have poor microfilaricidal effect; however, the adverse reactions are very benign. Surgical removal of the adult worm for relief of acute bulbar conjunctivitis is seldom indicated.

C. *Epidemic measures:* Not applicable.

D. *Disaster implications:* None.

E. *International measures:* None.

LYME DISEASE   ICD-9 695.9, 716.59
(Lyme borreliosis, Tick-borne meningopolyneuritis)

1. **Identification**—This tick-borne, spirochetal, zoonotic disease is characterized by a distinctive skin lesion, systemic symptoms, oligoarthritis, and neurologic and cardiac involvement occurring in varying combinations over a period of months to years. The illness typically begins in the summer and the usual first manifestation (the distinctive skin lesion called erythema migrans [EM] or erythema chronicum migrans [ECM]) appears as a red macule or papule which expands in an annular manner, sometimes with multiple similar lesions. To be considered diagnostically significant, a lesion must reach 5 cm in diameter. The lesions may be accompanied by malaise, fatigue, fever, headache, stiff neck, myalgia, migratory arthralgias or lymphadenopathy possibly lasting several weeks in untreated patients; these symptoms may precede the appearance of the skin lesions.

Within weeks to months after onset of the EM lesion, neurologic abnormalities (including the clinical picture of aseptic meningitis, encephalitis, chorea, cerebellar ataxia, cranial neuritis including facial palsy, motor or sensory radiculoneuritis and myelitis) may develop; symptoms fluctuate and may last for months or may become chronic. Cardiac abnormalities (including atrioventricular block, acute myopericarditis or cardiomegaly) may occur within a few weeks after onset of EM. Weeks to years after onset (mean=6 months), swelling and pain in large joints, especially the knees, may develop and recur for several years; chronic arthritis may occasionally result. A similar symptom complex occurs in Europe, but arthritis occurs less frequently there.

Diagnosis is currently based on clinical findings and serologic tests (which are poorly standardized) leading to variable results. Serologic tests (IFA, ELISA) are insensitive during the first several weeks of infection and may remain negative in persons treated early with antibiotics. Test sensitivity increases markedly when patients progress to later stages of the disease, but a small proportion of chronic Lyme disease patients may remain seronegative. Cross-reacting antibodies may cause false-positive reactions in patients with syphilis or relapsing fever. The etiologic agent grows at 33° C (91.4°F) in the Barbour, Stoenner, Kelly (BSK) medium; isolation from blood is difficult, but biopsies of the skin lesions may yield the organism more readily.

2. **Infectious agent**—The causative spirochete, *Borrelia burgdorferi*, was identified in 1982.

3. **Occurrence**—In the USA, endemic foci exist along the Atlantic coast from Massachusetts to Georgia, in the upper midwest in an expanding focus currently concentrated in Wisconsin and Minnesota, and in the West in California and Oregon. The etiologic organism has also been isolated in Ontario, Canada. Currently, increasing recognition of the

disease is redefining endemic areas, and sporadic cases have been reported from 46 states. Elsewhere, it occurs in Europe, the USSR, China, Japan and Australia. Initial infections occur primarily during summer, peaking in June and July but may occur in other seasons, depending on the life cyle of the tick in that area. The distribution of cases coincides with the distribution of *Ixodes dammini* ticks in eastern and midwestern USA, with *I. pacificus* in western USA, with *I. ricinus* in Europe, and with *I. persulcatus* in Asia. Dogs, cattle and horses develop systemic disease that may include the articular, neurologic and cardiac manifestations seen in human patients, depending on the species.

4. **Reservoir**—Certain *Ixodid* ticks through transstadial transmission. Wild rodents (especially *Peromyscus spp.*), deer (especially the white-tailed deer), and other animals maintain the cycle, with larval and nymphal ticks feeding on small mammals and adult ticks on deer.

5. **Mode of transmission**—Tick-borne; transmission does not occur until the tick has fed for several hours.

6. **Incubation period**—For EM, from 3-32 days after tick exposure. However, the early stages of the disease may be asymptomatic and the patient may present with later manifestations of the illness.

7. **Period of communicability**—No evidence of natural transmission from person to person. Rare cases of congenital transmission have been reported.

8. **Susceptibility and resistance**—All persons are probably suscepti-ble; known age range of cases is 2-88 years. Reinfection has occurred in those treated with antibiotics for early disease.

9. **Methods of control**—

    A. *Preventive measures:*

        1) Educate the public in mode of transmission by ticks and the means for personal protection.

        2) Avoid tick-infested areas when feasible; preferably wear light-colored clothing covering legs and arms; tuck pants into socks and apply tick repellent such as diethyltolua-mide (Deet®, Autan®) or permethrin repellents to pant legs and sleeves.

        3) If working or playing in an infested area, remove any surface ticks and search total body area every 3-4 hours for attached ticks. Remove any ticks promptly and care-fully without crushing, using gentle steady traction with forceps (tweezers) applied close to the skin to avoid leaving mouth parts in the skin; protect hands with gloves, cloth or tissue when removing ticks from man or animals.

        4) Measures designed to reduce tick populations are avail-

able (host management, habitat modification, chemical control), but are generally impractical on a large-scale basis.

B. *Control of patient, contacts and the immediate environment:*

1) Report to local health authority: Case report obligatory in most states (USA) and some countries, Class 3B (see Preface).
2) Isolation: None.
3) Concurrent disinfection: Carefully remove all ticks from patients.
4) Quarantine: None.
5) Immunization of contacts: None available.
6) Investigation of contacts and source of infection: Studies to determine source of infection are indicated when cases occur outside a recognized endemic focus.
7) Specific treatment: For adults, the EM stage can usually be treated effectively with tetracycline (250 mg 4 times daily) or doxycycline (100 mg twice daily) for 10 to 30 days. Children less than 8 years old can be treated with amoxicillin or phenoxymethyl penicillin, 50 mg/kg/day in divided doses, for 10 to 30 days. Erythromycin can be used in those who are allergic to penicillin or who cannot take tetracyclines. Later manifestations of the disease require longer courses of therapy and intravenous therapy. Ceftriaxone may prove to be a more effective antibiotic, especially for treatment of neurologic involvement at any age.

C. *Epidemic measures:* In hyperendemic areas, particular attention should be paid to identification of the tick species involved and of the areas infested, and to recommendations in 9A1, 2, and 3, above.

D. *Disaster implications:* None.

E. *International measures:* WHO Collaborating Centres (see Preface).

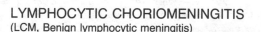

LYMPHOCYTIC CHORIOMENINGITIS ICD-9 049.0
(LCM, Benign lymphocytic meningitis)

1. **Identification**—A viral infection of animals, especially mice, transmissible to man, with a marked diversity of clinical manifestations. At

times, it begins with influenza-like symptoms, followed by complete recovery; in some cases, meningeal symptoms appear after a brief remission, or the illness may begin with meningeal or meningoencephalomyelitic symptoms. Orchitis and parotitis occur occasionally. The acute course is usually short; very rarely fatal, and even with extremely severe disease (e.g., coma with meningoencephalitis), prognosis for recovery without sequelae is usually good, but convalescence may be prolonged with fatigue and vasomotor instability. The CSF in cases with neurologic involvement typically shows a pleocytosis and, at times, a low glucose level. The primary pathologic finding in the rare human fatality is diffuse meningoencephalitis. A few fatal cases of hemorrhagic fever-like disease have been reported.

Laboratory diagnostic methods include isolation of virus from blood, nasopharynx or CSF early in the attack by intracerebral inoculation of LCM-free suckling mice or cell cultures; and rising titers of antibodies demonstrated by serologic testing of paired sera. Requires differentiation from other aseptic meningitides.

2. **Infectious agent**—Lymphocytic choriomeningitis virus, an arenavirus, serologically related to Lassa virus, Machupo and Junin viruses.

3. **Occurrence**—Not uncommon in Europe and the Americas; underdiagnosed. Loci of infection among feral mice often persist over long periods of time, resulting in sporadic clinical disease. Outbreaks have occurred from exposure to hamsters used as pets and laboratory animals. Nude mice, now extensively used in many research laboratories, are particularly susceptible to infection and may be prolific excretors of virus.

4. **Reservoir**—The infected house mouse, *Mus musculus,* is the natural reservoir; infected females transmit infection to the offspring, which become asymptomatic, persistent viral shedders. Infection also occurs in mouse and hamster colonies and in transplantable tumor lines.

5. **Mode of transmission**—Virus is excreted in urine, saliva and feces of infected animals, usually mice. Transmission to man is probably through oral or respiratory contact with virus-contaminated excreta, food or dust, or contamination of skin lesions or cuts; there is little evidence of person-to-person spread by ordinary contact. Handling bedding of naturally infected mice may place individuals at a high risk of infection.

6. **Incubation period**—Probably 8-13 days; 15-21 days until meningeal symptoms appear.

7. **Period of communicability**—Transmission from person to person has not been demonstrated and is unlikely.

8. **Susceptibility and resistance**—Persons who have recovered from the disease are immune, with cell-mediated as well as antibody-mediated

immunity. Demonstrable antibodies are markers of past infection, and do not necessarily indicate immunity.

9. **Methods of control—**

    A. *Preventive measures:* Clean home and place of work; eliminate mice and dispose of diseased animals. Virologic surveillance of commercial rodent breeding establishments, especially those producing hamsters and mice. Assure that laboratory mice are not infected, and that personnel handling mice follow established procedures to prevent infection from possibly infected animals.

    B. *Control of patient, contacts and the immediate environment:*

        1) Report to local health authority: Reportable in selected endemic areas, Class 3C (see Preface).

        2) Isolation: None.

        3) Concurrent disinfection: Of discharges from the nose and throat, urine, feces, and articles soiled therewith during acute febrile period. Terminal cleaning.

        4) Quarantine: None.

        5) Immunization of contacts: None.

        6) Investigation of contacts and source of infection: Search home and place of employment for presence of house mice or rodent pets.

        7) Specific treatment: None.

    C. *Epidemic measures:* Not applicable.

    D. *Disaster implications:* None.

    E. *International measures:* None.

LYMPHOGRANULOMA VENEREUM   ICD-9 099.1
(Lymphogranuloma inguinale, Climatic or tropical bubo, LGV)

    1. **Identification—**A sexually acquired chlamydial infection beginning with a small, painless, evanescent erosion, papule, nodule or herpetiform lesion on the penis or vulva, frequently unnoticed. Regional lymph nodes undergo suppuration followed by extension of the inflammatory process to the adjacent tissues. In the male, inguinal buboes are seen which may become adherent to the skin, fluctuate and result in sinus formation. In the female, inguinal nodes are less frequently affected, and involvement is mainly of the pelvic nodes with extension to the rectum

and rectovaginal septum, resulting in proctitis, stricture of the rectum and fistulae. Proctitis may result from rectal intercourse and LGV is a fairly common cause of severe proctitis in homosexual men. Elephantiasis of the genitalia may occur in either sex. Fever, chills, headache, joint pains and anorexia are present. The disease course is often long and disability great, but generally not fatal. A rare occurrence is generalized sepsis with arthritis and meningitis.

Diagnosis is made by demonstration of chlamydial organisms by IF or by culture of bubo aspirate, or by specific micro-IF serololgic test. CF testing is of diagnostic value if there is a fourfold rise or a single titer of ≥1:64. A negative CF test rules out the diagnosis.

2. **Infectious agent**—*Chlamydia trachomatis,* related to the organisms of trachoma and oculogenital chlamydial infections, but of immunotypes L-1, L-2 and L-3.

3. **Occurrence**—Worldwide, especially in tropical and subtropical areas; more common than ordinarily believed. Endemic in Asia and Africa, particularly among lower socioeconomic classes. Age incidence corresponds with sexual activity. Less commonly diagnosed in women, probably due to frequency of asymptomatic infections; however, sex differences are not pronounced in countries with high endemicity. All races are affected. In temperate climates, found predominantly among male homosexuals.

4. **Reservoir**—Man; often asymptomatic (particularly females).

5. **Mode of transmission**—Direct contact with open lesions of infected persons, usually during sexual intercourse.

6. **Incubation period**—Variable, with a range of 3-30 days for a primary lesion; if a bubo is the first manifestation, 10-30 days, to several months.

7. **Period of communicability**—Variable, from weeks to years, during presence of active lesions.

8. **Susceptibility and resistance**—Susceptibility is general; status of natural or acquired resistance unclear.

9. **Methods of control**—

    A. *Preventive measures:* Except for measures which are specific for syphilis, preventive measures are those for sexually transmitted diseases. See Syphilis, 9A.

    B. *Control of patient, contacts and the immediate environment:*

        1) Report to local health authority: A reportable disease in selected endemic areas; not a reportable disease in most countries, Class 3B (see Preface).

2) Isolation: None. Refrain from sexual contact until all lesions are healed.

3) Concurrent disinfection: None; care in disposal of discharges from lesions and of articles soiled therewith.

4) Quarantine: None.

5) Immunization of contacts: Not applicable; prompt treatment on recognition or clinical suspicion of infection.

6) Investigation of contacts and source of infection: Search for infected sexual contacts of patient. Recent contacts of confirmed active cases should receive specific therapy.

7) Specific treatment: Tetracycline antibiotics are effective for all stages, including buboes and ulcerative lesions. Administer orally for at least 2 weeks. Erythromycin or sulfonamides may be used when tetracycline is contraindicated. Do not incise buboes; drain by aspiration through healthy tissue.

C. *Epidemic measures:* Not applicable.

D. *Disaster implications:* None.

E. *International measures:* See Syphilis, 9E.

MALARIA   ICD-9 084

1. **Identification**—The four human malarias can be sufficiently similar in their early symptoms to make species differentiation difficult without laboratory studies. Furthermore, the fever pattern of the first few days of infection resembles that seen in early stages of many other illnesses (bacterial, viral and parasitic). Even the demonstration of parasites does not necessarily mean that malaria is all that the patient has (e.g., early yellow fever, Lassa fever, etc.). The most serious malarial infection, falciparum malaria (malignant tertian), may present a quite varied clinical picture, including fever, chills, sweats and headache, and may progress to icterus, coagulation defects, shock, renal and liver failure, acute encephalopathy, pulmonary and cerebral edema, coma and death. It is a possible cause of coma and other CNS symptoms, such as disorientation and delirium, in any person recently returned from a tropical area. Prompt treatment is essential, even in mild cases, since irreversible complications may appear suddenly; case fatality rates among untreated children and nonimmune adults exceeds 10% by a considerable margin.

The other human malarias, vivax (benign tertian), malariae (quartan), and ovale, generally are not life-threatening except in the very young, the very old and in patients with concurrent disease or immunodeficiencies. Illness may begin with indefinite malaise and a slowly rising fever of several days duration, followed by a shaking chill and rapidly rising temperature, usually accompanied by headache and nausea, and ending with profuse sweating. After an interval free of fever, the cycle of chills, fever and sweating is repeated, either daily, every other day or every third day. Duration of an untreated primary attack varies from a week to a month or longer. True relapses following periods with no parasitemia (seen with vivax and ovale infections) are common and may occur at irregular intervals for up to 2 and 5 years, respectively; malariae infections may persist for as many as 50 years with recurrent febrile episodes.

Individuals who are partially immune or who have been taking prophylactic drugs may show an atypical clinical picture and wide variations in the incubation period.

Laboratory confirmation is made by demonstration of malaria parasites in blood films. Repeated microscopic examinations may be necessary because of variation in density of *P. falciparum* parasitemia during the asexual cycle; furthermore, parasites are often not demonstrable in films from patients recently or actively under treatment. Several tests are under study involving the demonstration of parasite DNA in blood with probes, as are techniques permitting visual recognition of specific antigen-antibody interactions. Antibodies, demonstrable by IFA or other tests, appear after the first week of infection and may persist for years, indicating past malarial experience, and are not helpful for diagnosis of current illness.

2. Infectious agents—*Plasmodium vivax, P. malariae, P. falciparum* and *P. ovale.* Mixed infections are not infrequent in endemic areas.

3. Occurrence—Endemic malaria no longer occurs in many temperate zone countries and well-developed areas of tropical countries, but is a major cause of ill health in many parts of the tropics and subtropics where socioeconomic development is deficient; high transmission areas are also found on the fringes of forests in S America (i.e., Brazil) and SE Asia (i.e., Indonesia). Ovale malaria is seen mainly in sub-Saharan Africa where vivax malaria is absent. *P. falciparum,* refractory to cure with the 4-aminoquinolines (such as chloroquine), occurs in the tropical portions of both hemispheres. Current information on foci of drug-resistant malaria is published annually by the WHO and can be obtained from the Malaria Branch, CDC, Atlanta (see Preface). In the USA, several outbreaks of mosquito-transmitted malaria occurred in California in the late 1980s.

4. Reservoir—Man is the only important reservoir of human malaria. Nonhuman primates are naturally infected by many malarial species, including *P. knowlesi, P. cynomolgi, P. brasilianum, P. inui, P. schwetzi* and

P. simium, which can infect man, but natural transmission is extremely rare.

5. **Mode of transmission**—By the bite of an infective female anopheline mosquito. Most species feed at dusk and during early night hours; some important vectors have biting peaks around midnight or the early hours of the morning. When a female *Anopheles* mosquito ingests blood containing the sexual stages of the parasite (gametocytes), male and female gametes are set free in the mosquito stomach where they unite and enter the stomach wall to form a cyst in which thousands of sporozoites develop; this requires 8-35 days, depending on the species of parasite and the temperature to which the vector is exposed. These sporozoites migrate to various organs of the infected mosquito, and some that reach the salivary glands mature and are infective when injected into a person as the insect takes a blood meal.

In the susceptible host, the sporozoites enter hepatocytes and develop into exoerythrocytic schizonts. The hepatocytes rupture and asexual parasites (tissue merozoites) reach the bloodstream through the hepatic sinusoids and invade the erythrocytes to grow and multiply cyclically. Most will develop into asexual forms, from trophozoites to mature blood schizonts, which rupture to liberate erythrocytic merozoites, which invade other erythrocytes. Clinical symptoms are produced by the rupture of large numbers of erythrocytic schizonts. Within infected erythrocytes, some of the merozoites may develop into the male (microgametocyte) or the female (macrogametocyte) sexual forms.

The period between the infective bite and the appearance of the parasite in the blood is the "prepatent period," which varies from 6 to 9 days with *P. falciparum, P. vivax* and *P. ovale,* and 12-16 days in the case of *P. malariae.* Gametocytes usually appear within 3 days of parasitemia with *P. vivax* and *P. ovale,* and after 12-14 days in *P. falciparum.* Some exoerythrocytic forms of *P. vivax* and probably *P. ovale* exist as dormant forms (hypnozoites) which remain in hepatocytes to mature months later and produce relapses. This phenomenon does not occur in falciparum or malariae malaria, and reappearance of these forms of the disease is the result of inadequate treatment or of infection with drug-refractory strains. With *P. malariae,* low levels of erythrocytic parasites may persist for many years, to multiply at some future time to a level that may result again in clinical disease. Malaria may also be transmitted by injection or transfusion of blood of infected persons or by use of contaminated needles and syringes, as by drug users. Congenital transmission occurs rarely.

6. **Incubation period**—The time between the infective bite and the appearance of clinical symptoms is approximately 12 days for *P. falciparum,* 14 days for *P. vivax* and *P. ovale,* and 30 days for *P. malariae.* With some strains of *P. vivax,* mostly from temperate areas, there may be a protracted incubation period of 8-10 months; even longer with *P. ovale.* With infection by blood transfusion, incubation periods depend on the

number of parasites infused; they are usually short, but may range up to about 2 months.

7. Period of communicability—For infection of mosquitoes, as long as infective gametocytes are present in the blood of patients; this varies with species and strain of parasite and with response to therapy. Untreated or insufficiently treated patients may be a source of mosquito infection for more than 3 years in malariae, from 1-2 years in vivax, and generally not more than 1 year in falciparum malaria; the mosquito remains infective for life. Transmission by transfusion may occur as long as asexual forms remain in the circulating blood; with *P. malariae* this can continue for ≥40 years. Stored blood can remain infective for 16 days.

8. Susceptibility and resistance—Susceptibility is universal except in people with certain genetic traits. Tolerance or refractoriness to disease is present in adults in highly endemic communities where exposure to infective anophelines is continuous over many years. Most black Africans show a natural resistance to infection with *P. vivax,* possibly associated with the absence of Duffy factor on their erythrocytes. Persons with sickle cell trait have relatively low parasitemia when infected with *P. falciparum.*

9. Methods of control—

   A. Preventive measures:

     1)   Encourage sanitary improvements (such as filling and draining areas of impounded water) that will result in permanent elimination or reduction of anopheline breeding habitats. Larvicides and biological control with larvivorous fish may be useful.

     2)   Any use of a residual insecticide should be preceded by a careful appraisal of the particular problem area, the development of specific plans, and their approval by the government concerned. Where appropriate, apply residual insecticide on the inside walls of dwellings and on other surfaces upon which endophilic vector anophelines habitually rest; this will generally result in effective malaria control, except where vector resistance to these insecticides has developed or the vectors do not enter houses.

     3)   Nightly spraying of screened living and sleeping quarters with a liquid or aerosol preparation of pyrethrum or other insecticide is useful.

     4)   In endemic areas, install screens and use bed nets. The effectiveness of bed nets is greatly enhanced by impregnation with a synthetic pyrethroid (e.g., permethrin).

     5)   Insect repellents applied to uncovered skin of persons

exposed to bites of vector anophelines are useful when applied repeatedly. The most effective repellent presently available is diethyltoluamide (Deet®).

6) Blood donors should be questioned for a history of malaria or possible exposure to the disease. In the USA, blood donors who have not taken antimalarial drugs and have been free of symptoms may donate 6 months after return from an endemic area. If they have been on antimalarial prophylaxis, have had malaria, have immigrated, or are visiting from endemic areas, they may be accepted as donors 3 years after cessation of chemoprophylaxis or chemotherapy and departure from the endemic area, if they have remained asymptomatic. A migrant or visitor from an area where malariae malaria is or had been endemic may be a source of transfusion-induced infection for many years. Such areas include, but are not limited to, tropical Africa and countries such as Greece and Romania.

7) Prompt and effective treatment of acute and chronic cases is an important adjunct to malaria control.

8) Non-immune travelers who will be exposed to mosquitoes in malarious areas should regularly use suppressive drugs; in most endemic countries, chemoprophylaxis is recommended for pregnant women and young children as well. The possible side-effects of the drug or drug combination recommended for use in any particular area should be weighed against the actual likelihood of being bitten by an infected mosquito. The risk of exposure to those living in cities in most malarious areas is minimal, but it can be reduced further by the judicious use of supplementary methods of protection, such as nets and repellents.

a) In areas where travelers will be at risk of acquiring chloroquine-resistant *P. falciparum* (Asia, Africa, S America), mefloquine (a quinoline methanol) alone is recommended. The dose (250 mg for an adult) should be taken once each week for the first four weeks; subsequent doses are to be taken once every other week. Those taking mefloquine once every other week should take two doses after leaving the malarious area. Mefloquine is contraindicated in pregnant women, children under 30 lbs, individuals using beta-blockers or other drugs which may prolong or alter cardiac conduction, individuals with a history of psychiatric disorders or leprosy and individuals involved in tasks requiring fine coordination and spatial discrimination, such as airline crews.

Doxycycline alone, 100 mg once daily, is an alternative regimen for short-term travelers who are unable to take mefloquine. Doxycycline may cause diarrhea, monilial vaginitis, and photosensitivity. It should not be given to pregnant women and children less than 8 years old. Doxycycline prophylaxis can begin 1-2 days prior to travel to malarious areas, and should be continued daily during travel and for 4 weeks after leaving the malarious area.

Long-term travelers at risk of infection by chloroquine-resistant *P. falciparum* strains for whom mefloquine is contraindicated (including pregnant women, children under 30 lbs and those intolerant of the drug, etc.) should take once-weekly chloroquine alone. They should be given a treatment dose of Fansidar® (sulfadoxine 500 mg-pyrimethamine 25 mg) unless they have a history of sulfonamide intolerance. In the event of a febrile illness when professional medical care is not readily available, administer Fansidar® (adult dose 3 tablets) and obtain medical consultation as soon as possible. **It must be emphasized that such presumptive self-treatment is only a temporary measure and that prompt medical evaluation is imperative.**

b) For suppression of malaria in nonimmunes temporarily residing in or traveling through endemic areas where the plasmodia are chloroquine-sensitive (Middle America west of the Panama Canal, the island of Hispaniola and malarious areas of the Middle East), chloroquine (Aralen®), 5 mg base/kg body weight (300 mg base or 500 mg chloroquine phosphate for the average adult), once weekly. Pregnancy is not a contraindication. The drug must be continued on the same schedule for 4-6 weeks after leaving endemic areas.

c) These chemosuppressive drugs do not eliminate intrahepatic parasites, so that clinical relapses of vivax or ovale malaria may occur after the drug is discontinued. Primaquine, 0.25 mg base/kg/day for 14 days (15 mg base or 26.3 mg of primaquine phosphate for the average adult), is effective and may be given concurrently with or following the suppressive drug after leaving endemic areas; however, it can produce hemolysis in those with glucose-6-phosphate dehydrogenase (G-6-PD) deficiency. The decision to administer primaquine is made on an individual basis, considering the potential risk of adverse reactions. Larger daily doses (22.5 mg base) may be required for some SE Asian and southwest Pacific strains. Alternatively, primaquine, 0.75 mg base/kg, may be given once weekly for 8 doses (45 mg base or 79 mg primaquine phosphate for the average adult) after leaving endemic areas. If possible, prior to primaquine administration, the patient should be tested for possible G-6-PD deficiency. Primaquine should not be administered during pregnancy; chloroquine should be continued weekly for the duration of the pregnancy.

B. *Control of patient, contacts and the immediate environment:*

1) Report to local health authority: Obligatory case report as a Disease under Surveillance by WHO, Class 1A (see Preface), in nonendemic areas, preferably limited to smear-confirmed cases (USA); Class 3C is the more practical procedure in endemic areas.

2) Isolation: For hospitalized patients, blood precautions. Patients should be in mosquito-proof areas at night.

3) Concurrent disinfection: None.

4) Quarantine: None.

5) Immunization of contacts: Not applicable.

6) Investigation of contacts and source of infection: Determine history of previous infection or of possible exposure. If a history of needle sharing is obtained from the patient, investigate and treat all persons who shared the equipment. In transfusion-induced malaria, all donors must be located and their blood examined for malarial parasites and for antimalarial antibodies; parasite-positive donors should receive treatment.

7) Specific treatment for all forms of malaria:

a) The treatment of malarias due to infection with *P. vivax, P. malariae,* and *P. ovale* is the oral administration of a total of 25 mg of chloroquine base/kg administered over a 3-day period: 15 mg/kg the first day (10 mg/kg initially and 5 mg/kg 6 hours later; 600 and 300 mg doses for the average adult); 5 mg/kg the second day; and 5 mg/kg the third day.

b) For emergency treatment of adults with grave infections or for persons unable to retain orally administered medication, use quinine dihydrochloride, 20 mg base/kg, diluted in 500 ml of normal saline, glucose or plasma, administered by slow IV (over 2-4 hours); repeat in 8 hours at a lower dose (10 mg/kg) if needed, and then the same dose every 8 hours until it can be supplanted by oral quinine. The pediatric dosage is the same.

If there is evidence of renal failure, quinine dosage should be reduced. If parenteral quinine is not available, parenteral quinidine is equally effective in treatment of severe malaria. A loading dose of 15 mg quinidine gluconate base/kg body weight is administered by slow IV over 1-2 hours, followed by a constant IV infusion of 0.03 mg base/kg/minute controlled by a constant-infusion pump. The infusion may continue for a maximum of 72 hours. All parenteral drugs should be discontinued as soon as oral drug administration can be initiated. In extremely severe falciparum infections, particularly those with altered mental status or with a parasitemia approaching or exceeding 50% (some consider 10% adequate) exchange transfusion should be considered. All parenteral drugs should be discontinued as soon as oral drug administration can be initiated.

c) For *P. falciparum* infections acquired in areas where chloroquine-resistant strains are present, administer quinine, 25 mg/kg/day divided into 3 doses, for 7-10 days. (For grave infections, administer quinine as described above.) Along with quinine, administer tetracycline, 15 mg/kg given in 4 doses daily, for 7 days. Mefloquine has been in use for several years in SE Asia, and treatment failures have been reported. Every effort should be made to determine the therapeutic course producing the best results in the area where the disease was contracted, since drug-resistance patterns may vary in time and locale.

d) For prevention of relapses in mosquito-acquired *P. vivax* and *P. ovale* infections, administer primaquine, as described in 9A8b, above, upon completion of the treatment of an acute attack. It is desirable to test all patients (especially blacks, Asians and Mediterraneans) for G-6-PD deficiency to prevent drug-induced hemolysis. Many, particularly blacks, are able to tolerate the hemolysis, but consideration may have to be given to discontinuing primaquine, balancing the induced problem against the possible recurrence of malaria. Primaquine is not required in non-mosquito-transmitted disease (e.g., transfusion), since no liver phase occurs.

C. *Epidemic measures:* Determine the nature and extent of the epidemic situation. Intensify control measures directed against adult and larval stages of the important vectors, including elimination of breeding places, treatment of acute cases, use of personal protection and suppressive drugs. Mass treatment may be considered.

D. *Disaster implications:* Throughout history the malarias have been a concomitant or the result of wars and social upheavals. Any abnormal climatic or edaphic change which increases the availability of mosquito-breeding sites in endemic areas can lead to an increase in malaria.

E. *International measures:*

1) Disinsectization of aircraft before departure or in transit using a space-spray application of an insecticide of a type to which the vectors are susceptible.

2) Disinsectization of aircraft, ships and other vehicles on arrival if the health authority at the place of arrival has reason to suspect importation of malaria vectors.

3) Enforce and maintain rigid antimosquito sanitation within the mosquito flight range of all ports and airports.

4) In special circumstances, administer antimalarial drugs to potentially infected migrants, refugees, seasonal workers and persons taking part in periodic mass movement into an area or country where malaria has been eliminated. Primaquine, 30-45 mg base (0.5-0.75 mg/kg), given as a single dose, renders the gametocytes of falciparum malaria noninfectious.

5) Malaria is a Disease under Surveillance by WHO, as it is considered an essential element of the world strategy of primary health care. National health administrations are expected to notify WHO twice a year of: those areas originally malarious with no present risk of infection, those malaria cases imported into areas in the maintenance phase of eradication, those areas with chloroquine-resistant strains of parasites, and those international ports and airports free of malaria. WHO Collaborating Centres (see Preface).

MEASLES   ICD-9 055
(Rubeola, Hard measles, Red measles and Morbilli)

1. **Identification**—An acute, highly communicable viral disease with

prodromal fever, conjunctivitis, coryza, cough and Koplik spots on the buccal mucosa. A characteristic red blotchy rash appears on the third to seventh day, beginning on the face, becoming generalized, lasting 4-7 days, and sometimes ending in branny desquamation. Leukopenia is common. The disease is more severe in infants and adults than in children. Complications may result from viral replication or bacterial superinfection, and include otitis media, pneumonia, diarrhea and encephalitis. In the developed countries, death from uncomplicated measles is rare; deaths occur mainly in children less than 5 years old, from pneumonia, and occasionally from encephalitis. Measles is a more severe disease in the very young and in malnourished children, in whom it may be associated with hemorrhagic rash, protein-losing enteropathy, mouth sores, dehydration, diarrhea, blindness and severe skin infections; the case fatality rate may be 5-10% or more. Both acute and delayed mortality in infants and children have been documented. In children who are borderline nourished, measles often precipitates acute kwashiorkor and exacerbates vitamin A deficiency, leading to blindness. Subacute sclerosing panencephalitis (SSPE) develops very rarely (about 1/100,000) several years after infection, as a late sequel; over 50% of SSPE cases have had measles diagnosed in the first two years of life.

In those who received inactivated measles vaccine (prior to 1968 in the USA), infection with wild virus may cause severe atypical manifestations, with pneumonitis, pleural effusion, peripheral edema and an atypical rash with a predilection for the extremities resembling that of Rocky Mountain spotted fever.

Diagnosis is usually made on clinical and epidemiologic grounds. It can be confirmed by the presence of measles-specific IgM antibodies or a significant rise in antibody concentrations between acute and convalescent sera. Techniques used less commonly include identification of viral antigen in nasopharyngeal mucosal swab using FA techniques, or by virus isolation in cell culture from blood, conjunctiva, nasopharynx or urine specimens taken before the third day of rash.

2. **Infectious agent**—Measles virus, a member of the genus *Morbillivirus* of the family Paramyxoviridae.

3. **Occurrence**—Prior to widespread immunization, measles was common in childhood, so that over 90% of people had been infected by age 20; few persons went through life without an attack. Measles was endemic in large metropolitan communities, attaining epidemic proportions about every other year. In smaller communities and areas, outbreaks tended to be more widely spaced and somewhat more severe. With longer intervals between outbreaks, as in the Arctic and some islands, measles outbreaks often involved a large proportion of the population with a high case fatality rate. With effective childhood immunization programs, measles cases in the USA, Canada and other countries (Czechoslovakia) have dropped by 99% and are generally deferred to older age groups. In the

USA, there has been a marked increase in the last few years in the number of reported cases. These are now occurring in babies under 15 months of age (the previously recommended age for immunization), in unimmunized inner-city preschool children, and in the unvaccinated and vaccine failures among highly vaccinated school-age (including high school and college level) children. Sustained outbreaks have occurred in vaccinated school populations among the 2-5% who failed to seroconvert after one dose of vaccine. A second dose seroconverts 95% of these failures. Approximately 40% of cases now occurring in the USA have a history of previous vaccination. In temperate climates, measles occurs primarily in the late winter and early spring.

4. **Reservoir**—Man.

5. **Mode of transmission**—Airborne by droplet spread, direct contact with nasal or throat secretions of infected persons, and, less commonly, by articles freshly soiled with nose and throat secretions. Measles is one of the most highly communicable infectious diseases, and a herd immunity of 94% or more may be needed to interrupt community transmission.

6. **Incubation period**—About 10 days, varying from 7 to 18 days from exposure to onset of fever, usually 14 days until rash appears; rarely longer or shorter. IG, given for passive protection later than the third day of the incubation period, may extend the incubation to 21 days instead of preventing disease.

7. **Period of communicability**—From slightly before the beginning of the prodromal period to 4 days after appearance of the rash; communicability is minimal after the second day of rash. The vaccine virus has not been shown to be communicable.

8. **Susceptibility and resistance**—All persons who have not had the disease or who have not been successfully immunized are susceptible. Acquired immunity after disease is permanent. Infants born of mothers who have had the disease are immune for approximately the first 6-9 months or more, depending on the amount of residual maternal antibody at the time of pregnancy and the rate of antibody degradation. Maternal antibody interferes with response to vaccine. Vaccination at age 15 months produced immunity in 95-98% of recipients; revaccination may increase immunity levels to as high as 99%. It is not clear whether vaccine-induced immunity against clinical disease is lost over time; the majority of available evidence suggests that this does not occur.

9. **Methods of control**—

A. *Preventive measures:*

1) Vaccination: Live attenuated measles vaccine is the agent of choice and is indicated for all individuals susceptible to

measles, unless specifically contraindicated (see 9A1c, below). A single injection of live measles vaccine, which may be combined with other live vaccines (mumps, rubella) and can be administered concurrently with other vaccines, should induce active immunity in more than 95% of susceptible individuals, possibly for life, by producing a mild or inapparent, noncommunicable infection.

About 5-15% of non-immune vaccinees may develop malaise, fever to 39.4°C (103°F) 5-12 days post-vaccination, lasting 1-2 days, but with little disability. Rash, coryza, mild cough and Koplik spots may occasionally occur. Febrile seizures occur infrequently and without sequelae; the highest incidence is in children with a previous history, or a close family history (parents or siblings), of seizures. Encephalitis and encephalopathy have been reported following measles vaccination (approximately 1 case per 330,000 doses distributed).

In several recent outbreaks in the USA in which more than half the cases occurred among appropriately vaccinated children 5-19 years of age, primary vaccine failure (rather than waning of vaccine-induced immunity) may have been the major reason for the outbreaks. To reduce the number of primary vaccine failures in the USA, the current recommendation is a routine 2-dose measles vaccine schedule, with the initial dose administered at 15 months of age or as soon as possible thereafter. The second dose should be given at school entry (4-6 years of age), although localities can choose other ages, such as entry to middle or junior high school. Both doses should generally be given as a combined measles, mumps and rubella vaccine (MMR). Different schedules may be recommended in other countries; e.g., Canada recommends a single dose as soon as possible after the first birthday.

In counties with 5 or more cases in preschool children in each of the last 5 years, or with a recent outbreak among unvaccinated preschool children, initial vaccination with MMR at 12 months of age is recommended. During large community-wide outbreaks, the recommended age for vaccination may have to be further lowered to 6 or 9 months (monovalent measles vaccine), with the first dose of MMR at 15 months and the second at school entry.

Studies in Africa and Latin America indicate that the optimal age for immunization in developing countries, which depends on the persistence of maternal antibodies in the infant, would be at 9-10 months. Immunization should be carried out at any medical contact with an unimmunized child more than 9 months of age, unless contraindicated. The use of high-titered, immunogenic vaccines, such as the Edmonston-Zagreb strain, has been recommended by WHO to be given at 6 months of age in areas at high risk of significant morbidity and mortality from measles in infants <9 months of age.

a) Vaccine shipment and storage: Vaccination may not produce protection if the vaccine has been improperly handled or stored. Prior to reconstitution, freeze-dried measles vaccine is relatively stable and can be stored at refrigerator temperatures (2°-8°C; 35.6°-46.4°F) with safety for a year or more. Reconstituted vaccine should be kept at refrigerator temperatures and protected from light, which may inactivate the virus. Reconstituted vaccine unused after 8 hours should be discarded.

b) Revaccinations: In the USA, in addition to routine revaccination at school entry, revaccination should also be required of those entering educational institutions beyond high school, or entering hospital service, unless they have a documented history of measles or have received two doses of measles-containing vaccines. In those who received only inactivated measles vaccine before 1968, revaccination may produce more severe reactions, such as local edema and induration, lymphadenopathy and fever, but will protect against the atypical measles syndrome.

c) Contraindications to the use of live vaccines: Pregnancy, purely on theoretical grounds, vaccine should not be given to pregnant women; others should be advised of the theoretical risk of fetal wastage if they become pregnant within a month or two after vaccination. Patients with immune deficiency diseases or suppressed immune responses from leukemia, lymphoma or generalized malignancy, or from therapy with corticosteroids, irradiation, alkylating drugs or antimetabolites, should not receive live virus vaccine. Infection with HIV, or clinical AIDS, however, is not a contraindication because of the greater risk of severe measles in such individuals. Patients with a high fever or severe acute illness should have vaccination deferred until recovery; minor illnesses, such as diarrhea or respiratory infections, are not a contraindication. Measles vaccine should not be given to people who cannot eat eggs because of specific allergy. Vaccine should be given 14 days before, or deferred for 3 months after, IG or blood transfusion.

2) Public education by health departments and private physicians should encourage measles vaccination for all susceptible infants, children, adolescents and young adults born in 1957 or later. Those for whom vaccine is contraindicated, and unvaccinated persons identified more than 72 hours after exposure to measles in families or institutions, can be protected by measles IG given within 6 days after exposure.

3) The requirement for measles immunization for school attendance, from day-care centers through college, is an important and effective means of measles control in the USA and some provinces of Canada. Since sustained outbreaks have occurred in schools with immunization rates over 95%, even higher levels of immunity are needed to fully prevent outbreaks from occurring. This may be achieved by routine revaccination as a school-entry requirement.

B. *Control of patient, contacts and the immediate environment:*

1) Report to local health authority: Obligatory case report in most states (USA) and in many countries, Class 2B (see Preface). Early reporting provides opportunity for better outbreak control.

2) Isolation: Impractical in the community at large; children should be kept out of school for at least 4 days after appearance of the rash. In hospitals, respiratory isolation from onset of catarrhal stage of the prodromal period through fourth day of rash reduces the exposure of other patients at high risk.

3) Concurrent disinfection: None.

4) Quarantine: Usually impractical. Quarantine of institutions, wards or dormitories for young children is of value; strict segregation of infants if measles occurs in an institution.

5) Immunization of contacts: Live vaccine, if given within 72 hours of exposure, may provide protection. IG may be used within 6 days of exposure for susceptible household or other contacts for whom risk of complications is very high (contacts under 1 year of age), or for whom measles vaccine is contraindicated. The dose is 0.25 ml/kg (0.11 ml/lb) up to a maximum of 15 ml. For immunocompromised persons, 0.5 ml/kg is given, up to a maximum of 15 ml. Live measles vaccine should be given 3 months later

to those for whom vaccine is not contraindicated.

6) Investigation of contacts and source of infection: A search for and immunization of exposed susceptible contacts should be done to limit the spread of disease. Carriers are unknown.

7) Specific treatment: None.

C. Epidemic measures:

1) Prompt reporting of suspected cases and comprehensive immunization programs of all susceptibles to limit spread. In day-care, school and college outbreaks in the USA, all persons who have not received two doses of live vaccine at least one month apart on or after the first birthday should be immunized unless they have had prior physician-diagnosed measles or laboratory evidence of immunity.

2) In institutional outbreaks, new admissions should receive vaccine or measles IG.

3) In many less-developed countries, measles has a relatively high case fatality rate. If vaccine is available, prompt use at the beginning of an epidemic is essential to limit spread; if vaccine supply is limited, priority should be given to young children for whom the risk is greatest.

D. Disaster implications: Introduction of measles into refugee populations with a high proportion of susceptibles can result in devastating epidemics with high fatality rates.

E. International measures: None.

MELIOIDOSIS   ICD-9 025
(Whitmore disease, Rodent glanders)

1. **Identification**—An uncommon bacterial infection with a range of clinical manifestations from no disease to asymptomatic pulmonary consolidation to a rapidly fatal septicemia. It may simulate typhoid fever or, more commonly, tuberculosis, including pulmonary cavitation, empyema, chronic abscesses and osteomyelitis.

Diagnosis depends on isolation of the causative agent; a rising antibody titer in serologic tests is confirmatory. The possibility of melioidosis should be kept in mind in any unexplained suppurative disease, especially cavitating pulmonary disease, in a patient living in, or returned from SE Asia and other endemic areas.

2. **Infectious agent**—*Pseudomonas pseudomallei,* Whitmore's bacillus.

3. **Occurrence**—Clinical disease is uncommon, generally occurring in individuals who have had intimate contact with soil and surface water. It may appear as a complication of an overt wound or may follow aspiration of water. Cases have been recorded in, but probably are not restricted to, SE Asia, the Philippines, Vietnam, Thailand, Iran, Turkey, northeastern Australia, Papua New Guinea, Guam, Burkina Faso (Upper Volta), Ecuador, Panama, Mexico and Aruba. In certain of these areas, 5-20% of agricultural workers have demonstrable antibodies but no history of overt disease.

4. **Reservoir**—The organism is saprophytic in certain soils and waters. Various animals, including sheep, goats, horses, swine, monkeys and rodents (and a variety of animals and birds in zoological gardens) can become infected. There is no evidence that they are important reservoirs, except in the transfer of the agent to new foci.

5. **Mode of transmission**—Usually by contact with contaminated soil or water through overt or inapparent skin wounds, by aspiration or ingestion of contaminated water, or by inhalation of dust from soil.

6. **Incubation period**—Can be as short as 2 days. However, several months or years may elapse between the presumed exposure and the appearance of clinical disease.

7. **Period of communicability**—Person-to-person transmission is extremely rare; it has been reported only following sexual contact with an individual with prostatic infection. Laboratory-acquired infections are uncommon but do occur, especially if procedures produce aerosols.

8. **Susceptibility and resistance**—Disease in man is uncommon even among persons in endemic areas who have close contact with soil or water containing the infectious agent. Many chronically infected, asymptomatic patients develop clinical disease following severe injuries or burns, or have a history of a systemic disease such as diabetes. These conditions may precipitate disease or recrudescence of disease in asymptomatic infected individuals.

9. **Methods of control**—

   A. *Preventive measures:* Unknown.

   B. *Control of patient, contacts and the immediate environment:*

   1) Report to local health authority: No official report, Class 5 (see Preface).
   2) Isolation: Respiratory and sinus drainage precautions.
   3) Concurrent disinfection: Safe disposal of sputum and wound discharges.
   4) Quarantine: None.

5) Immunization of contacts: None.
6) Investigation of contacts and source of infection: Human carriers are not known.
7) Specific treatment: The most effective agent is co-trimoxazole. In vitro tests show susceptibility to sulfonamides, chloramphenicol, tetracyclines, many of the third generation cephalosporins and novobiocin. A favorable outcome may be expected in most subacute and chronic cases. The best treatment for septicemic cases has not been established, although recovery has been recorded following administration of multiple drugs; in chronic cases with positive cultures, pulmonary resection may be considered.

C. *Epidemic measures:* Not applicable to man; a sporadic disease.

D. *Disaster implications:* None.

E. *International measures:* None. Introduction should be considered when animals are moved to areas where the disease is unknown.

GLANDERS   ICD-9 024

Glanders is a highly communicable disease of horses, mules and donkeys; it has disappeared from most areas of the world, although enzootic foci are believed to exist in Asia and some eastern Mediterranean countries. Clinical glanders no longer occurs in the Western Hemisphere. Human infection has occurred rarely and sporadically, and almost exclusively in those whose occupations involve contact with animals or work in laboratories (e.g., veterinarians, equine butchers and pathologists). Infection with the etiologic organism, *Pseudomonas mallei (Malleomyces mallei)*, the glanders bacillus, cannot be differentiated serologically from *P. pseudomallei;* specific diagnosis can be made only by characterization of the isolated organism. Prevention depends on control of glanders in the equine species and care in handling causative organisms.

MENINGITIS
I. VIRAL MENINGITIS   ICD-9 047.9
(Aseptic meningitis, Serous meningitis, Nonbacterial or Abacterial meningitis)

1. **Identification**—A relatively common but rarely serious clinical

syndrome with multiple viral etiologies, characterized by sudden onset of febrile illness with signs and symptoms of meningeal involvement, CSF findings of pleocytosis (usually mononuclear but may be polymorphonuclear in early stages), increased protein, normal sugar and absence of bacteria. A rash resembling rubella characterizes certain types caused by echoviruses and coxsackieviruses; vesicular and petechial rashes may also occur. Active illness seldom exceeds 10 days. Transient paresis and encephalitic manifestations may occur; paralysis is unusual. Residual signs lasting a year or more may include weakness, muscle spasm, insomnia and personality changes. Recovery is usually complete. Gastrointestinal and respiratory symptoms may be associated with infection with enteroviruses.

Differential diagnosis: Various diseases caused by nonviral agents may mimic aseptic meningitis, such as inadequately treated pyogenic meningitis, tuberculous and cryptococcal meningitis, meningitis caused by other fungi, cerebrovascular syphilis and lymphogranuloma venereum. Postinfectious and postvaccinal reactions require differentiation, including sequelae to measles, mumps and varicella, and post-rabies and post-smallpox vaccination; these syndromes are usually encephalitic in type. Leptospirosis, listeriosis, syphilis, lymphocytic choriomeningitis, viral hepatitis, infectious mononucleosis, influenza and other diseases may produce the same clinical syndrome, and these are discussed in individual chapters.

Under optimal conditions, specific identification can be made in about half the cases using serologic and isolation techniques, and this is indicated in epidemics. Viral agents may be isolated in early stages from throat washings and stool, and occasionally from CSF and blood, by cell culture techniques and animal inoculation.

2. **Infectious agents**—A wide variety of infectious agents, many of which are associated with other specific diseases. Many viruses are capable of producing meningeal features. Half or more of the cases have no etiology demonstrated. In epidemic periods, mumps may be responsible for over 25% of cases of established etiology. In the USA, enteroviruses (picornaviruses) cause most cases of known etiology. Coxsackievirus group B, types 1-6, causes roughly one-third; and echovirus, types 2, 5, 6, 7, 9 (most), 10, 11, 14, 18 and 30, about one-half. Poliovirus, coxsackievirus (group A, types 2, 3, 4, 7, 9 and 10), arboviruses, measles, herpes simplex and varicella viruses, lymphocytic choriomeningitis virus, adenovirus and others are responsible for sporadic cases. The incidence of specific types varies with geographic location and time. Leptospira may be responsible for up to 20% of cases of "aseptic" meningitis in various areas of the world (see Leptospirosis).

3. **Occurrence**—Worldwide, as epidemics and sporadic cases. Actual incidence is unknown. Seasonal increases in late summer and early autumn are due mainly to arboviruses and enteroviruses, while late winter

outbreaks may be due mainly to mumps.

4., 5., 6., 7., and 8. Reservoir, Mode of transmission, Incubation period, Period of communicability, and Susceptibility and resistance—Vary with the specific infectious agent (refer to specific disease chapters).

9. **Methods of control**—

A. *Preventive measures:* Depend on etiology (see specific disease).

B. *Control of patient, contacts and the immediate environment:*

1) Report to local health authority: In selected endemic areas (USA); in many countries, not a reportable disease, Class 3B (see Preface). If confirmed by laboratory means, specify the infectious agent; otherwise, report as cause undetermined.

2) Isolation: Specific diagnosis depends on laboratory data not usually available until after recovery. Therefore, enteric precautions are indicated for 7 days after onset of illness unless a nonenteroviral diagnosis is established.

3) Concurrent disinfection: No special precautions are needed beyond routine sanitary practices.

4) Quarantine: None.

5) Immunization of contacts: See specific disease.

6) Investigation of contacts and source of infection: Not usually indicated.

7) Specific treatment: None for the usual causative viral agents.

C. *Epidemic measures:* See specific disease.

D. *Disaster implications:* None.

E. *International measures:* WHO Collaborating Centres (see Preface).

II. BACTERIAL MENINGITIS   ICD-9 320

The reported incidence of bacterial meningitis is 6/100,000 per year in the USA, and at least two-thirds of the cases are in children under 5. Any agent may cause infection at any age, but generally, *Haemophilus influenzae* serotype b is the predominant agent in children under five years of age; *Streptococcus pneumoniae* in people above that age. Meningococcal disease occurs sporadically and in epidemics; in many parts of the world, it is the leading cause of bacterial meningitis. The less common bacterial causes of meningitis, such as staphylococci, enteric bacteria, Group B streptococci and listeria, occur in persons with specific susceptibilities (such as neonates and patients with impaired immunity) or as the consequence of head trauma.

II A. MENINGOCOCCAL MENINGITIS   ICD-9 036.0
(Meningococcal infection, Cerebrospinal fever, Meningococcemia)

1. **Identification**—An acute bacterial disease characterized by sudden onset with fever, intense headache, nausea and often vomiting, stiff neck and, frequently, a petechial rash with pink macules or, very rarely, vesicles. Delirium and coma often appear; occasional fulminating cases exhibit sudden prostration, ecchymoses and shock at onset. Formerly, case fatality rates exceeded 50%, but with early diagnosis, modern therapy and supportive measures, the case fatality rate should be <10%.

Meningococcal infection may be asymptomatic, be restricted to the nasopharynx, or exhibit upper respiratory tract symptoms. It may cause meningococcal pneumonia, be invasive with acutely ill septicemic patients (two-thirds of whom show a petechial rash, sometimes with joint involvement), or be meningeal. In invasive disease, meningococcemia may occur without extension to the meninges and should be suspected in cases of otherwise unexplained acute febrile illness associated with petechial rash and leukocytosis. In fulminating meningococcemia, the death rate remains high despite prompt antibacterial treatment.

Diagnosis is confirmed by the demonstration of typical organisms in a Gram-stained smear of CSF and the recovery of meningococci from the CSF or blood. Microscopic examination of stained smears from petechiae may reveal organisms. Group-specific meningococcal polysaccharides may also be identified in CSF by LA, CIE, and coagglutination techniques.

2. **Infectious agent**—*Neisseria meningitidis*, the meningococcus. Group A organisms have caused the major epidemics in the USA (none since 1945) and elsewhere; presently, groups B and C are responsible for most cases in the USA. Certain serotypes (e.g., 2b and 15) have been associated with outbreaks of group B disease. Additional serogroups have been recognized as pathogens in recent years (e.g., groups W-135, X, Y and Z). Organisms belonging to some of these serogroups may be less virulent, but fatal infections and secondary cases have occurred with all.

3. **Occurrence**—Meningococcal infections are ubiquitous. Greatest incidence occurs during winter and spring; epidemics occur irregularly. Meningococcal disease, while primarily a disease of very small children, occurs commonly in children and young adults, in males more than in females, and more commonly among newly aggregated adults under crowded living conditions, such as in barracks and institutions. An area of high incidence has existed for many years in the sub-Saharan region of mid-Africa, caused by group A organisms. Epidemic group C disease was followed by a major group A epidemic in Brazil from 1974 to 1978. More recently, there have been group A epidemics in Nepal and India, as well

as in Ethiopia, Sudan and other African countries.

4. **Reservoir**—Man.

5. **Mode of transmission**—By direct contact, including respiratory droplets from nose and throat of infected persons; infection usually causes only an acute nasopharyngitis or a subclinical mucosal infection; invasion sufficient to cause systemic disease is comparatively rare. Carrier prevalence of ≥25% may exist without cases of meningitis. During epidemics, over half the men in a military unit may be healthy carriers of pathogenic meningococci. Fomite transmission is insignificant.

6. **Incubation period**—Varies from 2 to 10 days, commonly 3-4 days.

7. **Period of communicability**—Until meningococci are no longer present in discharges from nose and mouth. If the organisms are sensitive to sulfonamides, meningococci usually disappear from the nasopharynx within 24 hours after institution of treatment. Penicillin will temporarily suppress the organisms, but it does not usually eradicate them from the oro-nasopharynx.

8. **Susceptibility and resistance**—Susceptibility to the clinical disease is low and decreases with age; a high ratio of carriers to cases prevails. Those who are deficient in certain complement components are especially prone to recurrent disease. Group-specific immunity of unknown duration follows even subclinical infections.

9. **Methods of control**—

A. *Preventive measures:*

1) Educate the public on the need to reduce direct contact and exposure to droplet infection.

2) Reduce overcrowding in living quarters and workplaces, such as barracks, schools, camps and ships.

3) Vaccines containing group A, C, Y and W-135 meningococcal polysaccharides have been licensed in the USA and other countries for use in adults and older children; currently the quadrivalent vaccine is available in the USA. The vaccine is effective in adults and has been given to military recruits in the USA since 1971. Unfortunately, the C component is poorly immunogenic and ineffective in children under 2 years of age. Serogroup A vaccine is probably effective in younger children; however, for those 3 months to 2 years of age, 2 doses are given 3 months apart instead of the single dose given those over 2 years of age. The duration of protection is limited in children 1-3 years old. Routine immunization of civilians is not recommended. The risk to travelers planning to have prolonged contact with the local popu-

lace in countries experiencing epidemic meningococcal A or C diseases will be reduced by immunization. No vaccine effective against group B meningococci is currently available.

B. *Control of patient, contacts and the immediate environment:*

1) Report to local health authority: Obligatory case report in most states (USA) and countries, Class 2A (see Preface).

2) Isolation: Respiratory isolation for 24 hours after start of chemotherapy.

3) Concurrent disinfection: Of discharges from the nose and throat and articles soiled therewith. Terminal cleaning.

4) Quarantine: None.

5) Protection of contacts: Close surveillance of household and other intimate contacts for early signs of illness, especially fever, to initiate appropriate therapy without delay; prophylactic administration of an effective agent to intimate contacts, which can be defined as household contacts and persons socially close enough to have shared eating utensils (i.e., close friends at school but not the whole class).

Younger children in day-care centers are exceptions and, even if not close friends, should all be given prophylaxis after an index case is identified. If the organisms in the outbreak are sulfonamide-resistant or of unknown sulfonamide sensitivity, rifampin can be used, giving adults 600 mg twice a day for 2 days; children over 1 month old, 10 mg/kg; and for those less than 1 month old, 5 mg/kg. For adults, ceftriaxone, 250 mg IM, given in a single dose is effective; 125 mg IM for children under 15 years of age. Ciprofloxacin, 500 mg, may be given as a single oral dose to adults. If the organisms have been shown to be sensitive to sulfadiazine, it may be given to adults and older children at a dosage of 1.0 g every 12 hours for 4 doses; for infants and children, the dosage is 125-150 mg/kg/day divided into 4 equal doses, on each of 2 consecutive days. Health care personnel are rarely at risk even when caring for infected patients; only intimate exposure to nasopharyngeal secretions (e.g., as in mouth-to-mouth resuscitation) warrants prophylaxis. Vaccination of close household contacts is of no practical value.

6) Investigation of contacts and source of infection: Throat or nasopharyngeal cultures are of no value in control since carriage is variable and there is no consistent relationship between that found in the normal population and in an epidemic. The information derived can not be

used to decide who should receive prophylaxis.

7) Specific treatment: Penicillin given parenterally in adequate doses is the drug of choice for proven meningococcal disease; ampicillin and chloramphenicol are also effective. Treatment should begin immediately when the presumptive clinical diagnosis is made even before meningococci have been identified; in children, until the specific etiologic agent has been identified, the therapy must be effective against H. influenzae as well as S. pneumoniae.

While ampicillin is the drug of choice for both, as long as the organisms are ampicillin-sensitive, it should be combined with a third-generation cephalosporin or chloramphenicol in the many places where ampicillin-resistant H. influenzae strains are known to occur. The patient should be given rifampin prior to discharge from the hospital to assure elimination of the organism.

If the outbreak of meningococcal meningitis is caused by strains shown to be sulfonamide-sensitive, sulfadiazine IV may be given; however, sulfonamide-resistant strains of groups B and C, and recently group A meningococci, are commonplace in many parts of the world.

C. *Epidemic measures:*

1) When an outbreak occurs, major emphasis must be placed on careful surveillance, early diagnosis, and immediate treatment of suspected cases. A high index of suspicion is invaluable.

2) Separate individuals, and ventilate living and sleeping quarters of all persons who are exposed to infection because of crowding or congested living conditions, e.g., soldiers, miners and prisoners.

3) When the epidemic strain is sulfonamide-sensitive, mass chemoprophylaxis of a closed community with sulfadiazine (0.5 g for children, 1.0 g for adults, every 12 hours for 4 doses) reduces the carrier rate and limits spread of the infection. Because of the current widespread prevalence of sulfonamide-resistant meningococcal strains throughout the world, sulfonamide prophylaxis should not be instituted unless <5% of the strains obtained from cases or from a statistically valid sample of the carrier population show sulfonamide resistance (resistant strains are those resistant to more than 10 μg% of sulfadiazine). Rifampin reduces the carrier rate and limits spread of infection when the entire community is treated; however, since its use has been associated with the appearance of

resistant strains, this drug is not recommended for mass prophylaxis. It may be advisable to administer prophylaxis to all intimate contacts (see 9B5, above).

4) The use of vaccine should be considered for groups in which the cases are due to group A, C, W-135 or Y (see 9A3, above).

D. *Disaster implications:* Epidemics may develop in situations of forced crowding.

E. *International measures:* WHO Collaborating Centres (see Preface). While not covered by International Health Regulations, a valid certificate of vaccination against meningococcal meningitis may be required by some countries, as by Saudi Arabia for religious visitors.

II B. HAEMOPHILUS MENINGITIS ICD-9 320.0
(Meningitis due to *Haemophilus influenzae*)

1. **Identification**—This is the most common bacterial meningitis in children 2 months to 5 years of age in the USA. It is usually associated with a bacteremia. The onset can be subacute or (usually) sudden; symptoms are those of fever, vomiting, lethargy and meningeal irritation, with bulging fontanelle in infants or stiff neck and back in older children. Progressive stupor or coma is common. Occasionally, there is a low-grade fever for several days, with more subtle CNS symptoms.

Diagnosis may be made by isolation of organisms from blood or CSF. Specific capsular polysaccharide may be identified by CIE or LA techniques.

2. **Infectious agent**—Most commonly *Haemophilus influenzae* serotype b. This organism also may cause epiglottitis, pneumonia, septic arthritis, cellulitis, pericarditis, empyema and osteomyelitis. Other serogroups rarely cause meningitis.

3. **Occurrence**—Worldwide; most prevalent in the 2-month to 3-year age group; unusual over the age of 5 years. In developing countries, peak incidence is in children less than 6 months of age; in the USA, it is in children 6-12 months of age. Secondary cases may occur in families and day-care centers.

4. **Reservoir**—Man.

5. **Mode of transmission**—By droplet infection and discharges from nose and throat during the infectious period. The portal of entry is most commonly nasopharyngeal.

6. **Incubation period**—Unknown; probably short, 2-4 days.

7. **Period of communicability**—As long as organisms are present, which may be for a prolonged period even without nasal discharge.

Noncommunicable within 24-48 hours after starting effective antibiotic therapy.

8. Susceptibility and resistance—Assumed to be universal. Immunity is associated with the presence of circulating bactericidal and/or anticapsular antibody, acquired either transplacentally or from prior infection.

9. Methods of control—

A. *Preventive measures:*

1) Monitor for cases occurring in susceptible population settings, such as day-care centers and large foster homes.

2) Educate parents regarding the risk of secondary cases in siblings under 4 years old and the need for prompt evaluation and treatment if fever or stiff neck develops.

3) A protein-polysaccharide conjugate vaccine has been shown to prevent meningitis in children over 18 months of age and is licensed in the USA. It is recommended for routine use for all children at 18 months of age.

B. *Control of patient, contacts and the immediate environment:*

1) Report to local health authority: In selected endemic areas (USA), Class 3B (see Preface).

2) Isolation: Respiratory isolation for 24 hours after start of chemotherapy.

3) Concurrent disinfection: None.

4) Quarantine: None.

5) Protection of contacts: Rifampin prophylaxis (orally once daily for 4 days in a 20 mg/kg dose, maximal dose 600 mg/day) for all household contacts (including adults) in households where there are children (other than the index case) less than 4 years old. Rifampin prophylaxis of staff and children in day-care center classrooms can be considered when one case has occurred, but is recommended when 2 cases occur among the children, and children less than 2 years old have been exposed.

6) Investigation of contacts and source of infection: Observe contacts under 6 years old, and especially infants, including those in household, day-care centers and nurseries, for signs of illness, especially fever.

7) Specific treatment: Ampicillin has been the drug of choice (parenteral 200-400 mg/kg/day). However, since 10-35% of strains are now resistant due to β-lactamase production, chloramphenicol, ceftriaxone or other third-generation cephalosporins are recommended concurrently or singly until antibiotic sensitivities are known. The patient

should be given rifampin prior to discharge from the
hospital to assure elimination of the organism.

C. *Epidemic measures:* Not applicable.

D. *Disaster implications:* None.

E. *International measures:* None.

PNEUMOCOCCAL MENINGITIS ICD-9 320.1

Pneumococcal meningitis has a high case fatality rate. It is usually
fulminant and occurs with bacteremia but not necessarily with any other
focus, although there may be otitis media or mastoiditis. The onset is
usually sudden with high fever, lethargy or coma, and signs of meningeal
irritation. It is a sporadic disease in young infants, the elderly and in
certain high-risk groups, including asplenic and hypogammaglobulinemic
patients. Basilar fracture causing persistent communication with the
nasopharynx is a predisposing factor. (See Pneumonia, pneumococcal.)

NEONATAL MENINGITIS ICD-9 320.8

Infants with neonatal meningitis develop lethargy, seizures, apneic
episodes, poor feeding, hypo- or hyperthermia, and sometimes respiratory distress in their first week of life. The WBC count may be elevated
or depressed. Culture of the CSF yields either Group B streptococci,
Listeria monocytogenes (see Listeriosis) or *E. coli* K-1, acquired from the
birth canal. Infants 2 weeks to 2 months of age may develop similar
symptoms, with recovery from the CSF of Group B streptococci or
organisms of the *Klebsiella-Enterobacter-Serratia* group, acquired from the
nursery environment. The meningitis in both groups is associated with
septicemia. Treatment is with ampicillin, plus a third-generation cephalosporin or aminoglycoside, until the etiologic organism has been identified and its antibiotic susceptibilities determined.

MENINGOENCEPHALITIS DUE TO ICD-9 136.2
NAEGLERIA AND *ACANTHAMOEBA*
(Naegleriasis, Primary amebic meningoencephalitis,
Acanthamoebiasis)

1. Identification—A disease of the brain and meninges caused by
free-living amebae that ordinarily are found in water, soil and vegetation.

Two genera – *Naegleria* and *Acanthamoeba* – have been known to cause
meningoencephalitis. *Naegleria* organisms invade the brain and meninges

via the nasal mucosa and olfactory nerve, causing a typical syndrome of fulminating pyogenic meningoencephalitis with sore throat, severe frontal headache, occasional olfactory hallucinations, nausea, vomiting, high fever, nuchal rigidity and somnolence, and death within 10 days, usually on the fifth or sixth day. The disease occurs mainly in active young people of both sexes. *Acanthamoeba* can invade the brain and meninges, probably secondary to entry through a skin lesion, without involvement of the nasal and olfactory tissues, causing a disease characterized by insidious onset and prolonged course.

Diagnosis of the *Naegleria*-type syndrome is made by microscopic examination of wet mount preparations of fresh CSF in which motile amebae may be seen, or by culture on non-nutrient agar seeded with *Escherichia coli, Klebsiella aerogenes* or other suitable *Enterobacter* species. Amebae have been misidentified as macrophages or "gitter cells" and have been mistaken for *Entamoeba histolytica* when microscopic diagnosis is made under low magnification. The trophozoites of *Naegleria* may become flagellated after a few hours in water. The pathogenic *Naegleria* (*N. fowleri*) and *Acanthamoeba* species can be differentiated from each other morphologically and by immunologic tests on CSF and brain tissue.

2. Infectious agents—*Naegleria fowleri* and *Acanthamoeba culbertsoni,* and other species of *Acanthamoeba* (*A. polyphaga, A. castellanii, A. astronyxis*).

3. Occurrence—Over 100 cases of meningoencephalitis caused by *Naegleria* have been reported from the USA (predominantly Virginia, Florida, California, Georgia and Texas). Cases have been reported from Europe (Belgium, Czechoslovakia, England and Ireland), Australia, New Zealand, Papua New Guinea, Thailand, India, West Africa, Venezuela and Panama. Cases in which *Acanthamoeba* invaded the CNS have been reported from Africa, India, Korea, Japan, Peru, Venezuela and the USA (Arizona, California, Louisiana, New York, Pennsylvania, S Carolina, Texas, Utah and Virginia).

4. Reservoir—The organisms are free-living in aquatic and soil habitats.

5. Mode of transmission—*Naegleria* infection is acquired by exposure of the nasal passages to contaminated water, most commonly by diving or swimming in fresh water, especially somewhat stagnant ponds or lakes in areas of warm climate or during late summer, or in thermal springs or in bodies of water warmed by the effluent of industrial plants, or in hot tubs, spas, or inadequately maintained public swimming pools. The *Naegleria* trophozoites colonize the nasal tissues, then invade the brain and meninges by extension along the olfactory nerves. *Acanthamoeba* trophozoites reach the CNS by hematogenous spread, probably from a skin lesion or other site of primary colonization, frequently in chronically ill or immunosuppressed patients with no history of swimming or known source of infection.

6. **Incubation period**—From 3 to 7 days in documented cases of *Naegleria* infection; usually much longer in *Acanthamoeba* infection.

7. **Period of communicability**—No person-to-person transmission has been observed.

8. **Susceptibility and resistance**—Unknown. Apparently healthy individuals develop *Naegleria* infection; immunosuppressed individuals have increased susceptibility to infection with *Acanthamoeba*. *Naegleria* have not been found in asymptomatic individuals; *Acanthamoebae* have been found in the respiratory tract of healthy people.

9. **Methods of control**—

   A. *Preventive measures:*

   1) Educate the public to the dangers of swimming in lakes and ponds where infection is known or presumed to have been acquired, and of allowing such water to be forced into the nose by diving or underwater swimming.
   2) Protect the nasopharynx from exposure to water likely to contain *N. fowleri*. In practice, this is difficult to accomplish since the amebae may occur in a wide variety of aquatic bodies, including swimming pools.
   3) Swimming pools containing residual free chlorine of 1-2 parts/million are considered safe. No infection is known to have been acquired in a standard swimming pool in the USA.

   B. *Control of patient, contacts and the immediate environment:*

   1) Report to local health authority: Not reportable in most countries, Class 3B (see Preface).
   2) Isolation: None.
   3) Concurrent disinfection: None.
   4) Quarantine: None.
   5) Immunization of contacts: Not applicable.
   6) Investigation of contacts and source of infection: A history of swimming or introducing water into the nose within the week prior to onset of symptoms may suggest the source of *Naegleria* infection.
   7) Specific treatment: *N. fowleri* is sensitive to amphotericin B (Fungizone®); recovery has followed intravenous and intrathecal administration of amphotericin B and miconazole in conjunction with oral rifampin. Despite sensitivity of the organisms to antibiotics in laboratory studies, recoveries have been rare.

C. **Epidemic measures:** Multiple cases may occur following exposure to an apparent source of infection. Any grouping of cases warrants prompt epidemiologic investigation and the prohibition of swimming in implicated waters.

D. **Disaster implications:** None.

E. **International measures:** None.

ACANTHAMOEBIASIS OF THE EYE AND SKIN

Species of *Acanthamoeba* (*A. polyphaga*, *A. castellanii*) are widely distributed in the environment and have been associated with corneal lesions in the USA (Texas, New York, California, Ohio, Washington and Pennsylvania), England and the Netherlands. In soft contact lens wearers, home-made saline used as a cleaning or wetting solution, and exposure to spas or hot tubs have been implicated as sources of corneal infection. Chronic granulomatous lesions of the skin have been recorded in the USA (Arizona), Africa (Zambia) and Korea, with or without secondary invasion of the CNS. An infected mandibular bone graft has been recorded.

The amebae in eye and skin lesions usually have been demonstrated in stained smears of scrapings, swabs or aspirates; species identification has been based on immunodiagnostic tests on amebae in cultures, smears or tissue sections. Differentiation from *E. histolytica,* which can also cause skin lesions and eye infection, is necessary.

Prevention among soft contact lens wearers may be achieved by following strictly the wear and care procedures recommended by lens manufacturers and health care professionals. No reliable treatment has been reported, but topical propamidine was reported to be effective in one case; clotrimazole, miconazole and pimaricin have also been recommended.

MOLLUSCUM CONTAGIOSUM   ICD-9 078.0

1. **Identification**—A viral disease of the skin which results in a smooth-surfaced, firm and spherical papule with umbilication of the vertex. The lesions may be flesh-colored, white, translucent or yellow. Most molluscum papules are 2-5 mm in diameter, but giant cell molluscum papules (>15 mm in diameter) are occasionally seen. Lesions in adults are most often on the lower abdominal wall, pubis, genitalia or inner thighs; lesions on children are most often on the face, trunk and

proximal extremities. Lesions tend to disseminate in patients with HIV infection. Occasionally the lesions itch and a linear orientation is seen, suggesting autoinoculation by scratching. Also, in some patients, 50-100 lesions may become confluent and form a single plaque.

Without treatment, molluscum contagiosum persists for 6 months to 2 years. Any one lesion has a life span of 2-3 months. Lesions may resolve spontaneously or as a result of the inflammatory response following trauma or secondary bacterial infection. Treatment (i.e., mechanically removing the molluscum lesions) may shorten the course of the illness.

Diagnosis can be made clinically when multiple lesions are present. For confirmation, the core can be expressed onto a glass slide and examined by ordinary light microscopy for classic basophilic, Feulgen-positive, intracytoplasmic inclusions, the "molluscum bodies" or "Henderson-Paterson bodies." Histology can confirm the diagnosis.

2. Infectious agent—Taxonomic proposal is the genus *Molluscipoxvirus*, comprising two species differentiated by DNA endonuclease cleavage maps; they have not been grown in cell culture.

3. Occurrence—Worldwide. Serologic tests are not well standardized. Inspection of the skin is the only screening technique available. Therefore, epidemiologic studies of the disease have been limited. Population surveys have been conducted only in Papua New Guinea and Fiji, where the peak incidence of the disease is in childhood.

4. Reservoir—Man.

5. Mode of transmission—Usually by direct contact. Transmission is both sexual and nonsexual, the latter including spread via fomites. Autoinoculation is also suspected.

6. Incubation period—For experimental inoculation, 19-50 days; clinical reports, 7 days to 6 months.

7. Period of communicability—Unknown, but probably as long as lesions persist.

8. Susceptibility and resistance—Any age may be affected; more often seen in children. Disease is more common in patients with AIDS, in whom lesions may disseminate.

9. Methods of control—

    A. *Preventive measures:* Avoid contact with affected patients.

    B. *Control of patient, contacts and the immediate environment:*

        1) Report to local health authority: Official report not ordinarily justifiable, Class 5 (see Preface).

        2) Isolation: Generally not indicated. Infected children

should be excluded from close contact sports such as wrestling.

3) Concurrent disinfection: None.

4) Quarantine: None.

5) Immunization of contacts: None.

6) Investigation of contacts and source of infection: Examine sexual partners where applicable.

7) Specific treatment: Indicated to minimize risk of transmission. Curettage with local anesthesia. Freezing with liquid nitrogen has some advocates.

C. *Epidemic measures:* Suspend close contact activities.

D. *Disaster implications:* None.

E. *International measures:* None.

MONONUCLEOSIS, INFECTIOUS   ICD-9 075
(Gammaherpesviral mononucleosis, EBV mononucleosis, Glandular fever, Mono)

1. Identification—An acute viral syndrome characterized clinically by fever, sore throat (often with exudative pharyngotonsillitis) and lymphadenopathy (especially posterior cervical); hematologically by mononucleosis and lymphocytosis of 50% or more, including 10% or more atypical cells; and serologically by the presence of heterophile and EBV antibodies. In young children the disease is generally mild and more difficult to recognize. Jaundice occurs in about 4% of infected young adults although 95% will have abnormal liver function tests; splenomegaly occurs in 50%. Duration is from one to several weeks; the disease is rarely fatal. A chronic form of the disease has been suggested as one of the causes of a sub-set of the Chronic Fatigue Syndrome; this has not been proven.

The causal agent, Epstein-Barr virus (EBV), is also closely associated with the pathogenesis of African Burkitt's lymphoma and nasopharyngeal cancer (see Neoplasia, Malignant). Acute fatal immunoblastic sarcoma may occur, with or without initial features of infectious mononucleosis, in persons with an X-linked immunoproliferative disorder or an acquired defect in the immune system, including AIDS. It involves a polyclonal expansion of EBV-infected B-lymphocytes.

A syndrome resembling infectious mononucleosis clinically and hematologically is probably caused by herpesvirus type 6; it may also be due to cytomegalovirus (another member of the herpesvirus group; see Cytomegalovirus infections), toxoplasmosis (q.v.), and, rarely, certain other viral infections. Differentiation depends on laboratory results; only EBV elicits the heterophile antibody. EBV accounts for over 80% of both heterophile-positive and heterophile-negative cases of the "mono" syndrome.

Laboratory diagnosis is based on the finding of a lymphocytosis exceeding 50% (including 10% or more abnormal forms), abnormalities in liver function tests (SGOT) or an elevated heterophile antibody titer after absorption of the serum with guinea pig kidney. The most sensitive test is the absorbed horse-RBC test, the most specific of the common tests is the beef-cell hemolysin test, and the most frequently used procedure is a commercial, qualitative slide agglutination assay. An immune adherence hemagglutination assay is also a highly sensitive and specific test. Very young children may not show an elevation of the heterophile titer. If available, the IFA test for viral capsid IgM and IgA antibody or early antigen antibody against the causal virus is very helpful in diagnosis of heterophile-negative cases; anti-EB nuclear antibody (EBNA) is usually absent during the acute phase of illness.

2. **Infectious agent**—Epstein-Barr (EB) virus, human (gamma) herpesvirus 4, closely related to other herpes viruses morphologically, but distinct serologically; it infects and transforms B-lymphocytes.

3. **Occurrence**—Worldwide. Infection is common and widespread in early childhood in developing countries and in socioeconomically depressed population groups, where it is usually mild or asymptomatic. Clinically, typical infectious mononucleosis occurs primarily in developed countries where the age of infection is delayed until older childhood and young adulthood, so that it is most commonly recognized in high school and college students. About 50% of those infected will develop infectious mono.

4. **Reservoir**—Man.

5. **Mode of transmission**—Person-to-person spread by the oropharyngeal route, via saliva. Young children may be infected by saliva on the hands of nurses and other attendants, on toys, or by pre-chewing of baby food by the mother in developing countries; kissing facilitates spread among young adults. Spread may also occur via blood transfusion to susceptible recipients, but ensuing clinical disease is uncommon. Reactivated EBV may play a role in the interstitial pneumonia of HIV-infected infants and in B-cell tumors in HIV-infected adults.

6. **Incubation period**—From 4 to 6 weeks.

7. **Period of communicability**—Prolonged; pharyngeal excretion may persist for a year or more after infection; ≥15-20% of EBV antibody-positive healthy adults are long-term oropharyngeal carriers.

8. **Susceptibility and resistance**—Susceptibility is general. Infection confers a high degree of resistance; immunity from unrecognized child-

hood infection may account for low rates of clinical disease in lower socioeconomic groups. Reactivation of EBV may occur in immunodeficient individuals resulting in elevated antibody titers to EBV.

9. **Methods of control—**

A. *Preventive measures:* Undetermined. Use hygienic measures including handwashing to help prevent spread.

B. *Control of patient, contacts and the immediate environment:*

1) Report to local health authority: Official report not ordinarily justifiable, Class 5 (see Preface).
2) Isolation: None.
3) Concurrent disinfection: Of articles soiled with nose and throat discharges.
4) Quarantine: None.
5) Immunization of contacts: None.
6) Investigation of contacts and source of infection: For the individual case, of little value.
7) Specific treatment: None. Steroids may be of some value in severe toxic cases.

C. *Epidemic measures:* None.

D. *Disaster implications:* None.

E. *International measures:* None.

MUMPS
(Infectious parotitis)

ICD-9 072

1. **Identification**—An acute viral disease characterized by fever, swelling and tenderness of one or more salivary glands, usually the parotid and sometimes the sublingual or submaxillary glands. Orchitis, usually unilateral, occurs in 20-30% of postpubertal males and oophoritis in about 5% of females affected after puberty; sterility is an extremely rare sequel. The CNS is frequently involved, either early or late in the disease, usually as an aseptic meningitis, almost always without sequelae. Encephalitis reports range as high as 5/1000; case fatality rate has averaged 1.4%. Meningoencephalitis and orchitis may occur without salivary gland involvement. Permanent nerve deafness, usually unilateral, is a rare complication. Pancreatitis, neuritis, arthritis, mastitis, nephritis, thyroiditis and pericarditis may occur. Death is a rare outcome. Mumps infection during the first trimester of pregnancy may increase the rate of sponta-

neous abortions, but there is no firm evidence that mumps during pregnancy causes congenital malformations.

Serologic tests (CF, HI, EIA and neutralization) are of value in confirming diagnosis. Skin tests are unreliable. Virus may be isolated in chick embryo or cell cultures from saliva, blood, urine and CSF during the acute phase of the disease.

2. **Infectious agent**—Mumps virus, a member of the genus *Paramyxovirus*, antigenically related to the parainfluenza viruses.

3. **Occurrence**—Mumps is recognized less regularly than other common communicable diseases of childhood, such as measles and chickenpox, although serologic studies show that 85% or more of people have had mumps infection by adult life in the absence of immunization. About one-third of exposed susceptible persons have inapparent infections; most infections in children less than 2 years of age are subclinical. Winter and spring are seasons of greatest prevalence. In the USA, the incidence of mumps has declined dramatically since the wide use of mumps vaccine began after its licensure in 1967. This decline has occurred in all age groups, but with effective pediatric and preschool immunization programs, the greatest risk of infection has shifted toward older children, adolescents and young adults. However, in 1986 and 1987 an increase in reported mumps cases occurred in the USA.

4. **Reservoir**—Man.

5. **Mode of transmission**—By droplet spread and by direct contact with saliva of an infected person.

6. **Incubation period**—About 12 to 25 days, commonly 18 days.

7. **Period of communicability**—The virus has been isolated from saliva from 6-7 days before overt parotitis up to 9 days after; exposed nonimmune persons should be considered infectious from the 12th through 25th day after exposure. Maximum infectiousness occurs about 48 hours before onset of illness. Urine may be positive for as long as 14 days after onset of illness. Inapparent infections can be communicable.

8. **Susceptibility and resistance**—Susceptibility is general. Immunity is generally lifelong and develops after inapparent as well as clinical infections. Most adults, particularly those born before 1957, are likely to have been infected naturally and may be considered to be immune, even if they did not have recognized disease.

9. **Methods of control**—

    A.   *Preventive measures:* Live attenuated vaccine is available either as a single vaccine or in combination with rubella and measles live virus vaccines (MMR), the preparation most often used in the USA. Reported incidence of adverse reactions is dependent on the strain of mumps vaccine used. Fever may occur in 5% of recipients; parotitis, usually unilateral, has been reported in 1% of recipients of one commonly used vaccine about 2 weeks after immunization. Other reactions have been reported rarely. Immunization of persons already immune, either by wild or vaccine virus infection, is not associated with increased risk of adverse reactions. More than 95% of recipients develop a solid immunity which is long-lasting and may be lifelong. Vaccine may be administered any time after 1 year of age; if given in combination with measles vaccine, it should ordinarily be given at or after 15 months of age. Present recommendations for two-dose measles vaccination with MMR will protect against mumps. Special effort should be made to immunize before puberty all persons (especially males) with no definite history of mumps or vaccination. Vaccine is contraindicated in the immunosuppressed, women known to be pregnant should not be given live vaccines. Severe egg or neomycin sensitivity is a relative contraindication; vaccine should be given only under medical supervision. See Measles or Rubella for vaccine storage and transport, and for greater detail on contraindications.

B. *Control of patient, contacts and the immediate environment:*

   1) Report to local health authority: Selectively reportable, Class 3B (see Preface).

   2) Isolation: Respiratory isolation and private room for 9 days from onset of swelling; less if swelling has subsided. Exclusion from school or workplace until 9 days after onset of parotitis.

   3) Concurrent disinfection: Of articles soiled with nose and throat secretions.

   4) Quarantine: Exclusion of susceptibles from school or the workplace from the 12th through the 25th day after exposure.

   5) Immunization of contacts: While immunization after exposure to natural mumps does not protect contacts, it is not contraindicated under such conditions. IG is not effective when administered following exposure.

   6) Investigation of contacts and source of infection: Susceptible contacts should be immunized.

   7) Specific treatment: None.

C. *Epidemic measures:* Immunize susceptibles, especially those at risk of exposure; serologic screening to identify susceptibles is impractical and unnecessary since there is no risk in vaccinating those who are already immune.

D. *Disaster implications:* None.

E. *International measures:* None. Travelers should assure that they are immune to mumps.

MYALGIA, EPIDEMIC   ICD-9 074.1
(Epidemic pleurodynia, Bornholm disease, Devil's grip)

1. **Identification**—An acute viral disease characterized by paroxysms of severe pain localized in the chest or abdomen, which may be intensified by movement, usually accompanied by fever and frequently by headache. The pain tends to be more abdominal than thoracic in infants and young children, while the reverse applies to older children and adults. Most patients recover within one week of onset, but relapses do occur; no fatalities have been reported. Localized epidemics are characteristic. It is important to differentiate from more serious medical or surgical conditions. Complications occur relatively infrequently and include orchitis, pericarditis, pneumonia and aseptic meningitis. During outbreaks of epidemic myalgia, cases of group B coxsackievirus myocarditis of the newborn have been reported; while myocarditis in adults is a rare complication, the possibility should always be considered.

Diagnosis is supported by culture of the virus from throat secretions and feces, and by rise in titer of serum antibodies in paired sera obtained early and late in illness.

2. **Infectious agents**—Group B coxsackievirus types 1-3, 5 and 6, and echoviruses 1 and 6 are associated with the illness. Many group A and B coxsackieviruses and echoviruses have been reported in sporadic cases.

3. **Occurrence**—An uncommon disease, occurring in summer and early autumn; usually seen in children and young adults, ages 5-15, but all ages may be affected. Multiple cases in a household are frequent. Outbreaks have been reported in Europe, Australia, New Zealand and N America.

4. **Reservoir**—Man.

5. **Mode of transmission**—Directly by fecal-oral or respiratory droplet contact with an infected person, or indirectly by contact with articles freshly soiled with feces or throat discharges of an infected person who may or may not have symptoms. Group B coxsackieviruses have been found in sewage and flies, though the relationship to transmission of human infection is not clear.

6. **Incubation period**—Usually 3-5 days.

7. **Period of communicability**—Apparently during the acute stage of disease; stools may contain virus for several weeks.

8. **Susceptibility and resistance**—Susceptibility is probably general and type-specific immunity presumably results from infection.

9. **Methods of control**—

A. *Preventive measures:* None.

B. *Control of patient, contacts and the immediate environment:*

1) Report to local health authority: Obligatory report of epidemics, Class 4 (see Preface).

2) Isolation: Ordinarily limited to enteric precautions. Because of the possibility of serious illness in the newborn, if a patient in a maternity unit or nursery develops an illness suggestive of enterovirus infection, precautions should be instituted at once. Similarly, individuals (including medical personnel) with suspected enterovirus infections should be excluded from visiting maternity and nursery units, and from contact with infants and women near term.

3) Concurrent disinfection: Prompt and safe disposal of respiratory discharges and feces; wash or dispose of articles soiled therewith. Careful attention should be given to prompt handwashing when handling discharges, feces and articles soiled therewith.

4) Quarantine: None.

5) Immunization of contacts: None.

6) Investigation of contacts and source of infection: Of no practical value.

7) Specific treatment: None.

C. *Epidemic measures:* General notice to physicians of the presence of an epidemic and the necessity for differentiation of cases from more serious medical or surgical emergencies.

D. *Disaster implications:* None.

E. *International measures:* None.

MYCETOMA
ACTINOMYCETOMA
EUMYCETOMA
(Maduromycosis, Madura foot)

ICD-9 039
ICD-9 117.4

1. **Identification**—A clinical syndrome caused by a variety of aerobic actinomycetes (bacteria) and eumycetes (fungi), characterized by swelling and suppuration of subcutaneous tissues, and formation of sinus tracts with visible granules in the pus draining from the sinus tracts. Lesions are usually on the foot or lower leg, sometimes on the hand, shoulders and back, and rarely at other sites.

Mycetoma may be difficult to distinguish from chronic osteomyelitis and botryomycosis, the latter being a clinically and pathologically similar entity caused by a variety of bacteria, including staphylococci and Gram-negative bacteria.

Specific diagnosis depends on visualizing the granules in fresh preparations or histopathologic slides and isolation of the causative actinomycete or fungus in culture.

2. **Infectious agents**—Eumycetoma is caused principally by *Madurella mycetomatis, M. grisea, Pseudallescheria (Petriellidium) boydii, Scedosporium (Monosporium) apiospermum, Exophiala (Phialophora) jeanselmei, Acremonium (Cephalosporium) recifei, A. falciforme, Leptosphaeria senegalensis, Neotestudina rosatii,* and *Pyrenochaeta romeroi,* or several other species. Actinomycetoma is caused by *Nocardia brasiliensis, N. asteroides, N. otitidiscaviarum, Actinomadura madurae, A. pelletieri* or *Streptomyces somaliensis.*

3. **Occurrence**—Rare in continental USA; common in Mexico, northern Africa, southern Asia, and other tropical and subtropical areas, especially where people go barefoot (e.g., in Sudan).

4. **Reservoir**—Soil and decaying vegetation.

5. **Mode of transmission**—Subcutaneous implantation of conidia or hyphal elements from a saprophytic source by penetrating wounds (thorns, splinters).

6. **Incubation period**—Usually months.

7. **Period of communicability**—Not transmitted from person to person.

8. **Susceptibility and resistance**—While etiologic agents are widespread in nature, clinical infection is rare, suggesting intrinsic resistance.

9. **Methods of control**—

    A. *Preventive measures:* Protect against puncture wounds by wearing shoes and protective clothing.

B. **Control of patient, contacts and the immediate environment:**

1) Report to local health authority: Official report not ordinarily justifiable, Class 5 (see Preface).
2) Isolation: None.
3) Concurrent disinfection: None. Ordinary cleanliness.
4) Quarantine: None.
5) Immunization of contacts: None.
6) Investigation of contacts and source of infection: Not indicated.
7) Specific treatment: Some patients with eumycetoma may benefit from ketoconazole; some cases of actinomycetoma from sulfones, co-trimoxazole or long-acting sulfonamides. Penicillin and other antibiotics are not useful. Resection of small lesions may be helpful, while amputation of an extremity with advanced lesions may be required.

C. **Epidemic measures:** Not applicable, a sporadic disease.

D. **Disaster implications:** None.

E. **International measures:** WHO Collaborating Centres (see Preface).

NEOPLASIA, MALIGNANT

Infectious agents are now recognized as causes of, or risk factors in, malignant diseases. *Schistosoma haematobium* has been implicated in bladder cancer, *S. japonicum* in colorectal cancer in endemic areas in China, and *Clonorchis sinensis* and *Opisthorchis* in cholangiocarcinoma. Several viruses have been implicated in the pathogenesis of various human malignancies, either directly or indirectly; these malignancies usually represent the late outcome of the viral infection. Co-factors, both external (environmental) and internal (genetic and physiologic at the immunologic and molecular level), may play a role in each of these malignancies. Indeed, viruses and other causal factors appear to be part of a sequence of epidemiologic, immunologic and molecular events that ultimately lead to cancer. The virus is neither a necessary nor sufficient cause of all cases of virus-related malignancy; other causes are involved in some and co-factors are almost always involved. The implicated agents include both DNA and RNA viruses.

The 3 strongest DNA virus candidates as agents directly or indirectly involved in the pathogenesis of human malignancies are: (1) Hepatitis B virus (HBV) in relation to hepatocellular cancer (HCC); (2) Epstein-Barr virus (EBV) in relation to African Burkitt's lymphoma (BL), nasopharyngeal cancer (NPC), acute immunoblastic sarcoma and possibly Hodgkin's disease; some lymphomas occurring in immunosuppressed persons (renal transplant recipients, and X-linked lymphoproliferative disease) are also EBV-related; and (3) human papillomaviruses (HPV) and possibly herpes simplex virus (HSV) in relation to cervical and vulvar cancer. All these viruses are ubiquitous and common agents, worldwide in their distribution, and produce much more inapparent than apparent infection; most result in a latent virus state that is subject to reactivation. The associated malignancies are relatively rare events that occur in special geographic and host settings. Primary infection very early in life and/or reactivation of viral activity during immunosuppression are common features of most virus-related malignancies.

Among the RNA viruses, the retroviruses, including human T-cell lymphotropic virus (HTLV-I) and human immunodeficiency virus (HIV)-1 are associated with human T-cell leukemia/lymphoma and Kaposi sarcoma, respectively. In contrast to oncogenic DNA viruses, these viruses are less ubiquitous, and are more geographically localized; infection appears to occur later in life, but transmission via breast milk may set the stage for later malignancy.

The elements of proof relating these viruses to cancer include: (1) Serologic evidence of higher prevalence and/or higher titers of antibody (or of antigen in the case of HBV) in cases than in controls, with demonstration in prospective studies that these markers precede disease; (2) virologic evidence that the virus, its genome, or virus-specific sequences, are present in the malignant cells (and rarely, if ever, in normal cells or other forms of cancer); (3) demonstration of in vitro oncogenicity, as in transformation of normal cells; (4) experimental evidence that the virus or virus-infected cells can induce a similar malignant disease in animals (especially nonhuman primates) can be demonstrated in the malignant cells, and can be passed serially to other animals; and (5) protective evidence that removal of the virus, or immunization against it, reduces the incidence of tumors.

It cannot be expected that all morphologic examples of a single tumor will have the same cause in all geographic settings and age groups. This section provides brief summaries of the five more important associations.

I. HEPATOCELLULAR CARCINOMA   ICD-9 155.0
(HCC, Primary liver cancer, Primary hepatocellular carcinoma)

1. **Identification**—Primary hepatocellular cancer (PHC) or hepatocellular carcinoma (HCC) is recognized worldwide. It is among the most common malignant neoplasms in China, many parts of Asia, and Africa. It is relatively uncommon in the USA and Europe. Chronic infection with

hepatitis B virus (HBV) is an important risk factor in most cases; hepatitis C may be involved in other cases.

2. **Infectious agent**—There is a positive correlation between the prevalence rate of hepatitis B virus carriers in a geographic area and the incidence of HCC in that area. Prospective studies over 11 years in Taiwan have shown a hundredfold higher risk of HCC in persons chronically infected with HBV than in non-carriers. HBV DNA is demonstrable in HCC tumor cells. HBV viral sequences have been shown to be integrated into host hepatic DNA in patients with HCC. The tumor has not been experimentally reproduced in animals with human-derived virus. However, the woodchuck hepatitis virus, which is structurally and functionally related to HBV, produces a chronic infection which often leads to development of hepatocellular carcinoma. Aflatoxins (see Aspergillosis, section 1), genetic susceptibility, alcohol and other factors may be involved, but HBV appears to be the major risk factor in >85% of HCC cases in high-risk areas. Other cases of chronic hepatitis, cirrhosis, and hepatocellular cancer are probably due to hepatitis C virus.

3. **Occurrence**—HCC occurs with highest frequency in residents of areas with the highest prevalence of HBV carriers. These include Chinese (especially in coastal areas of China), Africans, Filipinos and Eskimos. In Taiwan and Mozambique, it is the most common tumor of young men; it may be the most common cancer overall. The geographic areas of high prevalence of the tumor, such as SE Asia and sub-Saharan Africa, have high prevalence of hepatitis B antigenemia, but there is variation from region to region.

4. **Reservoir**—Man.

5. **Mode of transmission**—HBV is transmitted through blood and body fluids (see Viral hepatitis B, section 5). Most patients go through a stage of liver cirrhosis before development of the tumor. Infection acquired during childhood has the greatest risk of progressing to the carrier state; presence of antigenemia (and especially of e antigen) in the mother results in early infection of the infant and is an important factor leading to chronic infection of the infant and later development of cirrhosis and HCC. Current evidence is that hepatitis C (HCV) is transmitted primarily by transfusions and intravenous drug abusers.

6. **Incubation (induction) period**—Variable. Studies of HBV infection occurring at birth leading to the appearance of the tumor in young adulthood suggest a 15-25 year induction period.

7. **Period of communicability**—Persons who become HBV carriers usually remain infected for life. The presence of hepatitis B e antigen correlates with HBV replication and infectivity. The tumor itself is not communicable.

8. Susceptibility and resistance—All are susceptible to HBV infection. The duration of the carrier state, aflatoxin exposure and alcohol consumption may increase the risk of tumor development.

9. Methods of control—See Viral hepatitis B. Interruption of transmission of HBV infection from mother to infant by administration of HB vaccine alone or HB vaccine plus HBIG to the newborn offers hope of prevention of the tumor. Cases should be reported to a tumor registry.

II. BURKITT'S LYMPHOMA   ICD-9 200.2
(African Burkitt's lymphoma, Endemic Burkitt's lymphoma, Burkitt's tumor)

1. Identification—Burkitt's lymphoma (BL) is a monoclonal tumor of B cells, usually involving African children, in whom jaw involvement is common. The pathologic and morphologic features have been strictly defined. The tumor may also develop in immunosuppressed patients (renal transplant patients, and those with familial and X-linked immunodeficiency, and AIDS). Tumors may be monoclonal, polyclonal or mixed; not all are Burkitt-type, but all are acute lymphoblastic sarcomas.

2. Infectious agent—Epstein-Barr virus (EBV), a herpesvirus that produces the clinical picture of infectious mononucleosis in young adults in developed countries, plays an important pathogenic role in about 97% of BL cases in Africa and Papua New Guinea, where EBV infection occurs in infancy, and malaria, a co-factor, is holoendemic. Both EBV and malaria are B-cell mitogens and induce a polyclonal B-cell proliferation; malaria depresses the T-cell control of B-cell proliferation. EBV is regarded as the initiator and malaria as the promotor of the tumor, but this sequence has not been proven. EBV is also associated with BL in about 30% of cases in low BL-endemic and nonmalarious areas (American BL).

The evidence for the relationship of EBV to African BL consists of: (1) Higher antibody titers against several EBV antigens in cases than in age- and sex-matched indigenous controls, but not against other herpesviruses. A prospective study has shown that the development of IgG antibody to viral capsid antigen precedes development of the tumor by 7-72 months, and that high antibody titers increase the risk of BL thirtyfold; (2) the presence of EBV genome in all tumor cells; (3) the in vitro "immortalization" or transformation of B cells by EBV; and (4) experimental reproduction by EBV of a malignant lymphoma in cotton-top marmosets and owl monkeys.

Chromosomal translocation, usually from chromosome 8 to 14, a characteristic of both EBV and non-EBV-related BL cells, is a genetic mechanism involved in the activation of the c-*myc* oncogene; this and perhaps other factors appear to be necessary for the malignant process.

The chromosomal changes and oncogene occur in both EBV-related and EBV-unrelated B-cell lymphoma.

3. Occurrence—Tumor is worldwide, but is hyperendemic in highly malarious areas, such as tropical Africa and lowland Papua New Guinea. These areas have heavy rainfall (usually >40 inches/year) and are below 3,000 feet elevation. In non-endemic areas only about 30% are EBV-related.

4. Reservoir—Man and perhaps other primates.

5. Mode of transmission—See Mononucleosis, Infectious, section 5. For the development of BL, primary infection usually occurs early in life, or later involves immunosuppression and reactivation of EBV. Malaria may be an important co-factor in Africa and Papua New Guinea.

6. Incubation (induction) period—Estimated at 2-12 years from primary EBV infection; peak onset of tumor after about 6 years. Much shorter in AIDS patients in whom an EBV-related lymphoma (especially of the brain) develops.

7. Period of communicability—See Mononucleosis, Infectious, section 7. The tumor is not communicable.

8. Susceptibility and resistance—Susceptibility to EBV is general; however, tumor development is rare and may occur when infection occurs early in life, usually in the presence of malaria, or in association with immunosuppression, or in genetically susceptible persons. In non-endemic areas, typical BL may occur unrelated to EBV and even in the absence of EBV infection.

9. Methods of control—Prevention of EBV infection early in life and malaria control (see Malaria) might reduce tumor incidence in Africa and Papua New Guinea. Subunit vaccines are in trial stage. Chemotherapy of the tumor is usually effective after the tumor develops. Cases should be reported to a tumor registry.

III. NASOPHARYNGEAL CARCINOMA ICD-9 147.9
(NPC)

1. **Identification**—This is a malignant tumor of the epithelial cells of the nasopharynx usually involving adults between 20 and 40 years of age. There is an approximate tenfold higher incidence in certain groups of Chinese descent from southern China and Taiwan, even in those who have moved elsewhere (including the USA), than in the general population.

IgA antibody to the viral capsid antigen of EBV in both serum and nasopharyngeal secretions is a characteristic feature of the disease, and has been used in China as a screening test for the tumor.

2. **Infectious agent**—The tumor is strongly associated with Epstein-Barr virus (EBV), but causality has not been established. The serologic and virologic evidence relating EBV to NPC is similar to that for African Burkitt's lymphoma (high EBV antibody titers, genome in tumor cells), and this relationship has been found without respect to the geographic origin of the patient. NPC has not been reproduced in experimental animals. Chromosomal changes such as those seen in Burkitt's lymphoma cells have not been found in NPC cells. Exposure to nitrosamines in certain foods may be an important co-factor.

3. **Occurrence**—Worldwide, but highest in southern China, SE Asia, North and East Africa, and in the Arctic. Males outnumber females about 2:1. Chinese persons with HLA-2 and SIN-2 antigen profiles have an approximate fivefold higher risk.

4. **Reservoir**—Only man is known to have the tumor.

5. **Mode of transmission**—EBV is probably transmitted via saliva. Infection occurs early in life in settings where NPC is most common, yet the tumor does not appear until age 20-40, suggesting the occurrence of some secondary, reactivating factor, with epithelial invasion later in life. Repeated respiratory infections or chemical irritants, such as nitrosamines in dried foods, may play a role. The tumor itself is not transmissible.

6. **Incubation period**—Unknown. The tumor occurs in adults; primary EBV infection probably in early childhood.

7. **Period of communicability**—For communicability of the etiologic virus, see Mononucleosis, Infectious, section 7.

8. **Susceptibility and resistance**—Persons of Chinese descent, especially with certain HLA haplotypes, are more susceptible to the tumor. The higher frequency of the tumor in persons of southern Chinese origin, without respect to later residence, and the association with certain HLA haplotypes suggest a genetic susceptibility; however, a lower incidence among those migrating to the USA and elsewhere suggests that possible environmental factor(s) may be associated co-factors.

9. **Methods of control**—None known. Early detection in highly endemic areas by screening for EBV IgA antibodies to viral capsid antigen permits early treatment. A subunit vaccine against EBV infection is under study. Chemotherapy after early recognition is the only specific therapy. Cases should be reported to a tumor registry.

IV. MALIGNANT NEOPLASM OF LYMPHATIC TISSUE   ICD-9 202
(Adult T-cell leukemia [ATL], T-cell lymphosarcoma [TLCL], peripheral T-cell lymphoma [Sézary's disease], Hairy cell leukemia)

1. **Identification**—Leukemias and lymphomas of T-cell origin exist

under the names adult T-cell leukemia (ATL) in Japan; T-cell lymphoma sarcoma-cell leukemia (TLCL) in the Caribbean; and peripheral T-cell lymphoma (Sézary's disease) in the USA. They involve primarily adults and seem to represent similar clinical syndromes, some cases of which are associated with the family of retroviruses called human T-cell lymphotrophic viruses (HTLV).

2. **Infectious agent**—HTLV-I has been implicated in the causation of leukemia/lymphoma by serologic, virologic and epidemiologic evidence. Antibody to HTLV-I in healthy adults is uncommon except in areas where the malignancy occurs. Both the time of acquisition of the antibody and the appearance of the tumors seem to be more common in adulthood, but early infection can occur via breast milk. In southern Japan, where ATL is common, antibody prevalence rates of 5-30% are present in the normal population; rates are higher in relatives of ATL patients, and highest in the cases themselves. The virus has been isolated from affected T-cells of cases, and viral sequences have been identified in such cells. HTLV-II was initially isolated from two cases of hairy cell leukemia; causality has not been established.

3. **Occurrence**—Human T-cell leukemia/lymphoma cases related to HTLV-I have been recognized most commonly in southern Japan and less commonly in the Caribbean Islands, Pacific coast of S America, equatorial Africa and southern USA. Adult Japanese and blacks are at highest risk; males are more often affected than females. Antibodies against HTLV-II are frequently found among intravenous drug abusers; pathogenicity has not been defined.

4. **Reservoir**—Human and probably other primates are infected with HTLV strains; the tumor has been found only in man.

5. **Mode of transmission**—Mother to child transmission through blood or breast milk is best established; transfer of blood or blood products by blood donation or intravenous drug abuse, and sexual transmission are probable.

6. **Incubation period**—Unknown.

7. **Period of communicability**—Unknown.

8. **Susceptibility and resistance**—The occurrence in Japanese and blacks suggests genetic susceptibility, but environmental causes have not been excluded.

9. **Methods of control**—In general, those for prevention of AIDS (q.v.). Effectiveness of screening donor blood for antibodies against HTLV-I and II has yet to be seen. Report to a tumor registry. In Japan, discontinuance of breast feeding by HTLV-I–infected mothers is under trial.

V. MALIGNANT NEOPLASM OF CERVIX UTERI

ICD-9 180

(Carcinoma of the uterine cervix, Cervical cancer)

1. **Identification**—Cervical cancer is the sixth most common cancer worldwide and occurs with a higher incidence in women who smoke and those with a history of early and frequent intercourse and multiple sexual partners, and often those who belong to the lower socioeconomic groups. Three-quarters of all patients are in developing countries. Human papillomavirus (HPV) and herpesvirus have been implicated in its causation; evidence implicating HPV suggests it may be a necessary but not sufficient factor in the causation of most cases of cervical carcinoma.

2. **Infectious agent**—Human papillomavirus (HPV) has been strongly implicated in the etiology of cervical cancer. While HPV is usually the cause of benign warts and verrucae (see Warts, Viral), evidence of HPV types 16 and 18 has been found in tumor tissue from cervical neoplasia, with the genome demonstrated inside the cells in 80-90% of the neoplasias; other types have been associated with acuminate warts, but only infrequently with true neoplasia. HPV is predominantly latent and non-lytic in stratified epithelial cells. However, HPV also occurs in normal tissues, so firm causal relationships are difficult to establish.

Herpes simplex virus types 1 and 2 (HSV 1, 2), especially in primary genital infections, have been implicated previously in a causal role, mostly on serologic grounds.

Recent cohort studies have failed to demonstrate that persons with HSV infection are at higher risk for cervical cancer than those without; these results cast doubt on the validity of earlier case-control studies. HSV may be a co-factor in some cases along with papillomavirus.

3. **Occurrence**—Worldwide, but higher in certain countries such as Colombia, Chile and Poland. Scandinavian countries and the USA are at intermediate risk; Israel and New Zealand are at low risk. Within each area, women with a history of early onset of sexual activity, frequent intercourse and multiple sexual partners are at highest risk. However, occurrence in nonpromiscuous women in some geographic areas suggests that sexual activity of males may be a critical determinant of the partner's risk of cancer. Persons of low socioeconomic status have more cervical cancer. In the USA, Jewish and Amish women have a lower incidence; black and Puerto Rican women, a higher incidence.

4., 5., 6., 7., 8., and 9. **Reservoir, Mode of transmission, Incubation period, Period of communicability, Susceptibility and resistance, and Methods of control**—See Herpes Simplex and Warts, Viral. Prevention of severe morbidity and mortality is based on screening programs for early detection by Papanicolaou (Pap) smears and surgical excision. Tumors should be reported to a tumor registry.

NOCARDIOSIS   ICD-9 039.9

1. **Identification**—A chronic bacterial disease usually originating in the lungs, which may spread by the blood to produce abscesses of the brain, subcutaneous tissue and other organs; the case fatality rate is high in cases with other than subcutaneous involvement. The frequent isolation of *Nocardia asteroides* from patients with other chronic pulmonary diseases may represent cases of a mild form of nocardiosis. The etiologic organisms also cause actinomycotic mycetomas (q.v.).

Microscopic examination of stained smears of sputum, pus or CSF reveals Gram-positive, weakly acid-fast, branching filaments; culture confirms the identity of the organism. Biopsy or autopsy establishes involvement in causing disease.

2. **Infectious agents**—*Nocardia asteroides, N. brasiliensis,* and *N. otitidiscaviarum;* aerobic actinomycetes.

3. **Occurrence**—An occasional sporadic disease in people and animals in all parts of the world. No evidence of age, sex, or racial differences.

4. **Reservoir**—Soil.

5. **Mode of transmission**—*Nocardia* species are presumed to enter the body principally by inhalation of contaminated dust.

6. **Incubation period**—Uncertain; probably a few days to a few weeks.

7. **Period of communicability**—Not directly transmitted from man or animals to man.

8. **Susceptibility and resistance**—Unknown. Endogenous or iatrogenic adrenal hypercorticism, lipoid pneumonia and pulmonary alveolar proteinosis probably predispose to infection. *Nocardia* species may cause opportunistic infection in patients with compromised immunity.

9. **Methods of control**—

   A. *Preventive measures:* None.

   B. *Control of patient, contacts and the immediate environment:*

   1) Report to local health authority: Official report not ordinarily justifiable, Class 5 (see Preface).
   2) Isolation: None.
   3) Concurrent disinfection: Of discharges and contaminated dressings.

4) Quarantine: None.

5) Immunization of contacts: None.

6) Investigation of contacts and source of infection: Not indicated.

7) Specific treatment: Co-trimoxazole, sulfisoxazole or sulfadiazine are effective in systemic infections if given early and for prolonged periods. Minocycline may be tried in sulfa-allergic patients who do not have brain abscess. Amikacin or high-dose ampicillin has been added to sulfonamides in patients failing to respond.

C. *Epidemic measures:* Not applicable, a sporadic disease.

D. *Disaster implications:* None.

E. *International measures:* None.

ONCHOCERCIASIS   ICD-9 125.3
(River blindness)

1. **Identification**—A chronic, nonfatal filarial disease with fibrous nodules in subcutaneous tissues, particularly of the head and shoulders (America) or pelvic girdle and lower extremities (Africa). The adult worms are found in these nodules which occur superficially and also in deep-seated bundles lying against the periosteum of bones or near joints. The female worm discharges microfilariae which migrate through the skin, often causing an intense pruritic rash, altered pigmentation, edema and atrophy of the skin. Pigment changes, particularly of the lower limbs, give the condition known as "leopard skin," while loss of skin elasticity and lymphadenitis may result in "hanging groin." Microfilariae frequently reach the eye where their invasion and subsequent death cause visual disturbances and blindness. Microfilariae may be found in organs and tissues other than skin and eye but the clinical significance of this is not yet clear; in heavy infections they may also be found in the blood, tears, sputum and urine.

Laboratory diagnosis is made by superficial skin biopsy with demonstration of microfilariae in fresh preparations by microscopic examination following incubation in water or saline; by excising nodules and finding adult worms; in ocular manifestations, by slit-lamp observation of microfilariae in the cornea, anterior chamber or vitreous body; or by finding microfilariae in the urine. In the provocative Mazzotti reaction (which may be dangerous in heavily infected individuals), oral administration of diethylcarbamazine citrate, 25 mg, or topical application of the drug, produces characteristic pruritis; this reaction may occur in low density infections when microfilariae are difficult to demonstrate. Differentiation of the microfilariae from those of other filarial diseases is required in endemic areas.

2. **Infectious agent**—*Onchocerca volvulus*, a filarial worm belonging to the class Nematoda.

3. **Occurrence**—Geographic distribution in the Western Hemisphere is limited to Guatemala (principally on the western slope of the Continental Divide), southern Mexico (states of Chiapas and Oaxaca), Venezuela, small areas in Ecuador, Brazil (states of Amazonas and Goias [new focus]); in Africa south of the Sahara in an area extending from Senegal to Ethiopia down to Angola in the west and Malawi in the east; also in Yemen. In some areas, in West Africa, until recent years, a high percentage of the population was infected in endemic areas, and visual impairment and blindness were serious problems. People abandoned the valleys and migrated to safer higher ground, but there the soils were far less fertile. The disease thus had grave socioeconomic consequences. This problem has now been largely overcome through the activities of the Onchocerciasis Control Programme in West Africa.

4. **Reservoir**—Man. The disease can be experimentally transmitted to chimpanzees, and has been found rarely in nature in gorillas. Other *Onchocerca* species found in animals cannot infect man, but may occur together with *O. volvulus* in the insect vector.

5. **Mode of transmission**—Only by the bite of infected female blackflies of the genus *Simulium:* in Central America mainly *S. ochraceum;* in S America, *S. metallicum* complex, *S. sanguineum/amazonicum* complex, *S. quadrivittatum* and other species; in Africa, *S. damnosum* complex and *S. neavei* complex, as well as *S. albivirgulatum* in Zaire. Microfilariae, ingested by a blackfly feeding on an infected person, penetrate thoracic muscles of the fly, develop into infective larvae, migrate to the cephalic capsule and are liberated on the skin and enter the bite wound during a subsequent bloodmeal.

6. **Incubation period**—Microfilariae are usually found in the skin only 1 year or more after the infective bite, but, in Guatemala, they have been found in children as young as 6 months of age. In Africa, vectors could be infective 7 days after a bloodmeal, but in Guatemala the extrinsic incubation period is measurably longer (up to 14 days) because of lower temperatures.

7. **Period of communicability**—People can infect flies as long as living microfilariae occur in their skin, i.e., for 10-15 years after last infection if untreated. The disease is not directly transmitted from person to person.

8. **Susceptibility and resistance**—Susceptibility is universal. Reinfection of infected persons may occur; severity of disease depends on cumulative effects of the repeated infections.

9. **Methods of control—**

A. *Preventive measures:*

1) Avoid bites of *Simulium* flies by wearing protective clothing and headgear as much as possible or by use of an insect repellent such as diethyltoluamide (Deet®).

2) Identify the vector species and their breeding sites; control the larvae, which usually develop in rapidly running streams and in artificial waterways, by use of biodegradable insecticides such as temephos (Abate®) at low concentrations, spraying 0.05 mg/liter for 10 minutes weekly in the wet season and 0.1 mg/liter for 10 minutes weekly in the dry season. Aerial spraying may be used to ensure coverage of breeding places in large-scale control operations such as in Africa; because of the mountainous terrain such procedures generally are not feasible in Central America. Elimination of *S. neavei,* which develop on crabs, has been effective.

3) Provide facilities for diagnosis and treatment.

B. *Control of patient, contacts and the immediate environment:*

1) Report to local health authority: Official report not ordinarily justifiable, Class 5 (see Preface).

2) Isolation: None.

3) Concurrent disinfection: None.

4) Quarantine: None.

5) Immunization of contacts: None.

6) Investigation of contacts and source of infection: A community problem.

7) Specific treatment: Ivermectin (Mectizan®) is being provided for treatment of onchocerciasis by Merck and Company. Given in a single oral dose of 150 µg/kg, with annual retreatment, this drug reduces the microfilarial load and morbidity; it kills microfilariae and also blocks the release of microfilariae from the uterus of the adult worm, effectively suppressing the number of microfilariae in the skin and eyes over a period of 6 to 12 months.

Diethylcarbamazine citrate (DEC, Banocide®, Hetrazan®, Notezine®) is effective against microfilariae but may cause severe adverse reactions which may respond to corticosteroids. DEC is no longer recommended for treatment of onchocerciasis other than in conjunction with suramin for full treatment of selected patients. Suramin (Bayer 205, Naphuride®, Antrypol®), which is available in the USA from CDC, Atlanta (see Preface), kills the adult worms and leads to gradual disappearance of microfilariae. Nephrotoxicity and other undesirable reactions may occur so its use requires close medical supervision. Neither drug is suited for mass treatment because of the possible serious side effects. In Central America where nodules commonly occur on the head, their excision is often carried out, as this may reduce symptoms and prevent blindness.

C. *Epidemic measures:* In areas of high prevalence, make concerted effort to reduce incidence, taking measures listed under 9A.

D. *Disaster implications:* None.

E. *International measures:* The Onchocerciasis Control Programme, a coordinated program in West Africa sponsored by the World Bank, UNDP, FAO and WHO, covers the area in 11 countries where the savanna form of the disease is endemic. Control has been based mainly on anti-blackfly measures, with insecticides applied systematically to the breeding sites in the rivers of the area. Ivermectin is now being distributed to communities on an ever-increasing scale as a supplement to larviciding.

ORF VIRUS DISEASE   ICD-9 051.2
(Contagious pustular dermatitis, Human orf, Ecthyma contagiosum)

1. **Identification**—A proliferative cutaneous viral disease transmissible to man by contact with infected sheep and goats, and occasionally wild ungulates (deer, reindeer). The lesion in man, usually solitary and located on hands, arms or face, is maculopapular or pustular, progressing to a weeping nodule with central umbilication. There may be several lesions, each measuring up to 3 cm in diameter, lasting 3-6 weeks. With secondary bacterial infection, lesions may become pustular. Regional adenitis occurs in a minority of cases. Erythema multiforme and erythema multiforme bullosum are rare complications. Disseminated disease and serious ocular damage have been reported. The disease has been confused with cutaneous anthrax and malignancy.

Diagnosis is made by a history of contact with sheep, goats or wild ungulates, and, in particular, their young; by EM demonstration of ovoid parapoxvirions in the lesion; by negative conventional bacteriology; by growth of the virus in cell cultures of ovine, bovine or primate origin; or by positive results of serologic tests.

2. **Infectious agent**—Orf virus, a DNA virus belonging to the genus *Parapoxvirus* of Poxviruses (family Poxviridae). The causative agent is closely related to other parapoxviruses which can be transmitted to humans as occupational diseases—milker's nodule virus of dairy cattle and bovine papular stomatitis virus of beef cattle. Contagious ecthyma parapoxvirus of domesticated camels may infect man on rare occasion.

3. **Occurrence**—Probably worldwide among farm workers, shepherds, veterinarians and abattoir workers in areas producing sheep and goats; an important occupational disease in New Zealand.

4. **Reservoir**—Probably in various ungulates (e.g., sheep, goats, reindeer and musk oxen). The virus is very resistant to physical factors, except UV light, and may persist in the environment and on animal skin and hair.

5. **Mode of transmission**—By direct contact with the mucous membranes of infected animals, with lesions on udders of nursing dams, or through intermediate passive transfer from apparently normal animals contaminated by contact, knives, shears, stall manger and sides, trucks and clothing. Person-to-person transmission is rare. Human infection may follow production and administration of vaccines to animals.

6. **Incubation period**—Generally 3-6 days.

7. **Period of communicability**—Unknown. Human lesions show a decrease in the number of virus particles as the disease progresses.

8. **Susceptibility and resistance**—Susceptibility is probably universal; recovery produces variable levels of immunity.

9. **Methods of control**—

   A. *Preventive measures:* Good personal hygiene and washing the exposed area with soap and water. Domestic and wild ungulates should be considered a potential source of infection. General cleanliness of animal housing areas. The efficacy and safety of parapoxvirus vaccines in animals has not been fully determined.

   B. *Control of patient, contacts and the immediate environment:*

      1) Report to local health authority: Not required, but desirable when a human case occurs in areas not previously known to have the infection, Class 5 (see Preface).

      2) Isolation: None.

3) Concurrent disinfection: Boil, autoclave or incinerate dressings.
4) Quarantine: None.
5) Immunization of contacts: None.
6) Investigation of contacts and source of infection: Important to secure history of contact.
7) Specific treatment: None.

C. *Epidemic measures:* None.

D. *Disaster implications:* None.

E. *International measures:* None for people.

PARACOCCIDIOIDOMYCOSIS   ICD-9 116.1
(South American blastomycosis, Paracoccidioidal granuloma)

1. **Identification**—A serious and at times fatal chronic mycosis characterized by patchy pulmonary infiltrates and/or ulcerative lesions of the mucosa (oral, nasal, GI) and of the skin. Lymphadenopathy is frequent. In disseminated cases all viscera may be affected; adrenal glands are especially susceptible.

Keloidal blastomycosis (Lobo's disease), a disease with only skin involvement, formerly confused with paracoccidioidomycosis, is caused by *Loboa loboi,* a fungus known only in its tissue form and not yet grown in culture.

Diagnosis is confirmed histologically or by cultivation of the infectious agent. Serologic techniques may assist in diagnosis.

2. **Infectious agent**—*Paracoccidioides brasiliensis,* a dimorphic fungus.

3. **Occurrence**—Endemic in the tropical and subtropical regions of S America and, to a lesser extent, of Central America and Mexico. Workers in contact with soil such as farmers, laborers and construction workers are especially at risk. Highest incidence is in adults aged 30-50 years; much more common in males than in females.

4. **Reservoir**—Presumably soil or fungus-laden dust.

5. **Mode of transmission**—Presumably acquired through inhalation of contaminated soil or dust.

6. **Incubation period**—Highly variable, from 1 month to many years.

7. **Period of communicability**—Direct transmission of clinical disease from person to person is not known.

8. Susceptibility and resistance—Unknown.

9. Methods of control—

A. *Preventive measures:* None.

B. *Control of patient, contacts and the immediate environment:*

1) Report to local health authority: Official report not ordinarily justifiable, Class 5 (see Preface).
2) Isolation: None.
3) Concurrent disinfection: Of discharges and contaminated articles. Terminal cleaning.
4) Quarantine: None.
5) Immunization of contacts: None.
6) Investigation of contacts and source of infection: Not indicated.
7) Specific treatment: Ketoconazole appears to be the drug of choice for all but the patients ill enough to require hospitalization, who should receive amphotericin B (Fungizone®) IV followed by prolonged therapy with ketoconazole. Sulfonamides are cheaper but less effective than ketoconazole.

C. *Epidemic measures:* Not applicable, a sporadic disease.

D. *Disaster implications:* None.

E. *International measures:* None.

PARAGONIMIASIS   ICD-9 121.2
(Pulmonary distomiasis, Lung fluke disease)

1. Identification—Clinically, the lungs are most frequently involved in this trematode disease. Symptoms are cough, hemoptysis, and occasionally, pleuritic chest pain. X-ray lesions may include diffuse and/or segmental infiltrates, nodules, cavities, ring cysts and/or pleural effusions. Localization in other organs is not infrequent, with worms in such sites as the CNS, subcutaneous tissues, intestinal wall, lymph nodes and genitourinary tract. Infection usually lasts for years and the infected person may appear essentially well. The disease may be mistaken for tuberculosis on chest x-rays of Asian immigrants.

The sputum generally contains orange-brown flecks, sometimes diffusely distributed, in which masses of eggs are seen microscopically, establishing the diagnosis. However, acid-fast staining for tuberculosis destroys the eggs and precludes diagnosis. Eggs are also swallowed and may be found in feces, especially when some concentration techniques are used. A highly sensitive and specific immunoblot serologic test has been developed.

2. Infectious agents—*Paragonimus westermani, P. skrjabini* and other species in Asia; *P. africanus* and *P. uterobilateralis* in Africa; *P. mexicanus (P. peruvianus)* and other species in the Americas; and *P. kellicotti* in the USA and Canada.

3. Occurrence—Extensive in Asia, particularly Korea and Japan; scattered foci in Laos, the Philippines and Taiwan, parts of mainland China, SE Asia, Liberia, West and Central Africa; and in S America (Brazil, Colombia, Ecuador, Peru, Venezuela), Central America (Costa Rica), Mexico and, less commonly, the USA and Canada.

4. Reservoir—Man, dog, cat, pig and wild carnivores are definitive hosts and act as reservoirs.

5. Mode of transmission—Infection occurs when the raw or partially cooked flesh of fresh water crabs, such as *Eriocheir* and *Potamon,* and of crayfish such as *Cambaroides,* containing infective larvae (metacercariae) are eaten. The larvae emerge in the duodenum, then penetrate the intestinal wall, migrate through the tissues, become encapsulated, usually in the lungs, and develop into egg-producing adults. Eggs leave the definitive host via sputum and feces, gain access to fresh water, and embryonate in 2-4 weeks. Larvae (miracidia) hatch, penetrate suitable fresh water snails (*Semisulcospira, Thiara, Aroapyrgus* or other genera) and undergo a cycle of development of approximately 2 months. Larvae (cercariae) emerge from the snail and penetrate and encyst in fresh water crabs and crayfish. Pickling of these crustaceans in wine, brine or vinegar, a common practice in Asia, frequently does not kill the encysted larvae.

6. Incubation period—Flukes mature and begin to lay eggs approximately 6 weeks after man ingests infective larvae. The interval until symptoms appear is long, variable, poorly defined, and depends on the organ invaded and the number of worms involved.

7. Period of communicability—Eggs may be discharged by infected people for up to 20 years; duration of infection in mollusc and crustacean hosts is not well defined. Not directly transmitted from person to person.

8. Susceptibility and resistance—Susceptibility is general. Increased resistance possibly develops as a result of infection.

9. Methods of control—

    A. Preventive measures:

        1) Educate the public in endemic areas about the life cycle of the parasite.

2) Stress thorough cooking of crustacea.
3) Dispose of sputum and feces in a sanitary manner.
4) Control snails by molluscicides where feasible.

B. *Control of patient, contacts and the immediate environment:*

1) Report to local health authority: Official report not ordinarily justifiable, Class 5 (see Preface).
2) Isolation: None.
3) Concurrent disinfection: Of sputum and feces.
4) Quarantine: None.
5) Immunization of contacts: None.
6) Investigation of contacts and source of infection: None.
7) Specific treatment: Praziquantel (Biltricide®).

C. *Epidemic measures:* In an endemic area, occurrence of small clusters of cases, or even sporadic infections, is an important signal for examination of local waters for infected snails, crabs and crayfish, and determination of reservoir mammalian hosts to establish appropriate controls.

D. *Disaster implications:* None.

E. *International measures:* WHO Collaborating Centres at Tulane University and in Beijing.

PEDICULOSIS   ICD-9 132

1. **Identification**—Infestation of the head, the hairy parts of the body and clothing (especially along the seams of inner surfaces), with adult lice, larvae and nits (eggs), which results in severe itching and excoriation of the scalp or body. Secondary infection may occur with ensuing regional lymphadenitis (especially cervical). Crab lice usually infest the pubic area; they may also infest hair of the face (including eye lashes), axillae and body surfaces.

2. **Infesting agents**—*Pediculus capitis,* the head louse; *P. humanus,* the body louse; and *Phthirus pubis,* the crab louse. Only the body louse is of major medical importance as the vector of epidemic typhus, trench fever and louse-borne relapsing fever. Lice of lower animals do not infest man, although they may be present transiently.

3. **Occurrence**—Worldwide. Outbreaks of head lice are common among children in schools and institutions.

4. **Reservoir**—People.

5. Mode of transmission—For head and body lice, direct contact with an infested person; for body lice and to a lesser extent for head lice, indirect contact with their personal belongings, especially shared clothing and headgear. While other means are possible, crab lice are most frequently transmitted through sexual contact. Lice leave a febrile host; fever and overcrowding increase transfer from person to person.

6. Incubation period—Under optimal conditions the eggs of lice hatch in a week, and sexual maturity is reached approximately 8-10 days after hatching.

7. Period of communicability—As long as lice or eggs remain alive on the infested person or in clothing.

8. Susceptibility and resistance—Any person may become louse-infested under suitable conditions of exposure. Repeated infestations often result in dermal hypersensitivity.

9. Methods of control

    A. Preventive measures:

        1) Avoid physical contact with infested individuals and their belongings, especially clothing and bedding.

        2) Health education of the public on the value of laundering clothing and bedding in hot water (55°C or 131°F for 20 min.) or dry cleaning to destroy nits and lice.

        3) Regular direct inspection of all primary school children for head lice and, when indicated, of body and clothing; this applies to children in schools, institutions, nursing homes and summer camps.

    B. Control of patient, contacts and the immediate environment:

        1) Report to local health authority: Official report not ordinarily justifiable; school authorities should be informed, Class 5 (see Preface).

        2) Isolation: Contact isolation until 24 hours after application of effective insecticide.

        3) Concurrent disinfection: With body lice among members of a family or group: Clothing, bedding and other appropriate vehicles of transmission (e.g., cosmetic articles) should be treated by laundering in hot water, dry cleaning or application of an effective chemical insecticide and ovicide (see 9B7, below). After chemical treatment has been completed, clothes and laundry facilities should be rinsed.

        4) Quarantine: None.

        5) Immunization of contacts: Does not apply.

        6) Investigation of contacts and source of infection: Exami-

nation of household and other close personal contacts, with concurrent treatment as indicated.

7) Specific treatment: For head and pubic lice: 1% permethrin (a synthetic pyrethroid) creme rinse (NIX®) is highly effective for control of both head lice and nits. It binds to the hair and remains effective for several weeks, so retreatment is not necessary. Other effective agents include pyrethrins synergized with piperonyl butoxide (A-200 Pyrinate®, RID® and XXX®), 1% gamma benzene hexachloride lotions (lindane, Kwell®; not recommended for infants, young children, and pregnant or lactating women), carbaryl and benzyl benzoate. With these agents, retreatment after 7-10 days is recommended to assure that no eggs have survived. The removal of all nits is recommended as a prerequisite for return to school of children previously found infested and treated.

For body lice: Clothing and bedding should be washed with the hot water cycle of an automatic washing machine or dusted with powders containing 1% lindane (if washer not available), or preferably 1% malathion or pyrethrins with piperonyl butoxide or carbaryl (in view of widespread resistance to lindane), and then laundered before using. Abate® (temephos) as a 2% dusting powder is also effective and is recommended by WHO for use in areas where strains of body lice are resistant to malathion.

C. *Epidemic measures:* Mass treatment as recommended in paragraph 9B7, above.

D. *Disaster implications:* Diseases for which *P. humanus* is a vector are particularly prone to occur at times of social upheaval (see Typhus fever, Epidemic).

E. *International measures:* None.

PERTUSSIS
PARAPERTUSSIS
(Whooping Cough)

ICD-9 033.0
ICD-9 033.1

1. **Identification**—An acute bacterial disease involving the respiratory tract. The initial catarrhal stage has an insidious onset with an irritating cough which gradually becomes paroxysmal, usually within 1-2 weeks, and lasts for 1-2 months or longer. Paroxysms are characterized by

repeated violent coughs; each series of paroxysms has many coughs without intervening inhalation and may be followed by a characteristic crowing or high pitched inspiratory whoop. Paroxysms frequently end with the expulsion of clear, tenacious mucus, often followed by vomiting. Infants less than 6 months old and adults often do not have the typical whoop or cough paroxysm. The number of fatalities in the USA is currently low; approximately 90% of deaths are among children under 1 year of age, and 75% are under 6 months. Case fatality rate is 0.5% in infants less than 6 months old in the USA. Morbidity and mortality are higher in females than males. In unimmunized populations, especially those with underlying malnutrition and multiple enteric and respiratory infections, pertussis is among the most lethal diseases of infants and young children. Pneumonia is the most common cause of death; fatal encephalopathy, probably hypoxic, and inanition from repeated vomiting occasionally occur.

In recent years in the USA, pertussis in adolescents and young adults, varying in severity from a mild, atypical respiratory illness to the full-blown syndrome, has been recognized with increasing frequency. Many of these cases occur in previously immunized persons, undoubtedly as a consequence of waning immunity.

Parapertussis is a similar but usually milder disease clinically indistinguishable from pertussis. It is usually seen in school-age children, and occurs relatively infrequently. Differentiation between *Bordetella parapertussis* and *B. pertussis* is based on culture, biochemical and immunologic differences. A similar clinical syndrome has been reported in association with viruses, especially adenoviruses.

Diagnosis is based on the recovery of the etiologic organism from nasopharyngeal swabs obtained during the catarrhal and early paroxysmal stages, or directly on cough plates. Direct FA staining of nasopharyngeal secretions may provide rapid presumptive diagnosis, but requires an experienced laboratory; false-positive and false-negative results can occur. Strikingly high total WBC counts with a strong preponderance of lymphocytes are found as the whooping stage develops; this may not occur in young infants.

2. **Infectious agents**—*Bordetella pertussis,* the pertussis bacillus; *B. parapertussis* causes parapertussis.

3. **Occurrence**—A disease common to children everywhere, regardless of race, climate, or geographic location. There has been a marked decline in incidence and mortality rates during the past four decades, chiefly in communities fostering active immunization and where good nutrition and medical care are available. From 1979-82, an average of 1,750 cases was reported annually in the USA. During 1983-87, reported cases increased to nearly 3,000 annually. In recent years, incidence rates have increased in countries where immunization levels have fallen (e.g., England, Japan and Sweden).

4. **Reservoir**—Man is the only host.

5. **Mode of transmission**—Primarily by direct contact with discharges from respiratory mucous membranes of infected persons by the airborne route, probably by droplets. Frequently brought home by an older sibling and sometimes by a parent.

6. **Incubation period**—Commonly 7 to 10 days, and rarely exceeding 14 days.

7. **Period of communicability**—Highly communicable in the early catarrhal stage before the paroxysmal cough stage. Thereafter, communicability gradually decreases and becomes negligible for ordinary non-familial contacts in about 3 weeks, despite persisting spasmodic cough with whoop. For control purposes, the communicable stage extends from the early catarrhal stage to 3 weeks after onset of typical paroxysms in patients not treated with antibiotics; when treated with erythromycin, the period of infectiousness usually extends only 5 days or less after onset of therapy.

8. **Susceptibility and resistance**—Susceptibility is universal; there is no clear evidence of effective transplacental immunity in infants. It is predominantly a childhood disease; incidence rates of reported (i.e., recognized) disease are highest under 5 years of age. Numerous milder and missed atypical cases occur in all age groups. One attack usually confers prolonged immunity, although second attacks can occasionally occur. Cases in adolescents and adults in the USA occur because of incomplete immunization and waning immunity.

9. **Methods of control**—

A. *Preventive measures:*

1) Educate the public, and particularly parents of infants, to the dangers of whooping cough and to the advantages of initiating immunization at 2 months of age and adhering to the immunization schedule. This is increasingly important because of the wide publicity of the relatively rare adverse reactions.

2) Active immunization is recommended with a vaccine consisting of a suspension of killed bacteria usually in combination with diphtheria and tetanus toxoids adsorbed on aluminum salts (Diphtheria and Tetanus Toxoids and Pertussis Vaccine Adsorbed USP). There is no advantage to nonadsorbed ("plain") preparations (not available in the USA), either for primary immunization or booster shots. In the USA, it is recommended that DTP be given at 2, 4, 6 and 15 to 18 months, with a booster at school entry, but not after the 7th birthday. Some coun-

tries recommend different ages of administration and/or number of doses; e.g., most developing countries use DTP vaccine at 6, 10 and 14 weeks of age. DTP can be given simultaneously with poliovirus (OPV), *Haemophilus influenzae* type b, and measles, mumps and rubella (MMR) vaccines at different sites. In the USA, a family history of convulsive seizures is not considered a contraindication to pertussis vaccine. Antipyretics prevent febrile seizure. Immunization with DTP should be delayed if the child has an intercurrent febrile infection; however, a mild illness without fever, such as a cold, is not a contraindication. In young infants with suspected neurologic disease, initiation of immunization may be delayed for some months (but no later than 1 year of age) to permit the disorder to become clarified, avoid possible confusion about the causation of symptoms, and determine whether the child should receive DT or DTP vaccine. Stable neurologic disorders, such as well-controlled seizures, are not contraindications.

In general, pertussis vaccine is not given to persons 7 years of age or older, since the disease is usually milder, and reactions to the vaccine are alleged to be increased in older children and adults; this has not been substantiated by available data. Vaccinees who experience severe reactions such as convulsions, persistent or unusually severe screaming, collapse, a temperature $>40.5°C$ ($>105°F$), or an encephalopathy should not receive further doses of pertussis-containing vaccines. Less serious systemic and local reactions follow a large proportion of DTP doses and are not contraindications to further pertussis vaccine doses. Pertussis vaccine may not provide complete or permanent immunity; active immunization started after exposure will not protect against disease resulting from that exposure but is not contraindicated. Best protection is obtained by adhering to the recommended schedule. Passive immunization is ineffective, and pertussis IG is no longer available.

3) When there is an outbreak, consider protection of health workers at high risk of exposure by using a 14-day course of erythromycin. Alternatively, the administration of a booster dose of 0.25 ml monovalent pertussis vaccine, if available, may be considered.

B. *Control of patient, contacts and the immediate environment:*

1) Report to local health authority: Case report obligatory in most states (USA) and countries, Class 2B (see Preface).

Early reporting permits better outbreak control.

2) Isolation: Respiratory isolation for known cases. Exclude suspected case from the presence of young children and infants, especially unimmunized infants, until the patient has received at least 5 days of a minimum 14-day course of antibiotics.

3) Concurrent disinfection: Discharges from nose and throat and articles soiled therewith. Terminal cleaning.

4) Quarantine: Inadequately immunized household contacts less than 7 years old should be excluded from schools, day-care centers and public gatherings for 14 days after last exposure or until the cases and contacts have received 5 days of a minimum 14-day course of antibiotics.

5) Protection of contacts: Passive immunization is not effective, and it is too late for the initiation of active immunization to protect against a prior exposure. Close contacts less than 7 years old who have not received 4 DTP doses or have not received a DTP dose within 3 years should be given a DTP dose as soon after exposure as possible. A 14-day course of erythromycin for household and other close contacts, regardless of immunization status, is recommended.

6) Investigation of contacts and source of infection: A search for early, missed and atypical cases is indicated where a nonimmune infant or young child is or might be at risk.

7) Specific treatment: Erythromycin shortens the period of communicability, but does not reduce symptoms except when given during the incubation period or early in the catarrhal stage of the disease.

C. *Epidemic measures:* A search for unrecognized and unreported cases is indicated to protect preschool children from exposure and to assure adequate preventive measures for exposed children less than 7 years old. Accelerated immunization with the first dose at 2 weeks of age, and the second and third doses at 4-week intervals, may be indicated; complete immunizations for those already started.

D. *Disaster implications:* Pertussis could become a problem if introduced into crowded refugee camps with many unimmunized children.

E. *International measures:* Assure completion of primary immunization of infants and young children before they travel to other countries; review need for a booster dose. WHO Collaborating Centres (see Preface).

PINTA
(Carate)

ICD-9 103

1. **Identification**—An acute and chronic nonvenereal treponemal skin infection. A scaling papule with satellite lymphadenopathy appears within 1-8 weeks after infection, usually on the hands, legs or dorsum of the feet. In 3-12 months a maculopapular, erythematous secondary rash appears and may evolve into tertiary splotches of altered skin pigmentation (dyschromic) of variable size. These treponema-containing macules pass through stages of blue to violet to brown pigmentation, finally becoming treponema-free depigmented (achromic) scars. Lesions are in different stages of evolution and are most common on the face and extremities. Organ systems are not involved; physical disability and death do not occur.

Spirochetes are demonstrable in dyschromic (but not achromic) lesions by darkfield or direct FA microscopic examination. Serologic tests for syphilis usually become reactive before or during the secondary rash, and thereafter behave as in venereal syphilis.

2. **Infectious agent**—*Treponema carateum,* a spirochete.

3. **Occurrence**—In the Western Hemisphere, found among isolated rural populations living under crowded unhygienic conditions in tropical areas of Central and S America. Predominantly a disease of older children and adults. Frequent in some Amazonian populations that wear little clothing in the hot humid climate.

4. **Reservoir**—Man.

5. **Mode of transmission**—Presumably person-to-person by direct and prolonged contact with initial and early dyschromic skin lesions; the location of primary lesions suggests that trauma provides a portal of entry. Lesions in children occur in body areas most scratched; various biting and sucking arthropods, especially blackflies, have been suspected but are not proven as biological vectors.

6. **Incubation period**—Usually 2-3 weeks.

7. **Period of communicability**—Unknown; potentially communicable while dyschromic skin lesions are active, sometimes for many years.

8. **Susceptibility and resistance**—Undefined; presumably as in other treponematoses.

9. **Methods of control**—

   A. *Preventive measures:* Those applicable to other nonvenereal treponematoses apply to Pinta; see Yaws, 9A.

B. *Control of patient, contacts and the immediate environment:*

1) Report to local health authority: In selected endemic areas; in most countries not a reportable disease, Class 3B (see Preface).

2), 3), 4), 5), 6), and 7) Isolation, Concurrent disinfection, Quarantine, Immunization of contacts, Investigation of contacts and source of infection, and Specific treatment: Same as for Yaws, 9B, 2) through 7).

C., D., and **E.** *Epidemic measures, Disaster implications* and *International measures:* See Yaws, C, D, and E.

PLAGUE   ICD-9 020
(Peste)

1. **Identification**—A specific zoonosis involving rodents and their fleas, which transfer the bacterial infection to various animals and to people. The initial response is commonly a lymphadenitis in those lymph nodes receiving drainage from the site of the flea bite. This is bubonic plague, and it occurs more often in lymph nodes in the inguinal area and less commonly in those in the axillary and cervical areas. The involved nodes become swollen, inflamed and tender and may suppurate. Fever is usually present. All forms, including instances in which lymphadenopathy is not apparent, may progress to septicemic plague with dissemination by the bloodstream to diverse parts of the body, including the meninges. Secondary involvement of the lungs results in pneumonia; mediastinitis or pleural effusion may develop. Secondary pneumonic plague is of special significance, since aerosolized droplets of sputum may serve as the source of primary pneumonic or of pharyngeal plague. Further person-to-person transfer can result in localized outbreaks or in devastating epidemics.

Untreated bubonic plague has a case fatality rate of about 50%; rarely, it is no more than a localized infection of short duration (pestis minor). Plague organisms have been recovered from throat cultures of asymptomatic contacts of pneumonic plague patients. Untreated primary septicemic plague and pneumonic plague are invariably fatal. Modern therapy markedly reduces fatality from bubonic plague; pneumonic and septicemic plague also respond if recognized and treated early.

A rapid presumptive diagnosis of plague can be made by visualizing bipolar-staining, ovoid, Gram-negative organisms in direct microscopic examination of material aspirated from a bubo, sputum or CSF. Examination by FA test is more specific and is particularly useful in sporadic cases. An antigen-capture ELISA test promises to permit an early rapid diagnosis in acute cases. Diagnosis is confirmed by culture and identification of the causal organism from fluid aspirated from buboes, blood, CSF or sputum, or by a ≥fourfold rise or fall in antibody titer. The passive hemagglutination test (PHA) using *Yersinia pestis* Fraction-1 antigen is most frequently used for serodiagnosis. Medical personnel in areas where the disease occurs often entertain the diagnosis of plague soon after seeing the patient. Visitors to endemic areas are often misdiagnosed when they develop the disease in localities where plague is seldom seen.

2. **Infectious agent**—*Yersinia pestis,* the plague bacillus.

3. **Occurrence**—Plague continues to be a threat because of vast areas of persistent wild rodent infection; contact of wild rodents with domestic rats occurs frequently in some enzootic areas. Wild rodent plague exists in the western third of the USA, large areas of S America, northcentral, eastern and southern Africa, central and SE Asia and Indonesia. There are several natural plague foci within the USSR. Urban plague has been controlled in most of the world; human plague has occurred recently in several countries in Africa (Angola, Kenya, Madagascar, Namibia, S Africa, Mozambique, Tanzania, Uganda, Zimbabwe, Zaire, Libya). Plague is endemic in Indonesia, Myanmar (Burma) and especially in Vietnam where thousands of cases of bubonic plague, both urban and rural, with scattered outbreaks of pneumonic plague, were reported between 1962 and 1972. In the Americas, foci in northeastern Brazil and the Andean region (Peru and Bolivia) continue to produce sporadic cases and occasional outbreaks. Human plague in the USA is sporadic, with only single cases or small common-source clusters in an area, usually following exposure to wild rodents or their fleas. In 1988, there were 15 cases reported; the largest numbers occurred in New Mexico and Colorado. No human-to-human transmission has occurred in the USA since 1924, although secondary plague pneumonia has occurred in about 20% of cases in recent years, and there have even been cases of primary plague pneumonia acquired from pets with secondary plague pneumonia.

4. **Reservoir**—Wild rodents (especially ground squirrels) are the natural reservoir of plague. Lagomorphs (rabbits and hares) and domestic cats may also be a source of infection to people.

5. **Mode of transmission**—Plague in people occurs as a result of human intrusion into the zoonotic (also termed sylvatic or rural) cycle during or following an epizootic, or by the entry of sylvatic rodents or their infected fleas into man's habitat. Domestic pets, particularly house cats, may carry plague-infected wild rodent fleas into homes and occa-

sionally transmit infection by their bites or scratches. Contact by commensal rodents and their fleas with plague among sylvatic rodents may
result in the development of a domestic rat epizootic and epidemic
plague.

The most frequent source of exposure resulting in human disease
worldwide has been the bite of infected fleas (especially *Xenopsylla
cheopis,* the oriental rat flea). Other important sources include the
handling of tissues of infected animals, especially rodents and rabbits, but
also carnivores; airborne droplets from human patients or household pets
(especially cats) with plague pharyngitis or pneumonia; and careless
manipulation of laboratory cultures. Certain occupations and lifestyles
carry an increased risk of exposure. Man-to-man transmission by *Pulex
irritans* fleas is important in the Andean region of S America and in other
places where plague occurs and this "human" flea is abundant.

6. **Incubation period**—From 2 to 6 days; may be a few days longer in
vaccinated individuals. For primary plague pneumonia, 1-6 days, usually
short.

7. **Period of communicability**—Fleas may remain infective for
months under suitable conditions of temperature and humidity. Bubonic
plague is not usually transmitted directly from person to person unless
there is contact with pus from suppurating buboes. Pneumonic plague
may be highly communicable under appropriate climatic conditions;
overcrowding facilitates transmission.

8. **Susceptibility and resistance**—Susceptibility is general. Immunity
after recovery is relative; it may not protect against a large inoculum.

9. **Methods of control**—

    A.   *Preventive measures:* The basic objective is to reduce the
likelihood of people being bitten by infected fleas or of being
exposed to pneumonic plague patients.

        1)   Educate the public in enzootic areas on the modes of
human exposure; the importance of preventing access to
food and shelter by peri-domestic rodents through appropriate storage and disposal of food, garbage and refuse;
and the importance of avoiding flea bites by use of
insecticides and repellents. In sylvatic or rural plague
areas, the public should be warned not to camp near
rodent burrows and to avoid handling, but to report, dead
or sick rodents to health authorities or park rangers. Dogs
and cats in such areas should be treated periodically with
appropriate insecticides.

        2)   Periodically survey rodent populations to determine the
effectiveness of sanitary programs or to evaluate the
potential for epizootic plague. Rat suppression by poison-

ing (see 9B6, below) may be necessary to augment basic environmental sanitation measures; rat control should always be preceded or accompanied by measures to control fleas. Maintain surveillance of natural foci by bacteriologic testing of sick or dead wild rodents and by serologic studies of wild carnivore and outdoor-ranging dog and cat populations in order to define areas of plague activity. Collection and testing of fleas from wild rodents and their nests or burrows may also be appropriate.

3) Control rats on ships and docks and in warehouses by rat-proofing or periodic fumigation, combined when necessary with destruction of rats and their fleas in vessels and in cargoes, especially containerized cargoes, before shipment and upon arrival from plague-endemic locations.

4) Active immunization with a vaccine of killed bacteria confers protection in most recipients for at least several months when administered in a primary series of 2 or 3 doses; booster injections are necessary. Vaccination of persons living in areas of high incidence and of laboratory and field workers handling plague bacilli or infected animals is justifiable but should not be relied upon as the sole preventive measure. Live attenuated vaccines are used in some countries, but they produce more reactions and there is no evidence that they are more protective.

B. *Control of patient, contacts and the immediate environment:*

1) Report to local health authority: Case report of suspected and confirmed cases universally required by International Health Regulations, Class 1 (see Preface).

2) Isolation: Rid patients, and especially their clothing and baggage, of fleas using an insecticide effective against local fleas and known to be safe for people; hospitalize if practical. For patients with bubonic plague, if there is no cough and the chest x-ray is negative, drainage/secretion precautions are indicated for 3 days after start of effective therapy. **For patients with pneumonic plague, strict isolation with precautions against airborne spread is required** until 3 full days of appropriate antibiotic therapy have been completed and there has been a favorable clinical response (see 9B7, below).

3) Concurrent disinfection: Of sputum and purulent discharges and articles soiled therewith. Terminal cleaning. Bodies of persons who died of plague should be handled with strict aseptic precautions.

4) Quarantine: Those who have been in household or face-

to-face contact with patients with pneumonic plague should be provided chemoprophylaxis (see 9B5) and placed under surveillance for 7 days; those who refuse chemoprophylaxis should be maintained in strict isolation with careful surveillance for 7 days.

5) Protection of contacts: In epidemic situations where human fleas are known to be involved, contacts of bubonic plague patients should be disinfested with an appropriate insecticide. All close contacts should be evaluated for chemoprophylaxis. Close contacts of confirmed or suspected plague pneumonia cases (including medical personnel) should be provided with chemoprophylaxis using tetracycline (15-30 mg/kg) or sulfonamides (40 mg/kg) daily in 4 divided doses for one week.

6) Investigation of contacts and source of infection: Search for persons with household or face-to-face exposure to pneumonic plague and for sick or dead rodents and their fleas. Flea control must precede or coincide with antirodent measures. Dust rodent runs, harborages and burrows in and around known or suspected plague areas with an insecticide labeled for flea control and known to be effective against local fleas. If nonburrowing wild rodents are involved, insecticide bait stations can be used. If urban rats are involved, disinfest by dusting the houses, outhouses and household furnishings; dust the persons and clothing of all residents in the immediate vicinity. Suppress rat populations by well-planned and energetic campaigns of poisoning and with vigorous concurrent measures to reduce rat harborages and food sources.

7) Specific treatment: Streptomycin, tetracyclines and chloramphenicol used early (within 8-24 hours after onset of pneumonic plague) are highly effective. After a satisfactory response to drug therapy, some patients will have a self-limited, brief febrile episode on the fifth or sixth day, unaccompanied by any other evidence of illness. Reappearance of fever may result from a secondary infection or a suppurative bubo which may require incision and drainage.

C. *Epidemic measures:*

1) Investigate all possible plague deaths with autopsy and laboratory examinations when indicated. Develop and carry out case-finding. Establish the best possible facilities for diagnosis and treatment. Alert existing medical facilities to report cases immediately and to utilize fully diagnostic and therapeutic services.

2) Attempt to mitigate public hysteria by appropriate informational and educational releases through the press and news media.

3) Institute intensive flea control in expanding circles from known foci.

4) Implement rodent destruction within affected areas **only after satisfactory flea control has been accomplished.**

5) Protect all contacts as noted in 9B5, above.

6) Protect field workers against fleas; dust clothing with insecticide powder and use insect repellents daily.

D. *Disaster implications:* Plague could become a significant problem in endemic areas when there are social upheavals, crowding and unhygienic conditions. See preceding and following paragraphs for appropriate actions.

E. *International measures:*

1) Telegraphic notification within 24 hours by governments to WHO and to adjacent countries of the first imported, first transferred or first nonimported case of plague in any area previously free of the disease. Report newly discovered or reactivated foci of plague among rodents.

2) Measures applicable to ships, aircraft, and land transport arriving from plague areas are specified in International Health Regulations (1969), Third Annotated Edition, 1983, WHO, Geneva.

3) All ships should be free of rodents or periodically de-ratted.

4) Ratproof buildings at seaports and airports; apply appropriate insecticide; de-rat with effective rodenticide.

5) International travelers: International regulations require that prior to their departure on an international voyage from an area where there is an epidemic of pulmonary plague, those suspected shall be placed in isolation for 6 days after last exposure. On arrival of an infested or suspected ship or an infested aircraft, travelers may be disinsected and kept under surveillance for a period of not more than 6 days from the date of arrival. Vaccination against plague cannot be required as a condition of admission to a territory.

6) WHO Collaborating Centres (see Preface).

PNEUMONIA
I. PNEUMOCOCCAL PNEUMONIA   ICD-9 481

1. **Identification**—An acute bacterial infection characterized typically by sudden onset with a shaking chill, fever, pleural pain, dyspnea, a cough productive of "rusty" sputum and leukocytosis. Onset may be less abrupt, especially in the elderly, and chest x-ray may provide the first evidence of pneumonia. In infants, vomiting and convulsions may be the initial manifestations. Consolidation may be bronchopneumonic, especially in children and the aged, rather than segmental or lobar. Pneumococcal pneumonia is an important cause of death in infants and the aged. The case fatality rate, formerly 20-40% among hospitalized patients, has fallen to 5-10% with antimicrobial therapy, but remains 20-40% among patients with substantial underlying disease.

Early etiologic diagnosis is important for treatment. The diagnosis can be suspected from the presence of many Gram-positive diplococci together with polymorphonuclear leukocytes in smears of sputum; it can be confirmed by isolation of pneumococci from blood or from secretions from the lower respiratory tract obtained by percutaneous transtracheal aspiration.

2. **Infectious agent**—*Streptococcus pneumoniae* (pneumococcus). Twenty-three capsular types out of 83 known account for approximately 90% of bacteremic infections in the USA.

3. **Occurrence**—A disease of continuing endemicity, particularly in infancy, old age and individuals with underlying medical conditions; more frequent in industrial cities and lower socioeconomic groups and in developing countries. It occurs in all climates and seasons; incidence is highest in winter and spring in temperate zones. Usually sporadic in the USA, it may occur in epidemics in closed populations and during rapid urbanization. Recurring epidemics have been described in South African miners; incidence is high in certain geographic areas (e.g., Papua New Guinea), and in children in many developing countries. An increased incidence often accompanies epidemics of influenza.

4. **Reservoir**—Man. Pneumococci are commonly found in the upper respiratory tract of healthy persons throughout the world.

5. **Mode of transmission**—By droplet spread, by direct oral contact, or indirectly, through articles freshly soiled with respiratory discharges. Person-to-person transmission of the organisms is common, but illness among casual contacts and attendants is infrequent.

6. **Incubation period**—Not well determined; may be as short as 1-3 days.

7. **Period of communicability**—Presumably until discharges of mouth and nose no longer contain virulent pneumococci in significant

numbers. Penicillin will render the patient noninfectious within 24-48 hours.

8. Susceptibility and resistance—Resistance against disease is generally high but may be lowered by any process affecting the anatomic or physiologic integrity of the lower respiratory tract, including influenza, pulmonary edema of any cause, aspiration following alcoholic intoxication or other causes, chronic lung disease, or exposure to irritants in the air. Resistance is also reduced in those who have anatomic or functional asplenia, chronic cardiovascular disease, diabetes mellitus, cirrhosis, Hodgkin's disease, lymphoma, multiple myeloma, chronic renal failure, nephrotic syndrome, recent organ transplantation and AIDS. Immunity, specific for the infecting capsular serotype, usually follows an attack and may last for years.

9. Methods of control—

    A. Preventive measures:

        1) Avoid crowding in living quarters whenever practical, particularly in institutions, barracks and ships.

        2) Administer polyvalent vaccine containing the capsular polysaccharides of the 23 pneumococcal types causing 90% of all bacteremic pneumococcal infection in the USA, to those at high risk of fatal infection, including individuals over 65 years of age.

           High-risk persons include those with anatomic or functional asplenia, sickle cell disease, human immunodeficiency virus (HIV) infection, and a variety of chronic systemic illnesses, including heart and lung disease, cirrhosis of the liver, renal insufficiency and diabetes mellitus. Because risk of infection and case fatality rates increase with age, benefits of immunization increase also. At the present time, it is recommended that the 23-valent pneumococcal vaccine be given only once to adults except those at highest risk for fatal pneumococcal infection (e.g., asplenic patients) for whom vaccine should be considered at ≥6-year intervals. Revaccination should also be considered for patients with diseases associated with a rapid decline in pneumococcal antibody levels (e.g., nephrotic syndrome, renal failure and transplant recipients). Revaccination after 3-5 years should be considered for children with nephrotic syndrome, asplenia, or sickle cell anemia who would be ≤10 years of age at revaccination. With the exception of those with anatomic or functional asplenia, those who have received the 14-valent vaccine need not be revaccinated with the 23-valent vaccine. Most of the pneumococcal antigen types in the 23-valent vaccine are poor immunogens in children under 2 years of age.

B. *Control of patient, contacts and the immediate environment:*

1) Report to local health authority: Obligatory report of epidemics; no individual case report, Class 4 (see Preface).
2) Isolation: None. If antimicrobial-resistant pneumococci are prevalent, contact isolation is warranted.
3) Concurrent disinfection: Of discharges from nose and throat. Terminal cleaning.
4) Quarantine: None.
5) Immunization of contacts: None. (See 9C, below.)
6) Investigation of contacts and source of infection: Of no practical value.
7) Specific treatment: Penicillin G, parenterally; use erythromycin for those hypersensitive to penicillin. Because pneumococci have been recognized that are relatively resistant to penicillin and other antimicrobials, the sensitivities of strains isolated from normally sterile sites including blood or CSF should be determined; infections with multiply-resistant strains may be treated with vancomycin.

C. *Epidemic measures:* In outbreaks in institutions or in other closed population groups, immunization with the 23-valent vaccine should be carried out unless it is known that the type causing disease is not included in the vaccine.

D. *Disaster implications:* Crowding of populations in temporary shelters bears a risk of disease, especially for the elderly.

E. *International measures:* None.

II. MYCOPLASMAL PNEUMONIA ICD-9 483
(Primary atypical pneumonia)

1. **Identification**—Predominantly a febrile bacterial lower respiratory infection; less often, a pharyngitis that sometimes progresses to bronchitis or pneumonia. Onset is gradual with headache, malaise, cough (often paroxysmal), and usually substernal pain (not pleuritic). Sputum, scant at first, may increase later. Early patchy infiltration of the lungs is often more extensive on x-ray than clinical findings suggest. In severe cases, the pneumonia may progress from one lobe to another. Leukocytosis occurs after the first week in approximately one-third of cases. Duration of illness varies from a few days to a month or more. Secondary bacterial

infection and other complications, such as CNS involvement, are infrequent and fatalities are rare.

Differentiation is required from pneumonitis due to many other agents: bacteria, adenoviruses, influenza, parainfluenza, measles, Q fever, psittacosis, certain mycoses and tuberculosis.

Diagnosis is based on a rise in antibody titers between acute and convalescent sera. The ESR is almost always high. Development of cold hemagglutinins (CA) supports the diagnosis and may occur in one-half to two-thirds of hospitalized cases. The level of CA titer reflects the severity of disease. The infectious agent may be cultured on special media.

2. **Infectious agent**—*Mycoplasma pneumoniae,* bacteria of the family of Mycoplasmataceae.

3. **Occurrence**—Worldwide; sporadic, endemic and occasionally epidemic, especially in institutions and military populations. Attack rates vary from 5 to >50/1000/year in military populations and 1-3/1000/year in civilians. Epidemics occur more often in late summer and fall, endemic disease is not seasonal but there can be much variation from year to year and in different geographic areas. There is no selectivity for race or sex. It occurs at all ages but is asymptomatic or very mild in children under 5 years; recognized disease is most frequent among school-age children and young adults.

4. **Reservoir**—Man.

5. **Mode of transmission**—Probably by droplet inhalation, direct contact with an infected person (probably including those with subclinical infections), or with articles freshly soiled with discharges of nose and throat from an acutely ill and coughing patient. Secondary cases of pneumonia among contacts, family members and attendants are frequent.

6. **Incubation period**—Six to 23 days.

7. **Period of communicability**—Probably less than 10 days; occasionally longer with persisting febrile illness or persistence of the organism in convalescence (as long as 13 weeks is known).

8. **Susceptibility and resistance**—Clinical pneumonia occurs in about 3 to 30% of infections with *M. pneumoniae,* depending on age. Disease varies from mild afebrile pharyngitis to febrile illness involving the upper or lower respiratory tract. Duration of immunity is uncertain. Second attacks of pneumonia may occur. Resistance has been correlated with humoral antibodies which remain for ≥1 year.

9. **Methods of control**—

    A. *Preventive measures:* Avoid crowded living and sleeping quarters whenever possible, especially in institutions, barracks and ships.

B. **Control of patient, contacts and the immediate environment:**

1) Report to local health authority: Obligatory report of epidemics; no individual case report, Class 4.
2) Isolation: None. Respiratory secretions may be infectious.
3) Concurrent disinfection: Of discharges from nose and throat. Terminal cleaning.
4) Quarantine: None.
5) Immunization of contacts: None.
6) Investigation of contacts and source of infection: Valuable in detecting treatable clinical disease among family members.
7) Specific treatment: Erythromycin or a tetracycline. Erythromycin is preferred for children less than 8 years of age to avoid tetracycline staining of immature teeth. Neither antibiotic eliminates organisms from the pharynx; during treatment erythromycin-resistant mycoplasmas may be selected.

C. **Epidemic measures:** No reliably effective measures for control are available.

D. **Disaster implications:** None.

E. **International measures:** WHO Collaborating Centres (see Preface).

III. PNEUMOCYSTIS PNEUMONIA   ICD-9 136.3
(Interstitial plasma-cell pneumonia, PCP)

1. Identification—An acute to subacute, often fatal pulmonary disease, especially in malnourished, chronically ill and premature infants. In older children and adults, it occurs as an opportunistic illness associated with the use of immunosuppressants and diseases of the immune system. It is a major disease problem for persons with acquired immunodeficiency syndrome (see AIDS). Clinically, there is progressive dyspnea, tachypnea and cyanosis; fever may not be present. Auscultatory signs, other than râles, are usually minimal or absent. Chest x-ray typically shows bilateral interstitial infiltrates. Postmortem examination reveals heavy airless lungs, thickened alveolar septa, and foamy material containing clumps of parasites in the alveolar spaces.

Diagnosis is established by demonstration of the causative agent in material from bronchial brushings, open lung biopsy, and lung aspirates or in smears of tracheobronchial mucus. Organisms can be identified by methenamine silver, toluidine blue O, Giemsa, Gram-Weigert, cresyl-echt-violet and IFA staining methods. There is no satisfactory culture method or serologic test in routine use at present.

2. **Infectious agent**—*Pneumocystis carinii*. Generally considered a protozoan parasite, recent studies have shown that the organism's DNA sequence closely resembles that of a fungus.

3. **Occurrence**—The disease has been recognized on all continents; may be endemic and epidemic in debilitated, malnourished or immuno-suppressed infants. It affects approximately 60% of patients with AIDS.

4. **Reservoir**—Man. Organisms have been demonstrated in rodents, cattle, dogs and other animals, but with the ubiquitous presence of the organism and its subclinical persistence in man and animals, there appears to be little public health significance of these potential animal sources of human infection.

5. **Mode of transmission**—Animal-to-animal transmission via the airborne route has been demonstrated in rats. The mode of transmission in man is not known. In one study, approximately 75% of normal individuals were reported to have humoral antibody to *P. carinii* by the age of 4 years, suggesting that subclinical infection is common. Pneumonitis in the compromised host may result from either a reactivation of latent infection or a newly acquired infection.

6. **Incubation period**—Unknown. Analysis of data from institutional outbreaks and animal studies indicates that the onset of disease often occurs 1 to 2 months after the establishment of the immunosuppressed state.

7. **Period of communicability**—Unknown.

8. **Susceptibility and resistance**—Susceptibility is enhanced by prematurity, by chronic debilitating illness, and by disease or therapy in which immune mechanisms are impaired. Infection with human immunodeficiency virus (HIV) is a predominant risk factor for PCP disease.

9. **Methods of control**—

   A. *Preventive measures:* Prophylaxis with either co-trimoxazole or pentamidine (oral or aerosolized) has proven to be effective (as long as the patient is on the drug) in preventing endogenous reactivation in immunosuppressed patients, especially those with HIV infection, those treated for lymphatic leukemia, and in organ transplant patients.

   B. *Control of patient, contacts and the immediate environment:*

   1) Report to local health authority: Official report not ordinarily justifiable, Class 5 (see Preface). When cases occur in persons with evidence of HIV infection, case report is required in most states, Class 2B (see Preface).
   2) Isolation: None.
   3) Concurrent disinfection: Insufficient knowledge.

4) Quarantine: None.
5) Immunization of contacts: None.
6) Investigation of contacts and source of infection: None.
7) Specific treatment: Co-trimoxazole is the drug of choice. Alternate drugs are pentamidine (oral or aerosolized) and trimetrexate with leucovorin; several drugs are currently under intensive evaluation.

C. *Epidemic measures:* Knowledge of source of the organism and mode of transmission is so incomplete that there are no generally accepted measures.

D. *Disaster implications:* None.

E. *International measures:* None.

IV. PNEUMONIAS DUE TO CHLAMYDIA   ICD-9 482.8

IV A. PNEUMONIA DUE TO CHLAMYDIA TRACHOMATIS   ICD-9 482.8
(Neonatal eosinophilic pneumonia)

1. **Identification**—A subacute chlamydial pulmonary disease occurring in early infancy among infants whose mothers have infection of the uterine cervix. Clinically, the disease is characterized by insidious onset, cough (characteristically staccato), lack of fever, patchy infiltrates on chest x-ray with hyperinflation, eosinophilia, and elevated IgM and IgG. A history of neonatal conjunctivitis is present in about 50% of cases. Duration of illness is commonly one to three weeks, but may extend as long as two months. No fatalities have been recorded.

Diagnosis is usually made by direct IF technique. Definition of the infecting immunotype is based on cell culture isolation of the causative agent from the posterior nasopharynx or demonstration of specific serum antibody at a titer of ≥1:32 by micro-IF. A high titer of specific IgG antibody supports the diagnosis.

2. **Infectious agent**—*Chlamydia trachomatis* of immunotypes D-K (excluding immunotypes that cause lymphogranuloma venereum).

3. **Occurrence**—Probably the worldwide distribution of genital chlamydial infection. The disease has been recognized in the USA and a number of European countries. Epidemics have not been recognized.

4. **Reservoir**—Man. Experimental infection with *C. trachomatis* has been induced in nonhuman primates and mice, but is not known to occur in nature.

5. **Mode of transmission**—Transmitted from the infected cervix to an infant during birth, with resultant nasopharyngeal infection (and occasionally chlamydial conjunctivitis). Respiratory transmission has not been established.

6. **Incubation period**—Not known, but pneumonia may occur in infants from one to 18 weeks of age (more commonly between four and 12 weeks). Nasopharyngeal infection is usually not recognized before two weeks of age.

7. **Period of communicability**—Unknown.

8. **Susceptibility and resistance**—Unknown. Maternal antibody does not protect the infant from infection.

9. **Methods of control**—

    A.   *Preventive measures:* Same as for Conjunctivitis, Chlamydial.

    B.   *Control of patient, contacts and the immediate environment:*

        1)   Report to local health authority: Official report not ordinarily justifiable, Class 5 (see Preface).

        2)   Isolation: Drainage/secretion precautions.

        3)   Concurrent disinfection: Of discharges from nose and throat.

        4)   Quarantine: None.

        5)   Immunization of contacts: None.

        6)   Investigation of contacts and source of infection: Examine parents for infection and treat if positive.

        7)   Specific treatment: Oral erythromycin (50 mg/kg/day) is the drug of choice. Sulfisoxazole is a possible alternative.

    C.   *Epidemic measures:* No epidemic occurrence recognized.

    D.   *Disaster implications:* None.

    E.   *International measures:* None.

IV B. PNEUMONIA CAUSED BY THE TWAR AGENT   ICD-9 482.8

1. **Identification**—An acute chlamydial respiratory disease with cough, frequently a sore throat and hoarseness, and fever at the onset. Sputum is scanty; few patients complain of chest pain. Pulmonary râles are usually present and x-ray usually discloses a single infiltrate in the middle or lower lung field. Illness is usually mild, but recovery is relatively slow with cough lasting for more than two weeks; in older

adults, bronchitis and sinusitis may become chronic. A fatal outcome is very rare in uncomplicated cases.

Laboratory diagnosis is primarily serologic: The CF test recognizes the chlamydial group antigens, and a specific micro-IF test for IgM (on sera obtained three weeks after initial infection) identifies the agent. In cases of reinfection, IgG antibody appears early and rises to a high level. Those treated with tetracycline may have a poor antibody response. The organism can be isolated from throat-swab specimens in the yolk sac of embryonated eggs, and can be cultured in HL cells.

2. **Infectious agent**—*Chlamydia pneumoniae*, strain TWAR, is the species name for the organism which has distinct morphologic and serologic differences from *C. psittaci* and *C. trachomatis*.

3. **Occurrence**—Presumably worldwide. Disease has been confirmed in Finland, Denmark, Norway, Sweden, the UK, Canada, Australia, Japan and the USA. The original isolate was made in Taiwan. Antibodies are rare in children below age 5, rising among teenagers and young adults to a plateau of about 50% by age 20-30, and remain high into old age. While clinical disease has been seen most frequently in young adults, disease has occurred in all ages; 8 of 18 cases reported from Canada were in people over 70 years of age and the oldest (with recovery) was 90. No seasonality has been noted.

4. **Reservoir**—Presumably man. No avian association has been found; no isolations or antibodies were found in pigeons and other birds captured at the site of an outbreak, nor in dogs or cats.

5. **Mode of transmission**—Not defined; possibilities include direct contact with secretions, via fomites, and airborne spread.

6. **Incubation period**—Relatively long; at least 10 days.

7. **Period of communicability**—Not defined but presumed to be prolonged based on military outbreaks lasting as long as 8 months.

8. **Susceptibility and resistance**—Susceptibility is presumed to be universal with increased likelihood of clinical disease in the presence of pre-existing chronic disease. Serologic evidence of recall type of immune response suggests immunity after infection; however, second episodes of pneumonia have been observed in military recruits, with a secondary type of serologic response to the second attack.

9. **Methods of control**—

    A. *Preventive measures:*

        1) Avoid crowding in living and sleeping quarters.
        2) Apply personal hygiene measures: cover mouth when coughing and sneezing, dispose of discharges from mouth and nose in a sanitary manner, and wash hands frequently.

B. *Control of patient, contacts and the immediate environment:*

1) Report to local health authority: Obligatory report of epidemics; no individual case report, Class 4 (see Preface).
2) Isolation: None. Respiratory secretions may be infectious.
3) Concurrent disinfection: Of discharges from nose and throat.
4) Quarantine: None.
5) Immunization of contacts: None.
6) Investigation of contacts and source of infection: Examine all members of the family for infection and treat if positive.
7) Specific treatment: Oral tetracycline or erythromycin, 2 g/day for 10-14 days.

C. *Epidemic measures:* Case finding and treatment.

D. *Disaster implications:* None.

E. *International measures:* None.

OTHER PNEUMONIAS   ICD-9 480, 482

Among the known viruses, the adenoviruses, respiratory syncytial virus, the parainfluenza viruses and probably others as yet unidentified, may produce a pneumonitis. Because these infectious agents cause upper respiratory disease more often than pneumonia, they are presented under Respiratory Disease, Acute Viral. Viral pneumonia occurs in measles, influenza and chickenpox. Pneumonia is also caused by infection with rickettsiae (Q fever) and *Legionella*. It can also be associated with the invasive phase of nematode infections, such as ascariasis, and with mycoses such as aspergillosis, histoplasmosis and coccidioidomycosis.

Various pathogenic bacteria commonly found in the mouth, nose and throat, such as *Staphylococcus aureus, Klebsiella pneumoniae, Haemophilus influenzae, Streptococcus pyogenes* (group A hemolytic streptococci), *Neisseria meningitidis* (notably group Y), *Bacteroides* spp., *Branhamella catarrhalis* and anaerobic cocci, may produce pneumonia, especially in association with influenza, as superinfection following broad-spectrum antibiotic therapy, as a complication of chronic pulmonary disease, and after aspiration of gastric contents or tracheostomy. With increased use of antimicrobial and immunosuppressive therapy, pneumonias caused by enteric Gram-negative bacilli have become more common, especially those caused by *Escherichia coli, Pseudomonas aeruginosa* and *Proteus* species. Management depends on the specific organism involved.

POLIOMYELITIS, ACUTE   ICD-9 045
(Polioviral fever, Infantile paralysis)

1. **Identification**—An acute viral infection with severity ranging from inapparent infection to nonspecific febrile illness, aseptic meningitis, paralytic disease and death. Symptoms of "minor illness" include fever, malaise, headache, nausea and vomiting; if the disease progresses, severe muscle pain and stiffness of neck and back with or without flaccid paralysis may occur. Paralysis of muscles of respiration and swallowing frequently threatens life. The site of paralysis depends upon the location of nerve cell destruction in the spinal cord or brain stem, but is characteristically asymmetrical. Case fatality rates for paralytic cases vary from 2 to 10% in different epidemics and increase markedly with age. Recent evidence indicates that further muscle weakness may infrequently occur many years after the acute attack; this is not related to persistence of the virus itself. Nonparalytic poliomyelitis is sometimes manifested as aseptic meningitis (q.v.). The incidence of inapparent infections and "minor illness" usually exceeds that of paralytic cases by a hundredfold or even greater, especially when infection occurs early in life.

Paralytic poliomyelitis can usually be recognized on clinical grounds but can be confused with post-infectious polyneuritis and other paralytic conditions. Other enteroviruses (enterovirus type 71, and sometimes type 70; coxsackieviruses, especially group A, type 7) can cause illness simulating paralytic poliomyelitis, though it is usually less severe, with fewer common signs and negligible residual paralysis. Tick-bite paralysis occurs uncommonly but worldwide; it is manifested by a flaccid ascending motor paralysis which usually disappears promptly when the tick is removed. Guillain-Barré syndrome may resemble paralytic poliomyelitis, but fever, headache, nausea, vomiting and pleocytosis are usually absent. Postencephalitic syndromes, cerebral palsy, trauma and some drugs may result in lameness or a flaccid paralysis simulating the residua of poliomyelitis.

The differential diagnosis of acute nonparalytic poliomyelitis includes other forms of acute nonbacterial meningitis, purulent meningitis, brain abscess, tuberculous meningitis, leptospirosis, lymphocytic choriomeningitis, infectious mononucleosis, the encephalitides and toxic encephalopathies.

The laboratory diagnosis is made by isolation of the virus by inoculating cell culture systems of human or monkey origin (primate cells) with fecal material or oropharyngeal secretions. Neutralizing antibodies may already be present when paralysis develops so that significant titer rises may not be demonstrable in paired sera; moreover, virus isolation from fecal material without antibody rise may occur, suggesting carriage rather than acute infection. Differentiation of "wild" from vaccine strains can be made in countries where molecular biology laboratory facilities are available.

2. **Infectious agent**—Poliovirus (genus *Enterovirus*) types 1, 2 and 3; all types can cause paralysis. Type 1 is isolated from paralytic cases most often, type 3 less so, and type 2 least commonly. Type 1 most frequently causes epidemics. Most vaccine-associated cases are due to types 3 or 2.

3. **Occurrence**—Worldwide. Before large-scale immunization programs were carried out, the highest incidence of clinically recognized disease was in temperate zones and in the more developed countries. Cases occurred sporadically and in epidemics, more commonly during summer and autumn, but with some variation from year to year and from region to region. Characteristically, poliomyelitis is a disease of children and adolescents. Improvement in living standards has been associated with emergence of paralytic cases in older individuals who did not acquire immunizing infections in childhood. Where poliovirus is highly endemic, antibodies to all 3 types of poliovirus are acquired through inapparent infection or minor illness before age 5. Before immunization programs were instituted in some developing countries, polio rates rose as infant mortality rates fell; epidemics, formerly rare in less developed areas, occurred with increasing frequency, mainly involving infants and young children. In such populations, most paralytic disease occurs before age 3.

In countries where polio vaccines have been used extensively, paralytic cases occur chiefly among groups not reached by immunization programs, mainly preschool children of lower social classes and members of religious groups who object to immunization. During 1978 and 1979, poliomyelitis appeared in one such religious group in the Netherlands, then spread to Canada, and finally affected members of a related religious group within the USA. The use of both live and killed virus vaccines has resulted in a marked decrease in worldwide overall incidence of paralytic disease. During 1986-1988, a yearly average of 227 cases was reported in industrialized Europe. Since 1979, no cases due to endemic "wild" virus have been reported in the USA, although from 1980 to 1987, an annual average of 9 paralytic cases was reported. In developed countries, where wild poliomyelitis transmission has been essentially eradicated, the few remaining cases have been associated with live virus vaccine or have been imported cases.

4. **Reservoir**—Man only, most frequently persons with inapparent infections, especially children. Long-term carriers have not been found.

5. **Mode of transmission**—Direct contact through close association. In rare instances milk, foodstuffs and other fecally contaminated materials have been incriminated as vehicles. There is no reliable evidence of spread by insects or virus-contaminated sewage; water is rarely involved.

Fecal-oral is the major route of transmission where sanitation is poor; during epidemics and where sanitation is good, pharyngeal spread becomes relatively more important. Virus is more easily detectable, and for a longer period, in feces than in throat secretions. Ingested virus multiplies first in the alimentary tract; viremia may then follow, leading to invasion of the CNS and selective involvement of motor neuron cells, resulting in flaccid paralysis, most commonly of the lower extremities.

6. **Incubation period**—Commonly 7-14 days for paralytic cases, with a reported range of 3 to possibly 35 days.

7. **Period of communicability**—Not accurately known. Poliovirus is demonstrable in throat secretions as early as 36 hours and in the feces 72 hours after exposure to infection in both clinical and inapparent cases. Virus persists in the throat for approximately 1 week and in the feces for 3-6 weeks or longer. Cases are most infectious during the first few days before and after onset of symptoms.

8. **Susceptibility and resistance**—Susceptibility to infection is general, but paralytic infections are rare, increasing in frequency with age at the time of infection. Type-specific immunity, apparently with lifelong duration, follows both clinically recognizable and inapparent infections. Second attacks are rare and result from infection with poliovirus of a different type. Infants born of immune mothers have transient passive immunity. Injection of other vaccines or certain other types of substances may provoke paralysis during the incubation period which is localized in the injected limb or appearing there first. Tonsillectomy increases the risk of bulbar involvement. Excessive muscular fatigue in the prodromal period may likewise predispose to paralytic involvement. An increased susceptibility to paralytic poliomyelitis is associated with pregnancy, but fetal abnormalities are rare.

9. **Methods of control**—

   A. *Preventive measures:*

      1) Educate the public on the advantages of immunization in early childhood.

      2) Currently, both injectable noninfectious inactivated poliovirus vaccine (IPV) and live attenuated oral poliovirus vaccine (OPV) preparations are commercially available and in wide use; they give excellent protection in most populations. Their use varies in different countries: Some use IPV alone, some OPV alone, a few use a combination. In the USA, OPV is preferred because it simulates natural infection and induces both circulating antibody and intestinal resistance, and protects susceptible contacts by secondary spread. In some developing countries, poor serologic response to OPV has been reported; this may

be due to breaks in the cold chain (so that the vaccine was permitted to warm and deteriorate), interference by intestinal infection by a variety of viruses or other agents, or unknown factors.

IPV blocks pharyngeal excretion but does not prevent intestinal infection, though it may limit the duration of viral excretion. Its use in combination with diphtheria-tetanus-pertussis (DTP) vaccine has been suggested as an alternative to or in addition to OPV. The WHO currently recommends OPV alone for routine use in the Expanded Programme on Immunization (EPI) in developing countries; vaccine is being contributed by Rotary International.

a) OPV—In the USA, trivalent, live, oral poliovirus vaccine (OPV) for primary immunization of infants is integrated with DTP immunization, so that the first dose is given with the first DTP inoculation at 2 months of age. A second dose should be given about 2 months later (a 6-week to 2-month interval is desirable) and a third dose at 15 months of age, together with the dose of MMR and (possibly) the fourth dose of DTP. In areas with a high risk of poliovirus exposure, the third dose is recommended at 6 months of age. This regimen usually provides protection against all 3 poliovirus types in close to 100% of recipients. An additional OPV dose is recommended for children on entry into elementary school to ensure that all are protected. No additional "boosters" are currently recommended except in situations of possible increased exposure to wild poliovirus, such as in travelers to endemic areas.

For children and adolescents (up to the 18th birthday) in nonendemic areas, primary immunization consists of two doses of OPV at 8-week intervals and a third dose 6 months to a year later. In endemic areas, such as tropical and developing countries, the basic course should be given to infants during the first 14 weeks of life, because true "infantile paralysis" usually occurs in the 6-21 month age group in these settings. Four doses are given: at birth, 6 weeks, 10 weeks and 14 weeks of age.

Contraindications to OPV include immune deficiency states (B-lymphocyte deficiency, thymic dysplasia), current immunosuppressive therapy, disease states associated with immunosuppresssion (AIDS, lymphoma, leukemia, generalized malignancy), and the presence of immunodeficient individuals in the household of potential vaccine recipients. (IPV can be used in such persons.) However, where polio is still a problem, WHO recommends the use of OPV for infants who may be human immunodeficiency virus (HIV)-infected. Diarrhea should not be considered a contraindication to OPV, but the dose should not be counted and another dose given at the first opportunity, since the diarrhea may have interfered with immunization. Rarely, cases of paralytic poliomyelitis have been associated with the vaccine strains in vaccine recipients or their healthy contacts. This occurs in about 1:2.6 million OPV doses distributed, usually after the first dose. In the USA, twice as many OPV-associated cases have occurred among contacts of the recipients as among the recipients themselves; the incidence is higher in adults than in children. Therefore, IPV is recommended for exposed non-vaccinated adults.

b) IPV—Formalin-inactivated poliovirus vaccine (IPV) containing all 3 polio types is given parenterally. In infancy, the primary schedule is usually integrated with DTP immunization by use of a combined vaccine or by concurrent injection. The first three doses are given at 1-2 month intervals, and a fourth dose 6-12 months after the third. IPV is indicated for those with contraindications to OPV (see 9A2a, above). Booster doses of IPV every 5 years have been recommended. A more potent IPV (E-IPV) is now in use in the USA, France and some other countries, with a 3-dose schedule similar to that for OPV, and is being used in developing countries alone or in combination with OPV in areas where response to OPV is poor. Almost 100% seroconversion occurs after 2-3 doses wherever tested.

c) Immunization of adults: Routine immunization for adults residing in the continental USA and Canada is not considered necessary, but a primary series of OPV or IPV is advised for adults traveling to developing countries, for members of communities or population groups in which poliovirus disease is present, for laboratory workers who may handle specimens containing poliovirus, and for health care workers who may be exposed to patients excreting polioviruses. Because of the slightly higher risk of vaccine-associated paralysis in adults, IPV is preferred for primary immunization; two doses of the current vaccine are given with a 1-2 month interval and a third dose given 6 to 12 months later. Those who have previously completed a course of immunization and now will be under increased risk of exposure may be given an additional dose of either IPV or OPV. If OPV is to be used for an infant or child in a household with documented nonimmune adults, consideration should be given to giving these adults at least one but preferably two doses of IPV one month apart before the infant is immunized, provided the delay does not compromise achieving full immunization of the infant.

d) When a combined product containing DTP and enhanced potency IPV becomes available, consideration should be given to a sequential schedule of two or more doses of IPV followed by two doses of OPV.

B. *Control of patient, contacts and the immediate environment:*

1) Report to local health authority: Obligatory case report of paralytic cases as a Disease under Surveillance by WHO, Class 1A. Each paralytic case will be so designated. If vaccine-associated, supplemental reports giving vaccine history and vaccine lot number, virus type, severity and persistence of residual paralysis 60 days or longer after onset are necessary measures for effective control. Nonparalytic cases are reported to the local health authority, Class 2A (see Preface).

2) Isolation: Enteric precautions in the hospital. Of little value under home conditions because the greatest risk of spread of infection was in the prodromal period.

3) Concurrent disinfection: Throat discharges, feces, and articles soiled therewith. In communities with modern and adequate sewage disposal systems, feces and urine can be discharged directly into sewers without preliminary disinfection. Terminal cleaning.

4) Quarantine: Of no community value because of large numbers of unrecognized infections in the population.

5) Protection of contacts: Vaccination of familial and other close contacts contributes little to immediate control; ordinarily the virus has already infected susceptible contacts by the time the first case is recognized. In countries with zero or near zero prevalence, occurrence of a single non-vaccine-associated paralytic case in a community should prompt an immediate investigation.

6) Investigation of contacts and source of infection: Thorough search for sick persons, especially children, to

assure early detection and to facilitate control and permit appropriate treatment of unrecognized and unreported cases. Foot drop, scoliosis and other deformities resulting in functional impairment may be late manifestations of initially mild illness.

7) Specific treatment: None; attention during the acute illness to the complications of paralysis requires expert knowledge, especially for patients in need of respiratory assistance.

C. *Epidemic measures:*

1) If wild poliovirus is implicated and at least two cases are associated in time, place and population group, an appropriate mass immunization program with trivalent OPV should be designed and initiated to prevent spread. Trivalent vaccines are effective in controlling outbreaks and should be put into use immediately. Seek to achieve the most rapid and complete immunization of epidemiologically relevant groups, especially younger children in developing countries. Establish vaccination centers in relation to population densities, taking advantage of normal social patterns; schools often meet these criteria.

2) With the use of mass immunization, it is no longer necessary to disrupt community activities by closing schools and other places of population aggregation.

3) Postpone elective surgery (especially nose and throat operations) and immunizations against other diseases until after the epidemic has ended.

4) Provide strategically located centers for specialized medical care of acutely ill patients and rehabilitation of those with significant paralysis.

D. *Disaster implications:* Overcrowding of nonimmune groups poses an epidemic threat.

E. *International measures:*

1) Poliomyelitis is a Disease under Surveillance by WHO. National health administrations are expected to inform WHO of outbreaks promptly by telegram or telex, and to supplement these reports as soon as possible with details of the source, nature and extent of the epidemic and of the identity of the type of epidemic virus involved.

The World Health Assembly has declared a goal to eradicate polio by the year 2000; the Pan American Health Organization has a goal of eradicating polio from the Americas by the end of the 1990s.

2) International travelers visiting areas of high prevalence should be adequately immunized.

3) WHO Collaborating Centres (see Preface).

PSITTACOSIS
(Ornithosis, Parrot fever)

ICD-9 073

1. **Identification**—An acute generalized chlamydial disease with variable clinical presentations; fever, headache, myalgia, chills and upper or lower respiratory tract disease are common. Respiratory symptoms are often disproportionately mild when compared with the extensive pneumonia demonstrable by x-ray. Cough is initially absent or non-productive; when present, sputum is mucopurulent and scant. Pleuritic chest pain and splenomegaly occur infrequently; the pulse is usually slow in relation to temperature. Lethargy, encephalitis, myocarditis and thrombophlebitis are occasional complications; occasional relapses occur. Although often mild or moderate in character, human disease can be severe, especially in untreated older persons.

Laboratory diagnosis is made by demonstrating a significant increase in specific antibodies during convalescence; or, under suitably safe laboratory conditions only, by isolation of the infectious agent from sputum, blood or postmortem tissues in mice, eggs or tissue culture. Recovery of the agent may be difficult, especially if the patient has received broad-spectrum antibiotics.

2. **Infectious agent**—*Chlamydia psittaci.*

3. **Occurrence**—Worldwide. Often associated with sick or apparently healthy pet birds. Outbreaks occasionally occur in individual households, pet shops, aviaries, avian exhibits in zoos and pigeon lofts. Processing and rendering plants, and turkey, geese, squab and duck farms have been sources of occupational disease. Most human cases are sporadic; infections are probably frequently not recognized.

4. **Reservoir**—Parakeets, parrots, pigeons, turkeys, ducks and other birds. Apparently healthy birds can be carriers and occasionally shed the infectious agent, particularly when subjected to the stresses of crowding and shipping.

5. **Mode of transmission**—Infection is usually acquired by inhaling

the agent from desiccated droppings and secretions of infected birds in an enclosed space, or directly from infected birds. Household birds, usually imported psittacine birds, are the most frequent source. Chlamydia may be aerosolized on turkey, squab and duck farms, and in poultry processing plants. Turkeys are commonly involved, but ducks, geese and pigeons are occasionally responsible for human disease. Laboratory infections have occurred. Transmission from person to person is rare; personnel attending patients with paroxysmal coughing may become infected.

6. **Incubation period**—From 4 to 15 days, commonly 10 days.

7. **Period of communicability**—Diseased as well as seemingly healthy birds may shed the agent intermittently, and sometimes continuously, for weeks or months. The rare person-to-person transmission can occur with paroxysmal coughing during the acute illness (however, these may have involved the newly described *C. pneumoniae* rather than *C. psittaci* organisms).

8. **Susceptibility and resistance**—Susceptibility is general; immunity following infection is incomplete and transitory. Older adults have a more severe illness. There is no evidence that those persons with antibodies at any given level are protected.

9. **Methods of control**—

   A. *Preventive measures:*

   1) Educate the public as to the danger of household or occupational exposure to infected pet birds. Medical personnel responsible for occupational health in processing plants should be aware that febrile headaches and pneumonic disease among the workers may be psittacosis.

   2) Regulate the importation, raising of and trafficking in birds of the parrot family. Prevent or eliminate infections of birds by quarantine and appropriate antibiotic treatment.

   3) Psittacine birds offered in commerce should be raised under psittacosis-free conditions and handled in such manner as to prevent infection. Tetracycline can be effective in controlling disease in parakeets, parrots and pigeons if properly administered to ensure adequate intake.

   4) Conduct surveillance of pet shops and aviaries where psittacosis has occurred or where birds epidemiologically linked to cases were obtained, and of farms or processing plants to which human psittacosis was traced epidemiologically. Infected birds should be treated or destroyed, and the room or area where they were housed thoroughly cleaned and disinfected with a phenolic compound.

B. *Control of patient, contacts and the immediate environment:*

1) Report to local health authority: Obligatory case report in most states (USA) and countries, Class 2A (see Preface).
2) Isolation: None. Coughing patients should be instructed to cough into disposable tissue.
3) Concurrent disinfection: Of all discharges. Terminal cleaning.
4) Quarantine: Of infected farms or premises with infected birds until diseased birds have been destroyed or adequately treated with tetracycline and the buildings disinfected.
5) Immunization of contacts: None.
6) Investigation of contacts and source of infection: Trace origin of suspected birds. Kill suspected birds and immerse bodies in 2% phenolic or equivalent disinfectant. Place in plastic bag, close securely, and ship frozen (on dry ice) to nearest laboratory capable of isolating chlamydia. If suspected birds cannot be killed, swab-cultures of their cloacae or droppings should be shipped to the laboratory in appropriate transport media and shipping container in compliance with postal regulations.
7) Specific treatment: Antibiotics of the tetracycline group, continued for 10-14 days after temperature returns to normal. Erythromycin is an alternative when tetracycline is contraindicated (pregnancy, children <8 years of age).

C. *Epidemic measures:* Epidemics related to infected aviaries or bird suppliers may be difficult to recognize, but may be extensive. Reported cases are usually sporadic or confined to family outbreaks, but should be investigated if more extensive outbreaks or epizootics among birds are to be recognized. Report outbreaks of psittacosis in flocks of turkeys to state agriculture and health authorities. Large doses of a tetracycline will suppress, but may not eliminate, infection in poultry flocks and may complicate investigations.

D. *Disaster implications:* None.

E. *International measures:* Reciprocal compliance with national regulations to control importation of psittacine birds.

Q FEVER
(Query fever)

ICD-9 083.0

1. **Identification**—An acute febrile rickettsial disease; onset may be sudden with chills, retrobulbar headache, weakness, malaise and severe sweats. There is considerable variation in severity and duration; infections may be asymptomatic. A pneumonitis occurs in some cases, with cough, scanty expectoration, chest pain and minimal physical findings. Abnormal liver function tests are common. Acute pericarditis and acute and chronic granulomatous hepatitis have been reported. Endocarditis can occur on native or prosthetic cardiac valves; these infections have an indolent course, extending over months or even years. Case fatality rate in untreated cases is <1%, and is negligible in treated cases, except in individuals who develop endocarditis. Organisms may survive for long periods within the heart valve vegetation with relapse years after the initial infection.

Laboratory diagnosis is made by demonstration of a rise in specific antibodies between acute and convalescent stages by IF, microagglutination, CF or ELISA tests; high titers of antibodies to phase I of the infective organism may indicate chronic infection, such as subacute endocarditis. Recovery of the infectious agent from blood of patients is diagnostic but poses a hazard to laboratory workers.

2. **Infectious agent**—*Coxiella burnetii,* an organism with two antigenic phases; phase I as found in nature and phase II after multiple laboratory passages in eggs or cell cultures. The organisms have an unusual stability in the environment and are relatively resistant to many disinfectants.

3. **Occurrence**—Reported from all continents; the incidence is greater than that reported because of the mildness of many cases, limited clinical suspicion and unavailability of testing laboratories. It is endemic in limited areas, affecting veterinarians, meat workers, dairy workers and farmers. Epidemics have occurred among workers in stockyards, meat packing and rendering plants, in diagnostic laboratories, in medical centers which use sheep in research and also where no direct animal contact can be demonstrated. Cases are common among researchers working with *C. burnetii;* casual visitors to research facilities often become infected.

4. **Reservoir**—Cattle, sheep, goats, cats, some wild animals (bandicoots and many species of feral rodents), and ticks are natural reservoirs. Infected domestic animals, including house cats, are usually asymptomatic, but shed massive numbers of organisms at parturition.

5. **Mode of transmission**—Commonly by airborne dissemination of rickettsiae in dust from premises contaminated by placental tissues, birth fluids and excreta of infected animals, in establishments processing infected animals or their by-products, and in necropsy rooms. Airborne

particles containing organisms may be carried downwind for a considerable distance (one-half mile or more). Also by direct contact with infected animals and other contaminated materials, such as wool, straw, fertilizer and the laundry of infected persons. Raw milk from infected cows may be responsible for some cases. Direct transmission by blood or marrow transfusion has been reported.

6. Incubation period—Depends on the size of the infecting dose; usually 2-3 weeks.

7. Period of communicability—Direct transmission from person to person rarely, if ever, occurs.

8. Susceptibility and resistance—Susceptibility is general. Immunity following recovery from clinical illness is probably lifelong, with cell-mediated immunity lasting longer than humoral.

9. Methods of control—

    A.   *Preventive measures:*

      1)   Educate the public on sources of infection and the necessity for adequate disinfection and disposal of animal products of conception and strict hygienic measures in cow and sheep sheds, barns and laboratories (dust, urine, feces, rodents and aerosols) and hygienic practices such as pasteurization of milk.

      2)   Pasteurizing milk from cows, goats and sheep at 62.8°C (145°F) for 30 minutes or at 71.7°C (161°F) for 15 seconds, or boiling, inactivates rickettsiae.

      3)   Immunization with inactivated vaccine prepared from *C. burnetii* (Phase I)-infected yolk sac is useful in protecting laboratory workers and is strongly recommended for those working with live *C. burnetii*. It might also be considered for abattoir workers and others in hazardous occupations, including those carrying out medical reasearh with sheep. To avoid severe local reactions, vaccine should not be used in individuals with a positive CF test or a history suggestive of Q fever, unless preceded by a sensitivity skin test with a small dose of vaccine. Vaccine may be obtained by contacting the Commanding Officer, US Army Medical Research Institute of Infectious Diseases, Frederick MD 21701, USA.

      4)   Research workers using sheep should consider immunization and should manage the animals and the research studies with the assumption that the sheep are excreting rickettsiae. Sheep-holding facilities should be away from populated areas and utilize precautions to prevent air flow to other occupied areas; no visitors should be permitted.

Sheep to be used as research animals should be quarantined and screened for *C. burnetii* infection prior to use. Vaccination of sheep has been reported to reduce markedly the shedding of rickettsiae.

B. **Control of patient, contacts and the immediate environment:**

1) Report to local health authority: In the USA, in areas where disease is endemic; in many countries not a reportable disease, Class 3B (see Preface).
2) Isolation: None.
3) Concurrent disinfection: Of sputum and blood and articles freshly soiled by these substances, using 0.05% hypochlorite, 5% peroxide or 1:100 Lysol. Use precautions at postmortem examination of suspected cases in humans or animals.
4) Quarantine: None.
5) Immunization of contacts: Unnecessary.
6) Investigation of contacts and source of infection: Search for history of contact with cattle, sheep or goats on farms or in research facilities, parturient cats, consumption of raw milk, or direct or indirect association with a laboratory which handles *C. burnetii*.
7) Specific treatment: Tetracyclines administered orally and continued for several days after the patient is afebrile; reinstitute if relapse occurs. For chronic endocarditis, tetracycline combined with rifampin has been used most widely recently; quinolones such as ciprofloxacin may be effective.

C. **Epidemic measures:** Outbreaks are generally of short duration; control measures are limited essentially to elimination of sources of infection, observation of exposed persons and antibiotic therapy for those becoming ill. Incriminated sheep-holding facilities should be disinfected thoroughly.

D. **Disaster implications:** None.

E. **International measures:** Control the importation of goats, sheep and cattle, and their products (wool, etc.). WHO Collaborating Centres (see Preface).

RABIES
(Hydrophobia, Lyssa)

ICD-9 071

1. **Identification**—An almost invariably fatal acute viral encephalomyelitis; onset is often heralded by a sense of apprehension, headache, fever, malaise, and indefinite sensory changes often referred to the site of a preceding animal bite wound. The disease progresses to paresis or paralysis; spasm of muscles of deglutition on attempts to swallow leads to fear of water (hydrophobia); delirium and convulsions follow. Without medical intervention, the usual duration is 2 to 6 days, sometimes longer; death is often due to respiratory paralysis.

Diagnosis is confirmed by specific FA staining of brain tissue or by virus isolation in mouse or cell culture systems. Presumptive diagnosis may be made by specific FA staining of frozen skin sections taken from the back of the neck at the hairline. Serologic diagnosis is based on neutralization tests in mice or cell culture.

2. **Infectious agent**—Rabies virus, a rhabdovirus of the genus *Lyssavirus*. All members of the genus are antigenically related, but use of monoclonal antibodies demonstrates differing nucleocapsid and surface protein patterns according to the animal species or the geographic location from which they originate. Rabies-related viruses that exist in Africa (Mokola and Duvenhage) and Europe (Duvenhage) have been associated rarely with fatal rabies-like human illness. Some of these illnesses may be diagnosed as rabies by the standard FA test.

3. **Occurrence**—Worldwide, with an estimated 30,000 deaths a year, almost all in developing countries. Uncommon in man in developed countries. In the ten years 1980-1989, 12 deaths occurred in the USA; 5 cases were acquired within the country, 7 were acquired elsewhere. The last case in the USA was diagnosed in February 1989, resulting from an unknown exposure outside the USA (Mexico).

Rabies is primarily a disease of animals. The only areas free of rabies in the animal population at present include Australia, New Zealand, New Guinea, Japan, Hawaii, Taiwan and Pacific islands, the UK, Ireland, mainland Norway, Sweden, Portugal, and some of the West Indies and Atlantic islands. Urban (or canine) rabies is transmitted by dogs, whereas sylvatic rabies is a disease of wild carnivores and bats (vampire, frugivorous, and insectivorous), with sporadic spillover to dogs, cats, and livestock. In Europe, fox rabies is widespread with a reduced number of cases since 1978 when oral rabies immunization was begun (Switzerland is now virtually rabies-free); since 1986, bat rabies cases have been regularly reported in Denmark, Holland and West Germany. In the USA and Canada, wildlife rabies most commonly involves skunks, raccoons, and bats. There has been a progressive epizootic among raccoons in the eastern USA for a decade.

4. **Reservoir**—Many wild and domestic Canidae, including dogs, foxes, coyotes, wolves and jackals; also skunks, raccoons, mongooses and other biting mammals. Vampire, frugivorous, and insectivorous bats are infected in Mexico, Central and S America; infected insectivorous bats are found in the USA, Canada and now Europe. In the developing countries, dogs remain the principal reservoir. Rabbits, squirrels, chipmunks, rats and mice are rarely infected, and their bites rarely, if ever, call for rabies prophylaxis.

5. **Mode of transmission**—Virus-laden saliva of a rabid animal is introduced by a bite or scratch (or, very rarely, into a fresh break in the skin or rarely through intact mucous membranes). Transmission from person to person is theoretically possible since the saliva of the infected human may contain virus, but has never been documented. Organ (corneal) transplants taken from persons dying of undiagnosed CNS disease have resulted in rabies in the recipients.

Airborne spread has been demonstrated in caves where millions of bats were roosting and in laboratory settings, but this occurs very rarely. In Latin America, transmission from infected vampire bats to domestic animals is common. In the USA, insectivorous bats rarely transmit rabies to man or other animals, wild or domestic.

6. **Incubation period**—Usually 2 to 8 weeks, occasionally as short as 5 days or as long as a year or more; depends on the severity of the wound, site of the wound in relation to the richness of the nerve supply and its distance from the brain, amount of virus introduced, protection provided by clothing and other factors.

7. **Period of communicability**—In dogs and cats, for 3 to 10 days before onset of clinical signs (rarely over 3 days) and throughout the course of the disease. Very rarely, longer periods of excretion before onset of symptoms have been observed; the significance of these observations is unknown. In one study, bats shed virus for 12 days before evidence of illness; in another study, skunks shed virus for at least 8 days before onset of symptoms. Some wild animals may shed virus for up to 18 days after onset of initial symptoms.

8. **Susceptibility and resistance**—All warm-blooded mammals are susceptible. Natural immunity in man is unknown.

9. **Methods of control**—

A. *Preventive measures:*

1) Register, license and vaccinate all dogs; collect and destroy ownerless animals and strays as indicated. Vaccinate all cats as prevention. Educate pet owners and the public that restrictions for dogs and cats are important (e.g., that pets be leashed in congested areas when not confined on

owner's premises; that strange-acting or sick animals of any species, domestic or wild, may be dangerous and should not be picked up or handled; that it is necessary to report such animals and animals that have bitten a person or another animal to the police and/or the local health department; that confinement and observation of such animals is a preventive measure against rabies); and that wild animals should not be kept as pets. Where this is sociologically impractical, repetitive total dog population vaccination has been effective.

2) Detain and clinically observe for 10 days any healthy-appearing dog or cat known to have bitten a person (unwanted dogs and cats may be killed immediately and examined for rabies by fluorescent microscopy); dogs and cats showing suspicious signs of rabies should be sacrificed and tested for rabies. Valuable dogs and cats need not be killed until existence of rabies is reasonably established by clinical signs. If the biting animal were infective at the time of the bite, signs of rabies will usually follow within 5-8 days, with a change in behavior, and excitability or paralysis, followed by death. All wild animals should be sacrificed immediately and the brain examined for evidence of rabies. In the case of bites by a normal-behaving, very valuable zoo animal, it may be appropriate to consider postexposure prophylaxis for the human victim and, instead of sacrificing the animal, hold it in quarantine for 6-12 months.

3) Submit immediately to a laboratory the intact heads, packed in ice (not frozen), of animals that die of suspected rabies, for testing for viral antigen by FA staining, or, if this is not available, by microscopic examination for Negri bodies.

4) Destroy immediately unvaccinated dogs or cats bitten by known rabid animals; if detention is elected, hold the animal in an approved pound or kennel for at least 6 months under veterinary supervision, and vaccinate against rabies 30 days before release. If previously vaccinated, revaccinate immediately and detain (leashing and confinement) for at least 90 days.

5) Cooperative programs with wildlife conservation authorities to reduce fox, skunk, raccoon, and other terrestrial wildlife hosts of sylvatic rabies have had limited effect, but may be used in circumscribed enzootic areas near campsites and areas of human habitation. If such focal depopulation is undertaken, it must be maintained to prevent repopulation from the periphery.

6) Individuals at high risk (e.g., veterinarians, wildlife conservation personnel and park rangers in enzootic areas, staff of quarantine kennels, laboratory and field personnel working with rabies, and long-term travelers to rabies endemic areas) should receive pre-exposure immunization. Two types of vaccine are currently available in the USA: Human Diploid Cell rabies Vaccine (HDCV), a commercially available inactivated vaccine prepared from virus grown in human diploid culture; and Rabies Vaccine, Adsorbed (RVA), an inactivated vaccine grown on rhesus diploid cells, prepared and distributed by the Michigan Department of Public Health, Division of Bio Products, 3500 N Logan St, Lansing MI (USA) 48909. For RVA, contact the Co-ordinating Physician at (517) 335-8050. Both vaccines are given in three 1.0-ml (IM) doses on days 0, 7 and 21 or 28; this regimen has also been so satisfactory that routine postvaccination serology is not routinely recommended but may be advisable for groups at high risk of exposure. If risk of exposure continues, either single booster doses are given, or preferably serum is tested for neutralizing antibody every 2 years, with booster doses given when indicated. The HDCV has also been approved for pre-exposure immunization at an intradermal dose of 0.1 ml given on days 0, 7 and 21 or 28. If the immunization is given in preparation for travel to a rabies-endemic area, 30 or more days must elapse after the three-dose series before departure; otherwise, the intramuscular regimen should be used. Results with intradermal vaccine have generally been good in the USA, but the mean antibody response is somewhat lower and may be of shorter duration than with the 1.0-ml dose given IM. However, the antibody response to intradermal vaccine given outside the USA has been erratic in some groups who were on chloroquine for antimalarial chemoprophylaxis; therefore, intradermal immunization should not be used in this situation unless facilities are available for testing sera for development of neutralizing antibodies. RVA should not be used intradermally.

7) Prevention of rabies after animal bites ("postexposure prophylaxis") consists of a) physical removal of the virus by proper cleansing of the bite wound and b) specific immunologic protection. No antirabies treatment is indicated unless the skin is broken or a mucosal surface has been contaminated by the animal's saliva.
a) Treatment of bite wound: The most effective rabies

prevention is immediate and thorough cleansing with soap or detergent and flushing with water of all wounds caused by an animal bite or scratch. The wound should not be sutured unless unavoidable for cosmetic or tissue support reasons. Sutures, if required, should be placed after local infiltration of antiserum (see 9A7b, below); they should be loose and not interfere with free bleeding and drainage.

b) Immunologic prevention of rabies in man is provided by administration of rabies immune globulin (RIG) as soon as possible after exposure to neutralize the virus in the bite wound, and then by giving vaccine to elicit active immunity.

Passive immunization: RIG should be used in a single dose of 20 I.U./kg; half should be infiltrated around the bite wound if possible, and the rest given IM. If serum of animal origin is used, an intradermal or subcutaneous test dose should precede its administration to detect allergic sensitivity, and the dose should be increased to a total of 40 I.U./kg.

Vaccine: Preferably HDCV in five 1.0-ml IM doses in the deltoid region; the first as soon as possible after the bite (at the same time as the single dose of RIG is given), and the other doses 3, 7, 14 and 28-35 days after the first dose. (The intradermal dose/route at multiple sites is being used in several countries for postexposure prophylaxis, but this has not been approved in the USA.) In individuals with possible immunodeficiency, a serum specimen should be collected at the time the last dose of vaccine is administered and tested for rabies antibodies. If sensitization reactions appear in the course of immunization, consult health department or infectious disease consultants for guidance. If the person has had a previous full course of antirabies inoculations with HDCV, or had developed neutralizing antibody after pre-exposure immunization (9A6, above) or after a postexposure regimen, only 2 doses of HDCV need to be given – one immediately and the second, 3 days later. With severe exposure (e.g., head bites), a dose may be given on day 7. No RIG is given with this regimen.

c) The following is a general guide to prophylaxis in different circumstances: If a bite were unprovoked, the animal not apprehended, and rabies is present in that species in the area, administer RIG and vaccine. Bites of wild carnivorous mammals and bats are considered potential rabies exposures unless negated by laboratory tests. If available, the biting animal may be killed immediately (with the owner's and health authorities' concurrence) and its brain examined by the FA technique to determine whether antirabies treatment is necessary. The decision whether to administer RIG and vaccine immediately after exposure to dogs and cats or during the observation period (see 9A2, above) should be based on the behavior of the animal, the presence of rabies in the area, and the circumstances of the bite. (See Guide, below.)

d) Vaccination with current rabies vaccines carries a very small risk of postvaccinal encephalitis; only 2 cases of transient neuroparalytic illness have been reported. Local reactions, such as pain, erythema, swelling or itching at the injection site, were reported in 25% of those receiving five 1.0-ml doses. Mild systemic reactions of headache, nausea, muscle aches, abdominal pain and dizziness were reported in about 20%. "Serum sickness-like" reactions, including primarily urticaria with generalized itching and wheezing, were reported infrequently.

However, among those receiving booster doses for pre-exposure prophylaxis, hypersensitivity reactions occur in approximately 6% of recipients, 2 to 21 days after HDCV, presenting as a generalized pruritic rash, urticaria, possible arthralgia, arthritis, angioedema, nausea, vomiting, fever and malaise. These symptoms have responded to antihistamines; a few have required corticosteroids or epinephrine. Persons exposed to rabies who develop these symptoms should complete the required number of injections but in a setting where reactions can be treated. Systemic allergic reactions in those receiving booster doses of RVA have been rare, reported in <1%. No significant reactions have been attributed to RIG (of human origin); however, antiserum from a nonhuman source produces serum sickness in 5-40% of recipients; newer purified animal globulins appear to have little risk. These risks must be weighed against the risk of contracting rabies.

e) Management of animal bites, adapted from the Seventh Report of the WHO Expert Committee on Rabies, 1984, and from the USPHS Advisory Committee on Immunization Practices (revision in process, 1990) should include:

CHECKLIST OF TREATMENTS FOR ANIMAL BITES

1. Clean and flush the wound immediately (first aid).
2. Thorough wound cleansing under medical supervision.
3. Rabies immune globulin and/or vaccine as indicated.
4. Tetanus prophylaxis and antibacterial treatment when required.
5. No sutures or wound closure advised unless unavoidable.

B. *Control of patient, contacts and the immediate environment:*

1) Report to local health authority: Obligatory case report required in most states (USA) and countries, Class 2A (see Preface).

2) Isolation: Contact isolation for respiratory secretions for duration of the illness.

3) Concurrent disinfection: Of saliva and articles soiled therewith. Although transmission to attending personnel has not been documented, immediate attendants should be warned of the potential hazard of infection from saliva, and should wear rubber gloves, protective gowns, and protection to avoid exposure from a patient coughing saliva in the attendant's face.

4) Quarantine: None.

5) Immunization of contacts: Contacts who have an open wound or mucous membrane exposure to the patient's saliva should receive antirabies specific treatment (see 9A7b, above).

6) Investigation of contacts and source of infection: Search for rabid animal and for persons and other animals bitten.

7) Specific treatment: For clinical rabies, intensive supportive medical care.

C. *Epidemic (epizootic) measures:* Applicable only to animals; a sporadic disease in man.

1) Establish area control under authority of state laws, public health regulations and local ordinances, in cooperation with appropriate wildlife conservation and animal health authorities.

2) Vaccinate dogs through officially-sponsored, intensified mass programs which provide immunizations at temporary and emergency stations. For protection of other domestic animals, approved vaccines appropriate for each animal species must be used.

3) In urban areas of the USA and other developed countries, strict enforcement of regulations requiring collection,

RABIES POSTEXPOSURE PROPHYLAXIS GUIDE*

The following recommendations are only a guide. In applying them, take into account the animal species involved, the circumstances of the bite or other exposure, vaccination status of the animal and presence of rabies in the region. Local or state health officials should be consulted if questions arise about the need for rabies prophylaxis.

SPECIES	CONDITION OF ANIMAL AT TIME OF ATTACK	TREATMENT
Domestic Dog and cat	Healthy and available for 10 days of observation	None, unless animal develops rabies[1]
	Rabid or suspected rabid	RIG[2] & HDCV[3]
	Unknown (escaped)	Consult public health official. If treatment is indicated, give RIG[2] & HDCV[3]
Wild Carnivores skunk, fox, bat, coyote, bobcat, raccoon	Regard as rabid unless proven negative by laboratory tests[4]	RIG[2] & HDCV[3]
Other livestock, rodents and lagomorphs (hares and rabbits)	Consider individually. Local and state public health officials should be consulted on questions about the need for rabies prophylaxis. Bites of squirrels, hamsters, guinea pigs, gerbils, chipmunks, rats, mice, other rodents, rabbits, and hares almost never call for antirabies prophylaxis.	

*All bites and wounds should immediately be cleansed thoroughly with soap and water. If antirabies treatment is indicated, both RIG and HDCV should be given as soon as possible, regardless of the interval from exposure.

[1] During the usual holding period of 10 days, begin treatment with RIG and HDCV at first sign of rabies in a dog or cat that has bitten someone. The symptomatic animal should be killed immediately and tested to confirm the diagnosis.

[2] If RIG is not available, use antirabies serum, equine. Do not use more than the recommended dosage.

[3] Local reactions to vaccines are common and do not contraindicate continuing treatment. Discontinue vaccine if FA tests of the animal are negative.

[4] The animal should be killed and tested as soon as possible. Holding for observation is not recommended.

Adapted from recommendations of the Immunization Practices Advisory Committee (ACIP), revision in process, 1990.

> detention and destruction of ownerless and stray dogs, and of unvaccinated dogs found off owners' premises, and control of the dog population by castration, spaying or drugs have been effective in breaking transmission cycles.

D. Disaster implications: A potential problem if the disease is freshly introduced or enzootic in an area where there are many stray dogs or wild reservoir animals.

E. International measures:

1) Strict compliance by common carriers and travelers with national laws and regulations requiring quarantine, vaccination of animals, certificates of health and origin, etc.

2) WHO Collaborating Centres (see Preface).

RAT-BITE FEVER ICD-9 026

Two bacterial diseases, rare in the USA, are included under the general term of rat-bite fever; streptobacillosis is caused by *Streptobacillus moniliformis,* and spirillosis by *Spirillum minus (minor).* Because they have clinical and epidemiologic similarities, only streptobacillosis is presented in detail; variations manifested by *Spirillum minus* infection (which is less common in the USA) are noted in a brief summary.

STREPTOBACILLOSIS ICD-9 026.1
(Streptobacillary fever, Haverhill fever, Epidemic arthritic erythema, Rat-bite fever due to *Streptobacillus moniliformis*)

1. **Identification**—An abrupt onset of chills and fever, headache and muscle pain, is followed shortly by a maculopapular or sometimes petechial rash most marked on the extremities. One or more large joints then usually become swollen, red and painful. There is usually a history of a rat bite within 10 days that healed normally. Relapses are common. Bacterial endocarditis and focal abscesses may occur late in untreated cases, with a case fatality rate of 7-10%.

Laboratory confirmation is made by isolation of the organism by inoculating material from the primary lesion, lymph node, blood, joint fluid or pus into the appropriate bacteriologic medium or laboratory animals (guinea pigs or mice which are not naturally infected). Serum antibodies may be detected by agglutination tests.

2. **Infectious agent**—*Streptobacillus moniliformis (Streptothrix muris rattus, Haverhillia multiformis, Actinomyces muris).*

3. **Occurrence**—Worldwide, but uncommon in N and S America and most European countries. Recent cases in the USA have followed bites by laboratory rats.

4. **Reservoir**—An infected rat, rarely other animals (squirrel, weasel).

5. **Mode of transmission**—Infection is transmitted by secretions of mouth, nose or conjunctival sac of an infected animal, most frequently introduced by biting. Sporadic cases occur without a history of a bite. Blood from an experimental laboratory animal has infected man. Direct contact with rats is not necessary; infection has occurred in persons working or living in rat-infested buildings. In outbreaks, contaminated milk or water has usually been suspected as the vehicle of infection.

6. **Incubation period**—Three to 10 days, rarely longer.

7. **Period of communicability**—Not directly transmitted from person to person.

8. **Susceptibility and resistance**—No information.

9. **Methods of control**—

   A. *Preventive measures:* Ratproof dwellings and reduce rat populations. Penicillin or doxycycline could be used as a prophylaxis in case of a rat bite.

   B. *Control of patient, contacts and the immediate environment:*

      1) Report to local health authority: Obligatory report of epidemics; no case report required, Class 4 (see Preface).
      2) Isolation: Blood/body fluid precautions for 24 hours after start of effective therapy.
      3) Concurrent disinfection: None.
      4) Quarantine: None.
      5) Immunization of contacts: None.
      6) Investigation of contacts and source of infection: Only to establish whether there are additional unrecognized cases.
      7) Specific treatment: Penicillin or tetracyclines. Treatment should continue for 7-10 days.

   C. *Epidemic measures:* A cluster of cases requires search for a common source, possibly a milk supply.

   D. *Disaster implications:* None.

   E. *International measures:* None.

SPIRILLOSIS   ICD-9 026.0
(Spirillary fever, Sodoku, Rat-bite fever due to *Spirillum minus*)

Rat-bite fever caused by *Spirillum minus (S. minor)* is the common form of sporadic rat-bite fever in Japan and Asia. Untreated, the case fatality rate is approximately 10%. Clinically, *Spirillum minus* disease differs from streptobacillary fever in the rarity of arthritic symptoms and the distinctive rash of reddish or purplish plaques. The incubation period is 1-3 weeks, and the previously healed bite wound reactivates when symptoms appear. Laboratory methods are essential for differentiation; animal inoculation is used for isolation of the spirillum.

RELAPSING FEVER   ICD-9 087

1. **Identification**—A systemic spirochetal disease in which periods of fever lasting 2-9 days alternate with afebrile periods of 2-4 days; the number of relapses varies from 1 to 10 or more. Each febrile period terminates by crisis. The total duration of the louse-borne disease averages 13-16 days; the tick-borne disease usually lasts longer. Transitory petechial rashes are common during the initial febrile period. The overall case fatality rate in untreated cases is between 2-10%; it has exceeded 50% in epidemic louse-borne disease.

Diagnosis is made by demonstration of the infectious agent in darkfield preparations of fresh blood or stained thick or thin blood films, or by intraperitoneal inoculation of laboratory rats or mice with blood taken during the febrile period.

2. **Infectious agents**—In louse-borne disease, *Borrelia recurrentis*. In tick-borne disease, many different strains have been distinguished by area of first isolation and/or vector rather than inherent biologic differences. Strains isolated during a relapse often show antigenic differences from those obtained during the immediately preceding paroxysm.

3. **Occurrence**—Characteristically, epidemic where it is spread by lice; endemic where it is spread by ticks. Louse-borne relapsing fever occurs in limited areas in Asia, eastern Africa (Ethiopia and the Sudan), northern and central Africa, and S America. The endemic tick-borne disease is widespread throughout tropical Africa; foci exist in Spain, northern Africa, Saudi Arabia, Iran, India, and parts of central Asia, as well as in N and S America. Epidemic louse-borne relapsing fever has not been reported in the USA for many years; human cases and occasional outbreaks of tick-borne disease occur in limited areas of several western states and western Canada.

4. Reservoir—For louse-borne disease, man; for tick-borne relapsing fevers, wild rodents and ticks through transovarian transmission.

5. Mode of transmission—Vector-borne; not directly transmitted from person to person. Epidemic relapsing fever is acquired by crushing an infective louse, *Pediculus humanus,* so as to contaminate the bite wound or an abrasion of the skin. Man also is infected by the bite or coxal fluid of an argasid tick, principally *Ornithodoros turicata* and *O. hermsi* in the USA, *O. rudis* and *O. talaje* in Central and S America, *O. moubata* and *O. hispanica* in Africa, and *O. tholozani* in the Near and Middle East. These ticks usually feed at night, rapidly engorge and leave the host; they have a longevity of 2-5 years and remain infective for their lifespan.

6. Incubation period—Five to 15 days; usually 8 days.

7. Period of communicability—The louse becomes infective 4-5 days after ingestion of blood from an infected person and remains so for life (20-40 days). Infected ticks can live for several years without feeding, remain infective during this period and pass the infection transovarially to their progeny.

8. Susceptibility and resistance—Susceptibility is general. Duration of immunity after clinical attack is unknown.

9. Methods of control—

A. Preventive measures:

1) Control lice by measures prescribed for louse-borne typhus fever (see Typhus fever, Epidemic Louse-Borne, 9A).

2) Control ticks by measures prescribed for Rocky Mountain spotted fever, 9A. Tick-infested human habitations present difficult problems and eradication is difficult or impossible. Spraying with approved acaricides such as diazinon, chlorpyrifos, propoxur or permethrin may be tried.

3) Use personal protection measures, including repellents and permethrin on clothing and bedding for persons with exposure in endemic foci.

4) Antibiotic chemoprophylaxis with tetracyclines may be taken after exposure (arthropod bites) when risk of acquiring the infection is high.

B. Control of patient, contacts and the immediate environment:

1) Report to local health authority: Report of louse-borne relapsing fever required as a Disease under Surveillance by WHO, Class 1A; tick-borne disease, in selected areas, Class 3B (see Preface).

2) Isolation: Blood/body fluid precautions. The patient, his clothing, all household contacts and the immediate environment should be deloused or freed of ticks.

3) Concurrent disinfection: None, if proper disinfestation has been carried out.

4) Quarantine: None.

5) Immunization of contacts: None.

6) Investigation of contacts and source of infection: For the individual tick-borne case, search for sources of infection; for louse-borne disease, application of appropriate lousicidal preparation to infested contacts (see Pediculosis, 9B6).

7) Specific treatment: Tetracyclines.

C. *Epidemic measures:* When reporting has been good and cases are localized, apply 1% permethrin dust or spray (an insecticide with residual effect) to contacts and their clothing, and permethrin spray at 0.003-0.3 kg/hectare (2.47 acres) to the immediate environment of all reported cases. Where infection is known to be widespread, apply permethrin systematically to all persons in the community, or to outdoor target areas where ticks are prevalent. For sustained control, a treatment cycle of one month is recommended during the transmission season.

D. *Disaster implications:* A serious potential hazard among louse-infested populations. Epidemics are common in wars, famine, and other situations where the prevalence of pediculosis is enhanced, as among overcrowded, malnourished populations with poor personal hygiene.

E. *International measures:*

1) Telegraphic notification by governments to WHO and adjacent countries of the occurrence of an outbreak of louse-borne relapsing fever in an area previously free of the disease.

2) Louse-borne relapsing fever is not a disease subject to the International Health Regulations, but the measures outlined in 9E1, above, should be followed since it is a Disease under Surveillance by WHO.

RESPIRATORY DISEASE, ACUTE VIRAL (EXCLUDING INFLUENZA)
(Acute viral rhinitis, A.v. pharyngitis, A.v. laryngitis, etc.)

Numerous acute respiratory illnesses of known and presumed viral etiology are grouped here under the general title of Respiratory Disease, Acute Viral. Clinically, and by CIOMS taxonomy, infections of the upper respiratory tract can be designated as acute viral rhinitis (upper respiratory infections, URI), acute viral pharyngitis, and acute viral laryngitis; and infections involving the lower respiratory tract can be designated as acute viral tracheobronchitis, bronchitis, bronchiolitis or acute viral pneumonia. These respiratory syndromes are associated with a large number of viruses, each of which is capable of producing a wide spectrum of acute respiratory illnesses. The illnesses caused by known agents have important epidemiologic attributes in common, such as reservoir and mode of transmission. Many of the viruses invade any part of the respiratory tract; others show a predilection for certain anatomic sites. Some predispose to bacterial complications. Morbidity and mortality from acute respiratory diseases are especially significant in pediatric practice; in adults, the relatively high incidence and resulting disability, with consequent economic loss, make diseases of this group a major health problem worldwide.

Several other nonbacterial infections of the respiratory tract are recognized as disease entities and are presented as separate chapters because they are sufficiently uniform in their clinical and epidemiologic manifestations and occur in such regular association with specific infectious agents: influenza, ornithosis, enteroviral vesicular pharyngitis (herpangina) and epidemic myalgia (pleurodynia) are examples. Particularly in pediatric practice, influenza must be considered in cases of acute respiratory tract disease.

Symptoms of upper respiratory tract infection, mainly pharyngotonsillitis, can be produced by bacterial agents, of which group A streptococcus is the most common. Practical management of acute respiratory disease depends on the differentiation of viral infections from disease entities for which specific antimicrobial measures are available; thus, it is important to rule out group A streptococcal infection, especially in children over 2 years, by appropriate culture even though more illnesses are caused by viruses. In addition, in outbreaks or epidemics of continuing high incidence not due to streptococci, it is important to identify the cause in a representative sample of typical cases by appropriate clinical and laboratory methods to rule out other diseases, e.g., mycoplasmal pneumonia and Q fever, for which specific treatment may be effective.

I. ACUTE FEBRILE RESPIRATORY DISEASE

ICD-9 461-466; 480

1. **Identification**—Viral diseases of the respiratory tract may be characterized by fever and one or more constitutional reactions such as chills or chilliness, headache, general aching, malaise and anorexia; occasionally in infants by GI disturbances. Localizing signs also occur at various sites in the respiratory tract, either alone or in combination, such as rhinitis, pharyngitis or tonsillitis, laryngitis, laryngotracheitis, bronchitis, bronchiolitis, pneumonitis or pneumonia. There may be associated conjunctivitis. Symptoms and signs usually subside in 2-5 days without complications; infection may, however, be accompanied by laryngitis, bronchiolitis or pneumonitis, or be complicated by bacterial sinusitis, otitis media or pneumonia. WBC counts and respiratory bacterial flora are within normal limits unless modified by complications.

Specific diagnosis depends on isolation of the etiologic agent from respiratory secretions in appropriate cell or organ cultures, identification of viral antigen in nasopharyngeal cells by FA, ELISA and RIA tests, and/or antibody studies of paired sera.

2. **Infectious agents**—Parainfluenza virus, types 1, 2, 3 and rarely type 4; respiratory syncytial virus (RSV); adenovirus, especially types 1-5, 7, 14, and 21; rhinoviruses; certain coronaviruses; certain types of coxsackievirus groups A and B; and echoviruses are considered etiologic agents of acute febrile respiratory illnesses. Influenza virus (q.v.) can produce the same clinical picture, especially in children. Some of these agents have a greater tendency to cause more severe illnesses; others have a predilection for certain age groups and populations. RSV, the major viral respiratory tract pathogen of early infancy, produces illness with greatest frequency during the first 2 years of life; it is the major known etiologic agent of bronchiolitis, and is a cause of pneumonia, croup, bronchitis, otitis media and febrile upper respiratory illness. The parainfluenza viruses are the major known etiologic agents of croup and also cause bronchitis, pneumonia, bronchiolitis and febrile upper respiratory illness in pediatric populations. Adenoviruses are associated with several forms of respiratory disease; types 4, 7 and 21 are common causes of acute respiratory disease (ARD) in unimmunized military recruits.

3. **Occurrence**—Worldwide. Seasonal in temperate zones, with greatest incidence during fall and winter and occasionally spring. In tropical zones, respiratory infections tend to be more frequent in wet and colder weather. In large communities, some viral illnesses are constantly present, usually with little seasonal pattern (e.g., adenovirus type 1); others tend to occur in sharp outbreaks (e.g., RSV).

Annual incidence is high, particularly in infants and children, and depends upon the number of susceptibles and the virulence of the agent.

During autumn, winter and spring, attack rates for preschool children may average 2%/week as compared to 1%/week for school-age children and 0.5%/week for adults. Under special host and environmental conditions, certain viral infections may disable more than half of a closed community within a few weeks, e.g., outbreaks of adenovirus types 4 or 7 in military recruits.

4. **Reservoir**—Man. Many known viruses produce inapparent infections; adenoviruses may remain latent in tonsils and adenoids. Viruses of the same groups cause similar infections in many animal species but are of minor importance as sources of human infections; RSV and parainfluenza are occasionally transmitted from animals to man.

5. **Mode of transmission**—Directly by oral contact or by droplet spread; indirectly by hands, handkerchiefs, eating utensils or other articles freshly soiled by respiratory discharges of an infected person. Viruses discharged in the feces, including enteroviruses and adenoviruses, may be involved. Outbreaks of illness due to adenovirus type 3, 4 and 7 have been related to swimming pools.

6. **Incubation period**—From 1 to 10 days.

7. **Period of communicability**—Shortly prior to and for the duration of active disease; little is known about subclinical or latent infections. Especially in infants, RSV shedding may very rarely persist for several weeks or longer after clinical symptoms subside.

8. **Susceptibility and resistance**—Susceptibility is universal. Illness is more frequent and more severe in infants, children and the elderly. Infection induces specific antibodies which are usually short-lived. Reinfection with RSV and parainfluenza viruses is common, but the illness is generally milder. Individuals with compromised cardiac, pulmonary or immune systems are at increased risk of severe illness.

9. **Methods of control—**

    A. *Preventive measures:*

      1) Educate the public in personal hygiene, as in covering the mouth when coughing and sneezing, in sanitary disposal of discharges from mouth and nose and in frequent handwashing.

      2) When possible, avoid crowding in living and sleeping quarters, especially in institutions, in barracks and on shipboard.

      3) Oral live adenovirus vaccines have proven effective against adenovirus 4, 7 and 21 infections in military recruits, but are not indicated in civilian populations because of the low incidence of specific disease.

B. **Control of patient, contacts and the immediate environment:**

1) Report to local health authority: Obligatory report of epidemics; no individual case report, Class 4 (see Preface).

2) Isolation: Contact isolation is desirable in childrens' hospital wards. Outside of hospitals, ill persons should avoid direct and indirect exposure of young children, debilitated or aged persons or patients with other illnesses.

3) Concurrent disinfection: Of eating and drinking utensils; sanitary disposal of oral and nasal discharges.

4) Quarantine: None.

5) Immunization of contacts: None.

6) Investigation of contacts and source of infection: Not generally indicated.

7) Specific treatment: None. Indiscriminate use of antibiotics is to be discouraged; they should be reserved for patients with group A streptococcal pharyngitis and for patients with identified bacterial complications such as otitis media, pneumonia and sinusitis. Aerosolized ribavirin has shown promise of effectiveness in treatment of RSV.

C. **Epidemic measures:** No effective measures known. Good infection control procedures can prevent nosocomial transmission; procedures such as ultraviolet irradiation, aerosols and dust control have not proven useful. Avoid crowding (see 9A2, above).

D. **Disaster implications:** None.

E. **International measures:** WHO Collaborating Centres (see Preface).

II. THE COMMON COLD ICD-9 460
(Acute viral rhinitis, Acute coryza)

1. **Identification**—Acute catarrhal infection of the upper respiratory tract characterized by coryza, sneezing, lacrimation, irritated nasopharynx, chilliness and malaise lasting 2-7 days. Fever is uncommon in children over 3 years old and rare in adults. No fatalities reported, but disability is important because it affects work performance, and industrial and school absenteeism; illness may be accompanied by laryngitis, tracheitis and bronchitis and may predispose to more serious complications such as sinusitis and otitis media. WBC counts are usually normal and bacterial flora of the respiratory tract are within normal limits in the absence of complications.

Cell or organ culture studies of nasal secretions may demonstrate a known virus in 20-35% of cases. Specific clinical, epidemiologic and other manifestations aid differentiation from similar diseases due to toxic, allergic, physical or psychological stimuli.

2. **Infectious agents**—Rhinoviruses, of which there are more than 100 recognized serotypes, are the major known etiologic agents of the common cold in adults, especially in the fall season. Coronaviruses, such as 229E, OC43 and B814, are also responsible for the common cold in adults, they appear to be especially important in the winter and early spring when the prevalence of rhinoviruses is low. Other known respiratory viruses account for a small proportion of common colds in adults. In infants and children, parainfluenza viruses, RSV, influenza, adenoviruses, certain enteroviruses and coronaviruses cause common cold-like illnesses. The etiology of over half of common colds has not been identified.

3. **Occurrence**—Worldwide, both endemic and epidemic. In temperate zones, incidence rises in fall, winter and spring. Many persons, except in small isolated communities, have 1-6 colds yearly. Incidence is highest in children under 5 years; gradual decline with increasing age.

4. **Reservoir**—Man.

5. **Mode of transmission**—Presumably by direct contact or by inhalation of airborne droplets; indirectly by hands and articles freshly soiled by discharges of nose and throat of an infected person. Rhinovirus, RSV, and probably other similar viruses, are transmitted by contaminated hands carrying virus to the mucous membranes of the eye or nose.

6. **Incubation period**—Between 12 and 72 hours, usually 48 hours.

7. **Period of communicability**—Nasal washings taken 24 hours before onset and for 5 days after onset have produced symptoms in experimentally infected volunteers.

8. **Susceptibility and resistance**—Susceptibility is universal. Inapparent and abortive infections occur; frequency of healthy carriers is undetermined, but known to be rare with some viral agents, notably rhinoviruses. The frequently repeated attacks may be due to short duration of homologous immunity, to the multiplicity of agents or to other causes.

9. **Methods of control**—

   A. *Preventive measures:* See I, 9A, above.

   B. *Control of patient, contacts and the immediate environment:*

      1) Report to local health authority: Official report not ordinarily justifiable, Class 5 (see Preface).

2), 3), 4), 5), 6), and 7): Isolation, Concurrent disinfection, Quarantine, Immunization of contacts, Investigation of contacts and source of infection, and Specific treatment: See I, 9B, 2) through 7), above.

C., D., and **E. Epidemic measures, Disaster implications,** and **International measures:** See I, 9C, 9D, and 9E, above.

RICKETTSIOSES, TICK-BORNE   ICD-9 082
(Spotted fever group)

These are a group of clinically similar diseases caused by closely related rickettsiae. They are transmitted by *Ixodid* (hard) ticks, which are widely distributed throughout the world; tick species differ markedly by geographic area. For all of these rickettsial fevers similar control measures are applicable, and the tetracyclines and chloramphenicol are effective therapeutically.

The sensitive and specific micro-IFA tests become positive in the second week of illness, and CF tests using group-specific spotted fever antigens somewhat later. The Weil-Felix reactions with Proteus OX-19 and Proteus OX-2 are much less sensitive and specific.

I. ROCKY MOUNTAIN SPOTTED   ICD-9 082.0
FEVER
(New World spotted fever, Tick-borne typhus fever, São Paulo fever)

1. **Identification**—This prototype disease of the spotted fever group is characterized by sudden onset with moderate to high fever, which ordinarily persists for 2-3 weeks in the untreated cases, significant malaise, deep muscle pain, severe headache, chills and conjunctival injection. In about half the cases, a maculopapular rash appears on the extremities on about the third day; this soon includes the palms and soles and spreads rapidly to much of the body; petechiae and hemorrhages are common. The case fatality rate is about 15-20% in the absence of specific therapy; with prompt recognition and treatment, death is uncommon, yet 4% of cases reported in the USA during recent years have been fatal. Absence or delayed appearance of the typical rash contributes to delay in diagnosis and increased fatality.

This clinical syndrome, especially early Rocky Mountain spotted fever (RMSF), may be confused with meningococcemia (see Meningitis) and enteroviral infection.

Diagnosis is based on serologic response to specific antigens. The rickettsiae have been identified in skin biopsies using IF antisera.

2. Infectious agent—*Rickettsia rickettsii.*

3. Occurrence—Throughout the USA during spring, summer and fall. Two-thirds of cases reported in recent years have been in N and S Carolina, Virginia, Maryland, Georgia, Tennessee and Oklahoma. In 1988, the highest incidence rates were seen in Oklahoma, N Carolina, Arkansas, Missouri and Kansas. Few cases have been reported from the Rocky Mountain region. In the western USA, adult males are infected most frequently, while in the East, the incidence is higher in children; the difference relates to conditions of exposure to infected ticks. The case fatality rate increases with age. Infection also occurs in Canada, western and central Mexico, Panamá, Costa Rica, Colombia and Brazil.

4. Reservoir—Maintained in nature in ticks by transovarian and transstadial passage. The rickettsiae can be transmitted to dogs, various rodents and other animals; animal infections are usually subclinical, but disease in dogs has been observed.

5. Mode of transmission—Ordinarily by bite of an infected tick. Several hours (4-6) of attachment of the tick and feeding on blood are required before the rickettsiae become reactivated to become infectious for man. Contamination of skin with crushed tissues or feces of the tick may also cause infection. In eastern and southern USA, the common vector is the dog tick, *Dermacentor variabilis;* in northwestern USA, the wood tick, *D. andersoni;* in southwestern USA, occasionally the Lone Star tick, *Amblyomma americanum.* The principal vector in Latin America is *A. cajennense.*

6. Incubation period—From 3 to about 14 days.

7. Period of communicability—Not directly transmitted from person to person. The tick remains infective for life, commonly as long as 18 months.

8. Susceptibility and resistance—Susceptibility is general. One attack probably confers lasting immunity.

9. Methods of control—

   A. *Preventive measures:*

   1) See Lyme disease, 9A.
   2) Deticking dogs and using tick repellent collars on them minimizes the tick population near residences. Indoor treatment of baseboards, wall crevices, especially in dog quarters, with residual insecticide may help.
   3) No vaccine is presently licensed in the USA for public use.

B. *Control of patient, contacts and the immediate environment:*

1) Report to local health authority: Case report obligatory in all states (USA) and most countries, Class 2B (see Preface).
2) Isolation: None.
3) Concurrent disinfection: Carefully remove all ticks from patients.
4) Quarantine: None.
5) Immunization of contacts: Unnecessary.
6) Investigation of contacts and source of infection: Not profitable except as a community measure. (See Lyme disease, 9C.)
7) Specific treatment: Tetracyclines or chloramphenicol (the latter is preferred for children under 8 and pregnant women) in daily oral doses until the patient is afebrile (usually 3 days) and for 1-2 additional days. Treatment should be initiated on clinical and epidemiologic considerations without waiting for laboratory confirmation of the diagnosis.

C. *Epidemic measures:* See Lyme disease, 9C.

D. *Disaster implications:* None.

E. *International measures:* WHO Collaborating Centres (see Preface).

II. BOUTONNEUSE FEVER   ICD-9 082.1
(Mediterranean tick fever, Mediterranean spotted fever, Marseilles fever, African tick typhus, Kenya tick typhus, India tick typhus)

1. Identification—A mild to severe febrile illness of a few days to 2 weeks; there may be a primary lesion at the site of a tick bite. This lesion (tâche noire), often evident at the onset of fever, is a small ulcer 2-5 mm in diameter with a black center and red areola; regional lymph nodes are enlarged. In some areas, such as the Negev in Israel, primary lesions are rarely seen. A generalized maculopapular erythematous rash usually involving palms and soles appears about the 4th-5th day and persists 6-7 days; with antibiotic treatment, fever lasts no more than 2 days. The case fatality rate is very low (< 3%) even without specific therapy.

Culturing blood on human fibroblast monolayers permits demonstration of the organisms by IF.

2. Infectious agent—*Rickettsia conorii.*

3. Occurrence—Widely distributed throughout the African Continent, in India and in those parts of Europe and the Middle East adjacent to the Mediterranean, Black and Caspian Seas, and possibly in Mexico.

Expansion of the European endemic zone to the north is occurring because tourists often carry their dogs with them; they acquire infected ticks, which establish tick colonies when they return home, and transmission occurs. In more temperate areas, highest incidence is during warmer months when ticks are numerous; in tropical areas, throughout the year. Outbreaks may occur when groups of travelers are bitten by ticks, such as people on safari in Africa.

4. **Reservoir**—As in RMSF, above.

5. **Mode of transmission**—In the Mediterranean area, by bite of infected *Rhipicephalus sanguineus,* a dog tick. In South Africa, ticks infected in nature and presumed to be vectors include *Haemaphysalis leachi, Amblyomma hebraeum, R. appendiculatus, Boophilus decoloratus,* and *Hyalomma aegyptium.*

6. **Incubation period**—Usually 5-7 days.

7., 8., and 9. **Period of communicability, Susceptibility and resistance,** and **Methods of control**—As in RMSF, above.

III. QUEENSLAND TICK TYPHUS   ICD-9 082.3

1. **Identification**—Clinically similar to Boutonneuse fever.

2. **Infectious agent**—*Rickettsia australis.*

3. **Occurrence**—Queensland, Australia.

4. **Reservoir**—As in RMSF, above.

5. **Mode of transmission**—As in RMSF, above. *Ixodes holocyclus,* infesting small marsupials and wild rodents, is probably the major vector.

6. **Incubation period**—About 7-10 days.

7., 8., and 9. **Period of communicability, Susceptibility and resistance,** and **Methods of control**—As in RMSF, above.

IV. NORTH ASIAN TICK FEVER   ICD-9 082.2
(Siberian tick typhus)

1. **Identification**—Clinically similar to Boutonneuse fever.

2. **Infectious agent**—*Rickettsia sibirica.*

3. **Occurrence**—Asiatic USSR, north China and the Mongolian People's Republic.

4. **Reservoir**—As in RMSF, above.

5. **Mode of transmission**—By the bite of ticks in the genera *Dermacentor* and *Haemaphysalis,* which infest certain wild rodents.

6. **Incubation period**—Two to 7 days.

7., 8., and 9. **Period of communicability, Susceptibility and resistance, and Methods of control**—As in RMSF, above.

RICKETTSIALPOX   ICD-9 083.2
(Vesicular rickettsiosis)

An acute febrile illness transmitted by mites. An initial skin lesion at the site of a mite bite, often associated with lymphadenopathy is followed by fever; then a disseminated skin rash appears, generally not involving the palms and soles, and lasting only a few days. It may be confused with chickenpox. Death is uncommon and the infection is responsive to tetracyclines. Diagnosis is made by CF or IFA testing. The disease is caused by *Rickettsia akari,* a member of the spotted fever group of rickettsiae close to *R. australis,* transmitted to man from mice *(Mus musculus)* by a mite *(Liponyssoides sanguineus).* It has occurred in urban areas of the eastern USA, primarily in New York, and in the USSR. The incidence has been markedly reduced by changes in management of garbage in tenement housing, so that only six cases have been diagnosed in New York since 1971. In the USSR, commensal rats are reported to be sources of infection. Rickettsial isolations have been made in Africa and Korea. Prevention is by rodent elimination, followed by mite control.

RUBELLA   ICD-9 056
(German measles)
CONGENITAL RUBELLA   ICD-9 771.0
(Congenital rubella syndrome)

1. **Identification**—Rubella is a mild febrile viral disease with a diffuse punctate and maculopapular rash sometimes resembling that of measles or scarlet fever. Children usually present few or no constitutional symptoms, but adults may experience a 1-5 day prodrome of low-grade fever, headache, malaise, mild coryza and conjunctivitis. Postauricular, occipital and posterior cervical lymphadenopathy is characteristic and precedes the rash by 5-10 days.

Up to half the infections occur without evident rash. Leukopenia is common and thrombocytopenia can occur, but hemorrhagic manifestations are rare. Arthralgia and, less commonly, arthritis complicate a substantial proportion of infections, particularly among adult females. Encephalitis is a rare complication, occurring more frequently in adults than in children.

Rubella is important because of its ability to produce anomalies in the developing fetus. Congenital rubella syndrome occurs in ≥25% of infants born to women who acquired rubella during the first trimester of pregnancy; the risk of a single congenital defect falls to approximately 10-20% by the 16th week, and defects are rare when the maternal infection occurs after the 20th week of gestation.

Fetuses infected early are at greatest risk of intrauterine death, spontaneous abortion and congenital malformations of major organ systems. These include single or combined defects: deafness, cataracts, microphthalmia, congenital glaucoma, microcephaly, meningoencephalitis, mental retardation, patent ductus arteriosus, atrial or ventricular septal defects, purpura, hepatosplenomegaly, jaundice and radiolucent bone disease. Moderate and severe cases of congenital rubella are recognizable at birth; mild cases with only slight cardiac involvement or partial deafness may not be detected for months or even years after birth. Insulin-dependent diabetes mellitus is recognized as a frequent late manifestation of congenital rubella in certain geographic areas. Congenital malformations and even fetal death may occur following inapparent maternal rubella.

Differentiation of rubella from measles (q.v.), scarlet fever (see Streptococcal diseases), and other similar exanthems is often necessary (e.g., Erythema infectiosum (q.v.) and Exanthem subitum, below). Macular and maculopapular rashes occur in 1-5% of patients with infectious mononucleosis (especially if given ampicillin), in infections with certain enteroviruses, and after certain drugs.

Clinical diagnosis of rubella is often inaccurate, so laboratory confirmation is important. Rubella, especially in pregnant women, can be confirmed by a fourfold rise in specific antibody titer between acute and convalescent phase serum specimens by HAI, passive HA, LA or ELISA testing, or by the presence of rubella-specific IgM indicating a recent infection.

Sera should be collected as early as possible (within 7-10 days) after onset of illness, and again at least 7-14 days (preferably 2-3 weeks) later. Virus may be isolated from the pharynx 1 week before until 2 weeks after onset of rash. Blood, urine or stool specimens may yield virus. The diagnosis of congenital rubella in the newborn is confirmed by the presence of specific IgM antibodies in a single specimen, the persistence of an HAI titer beyond the time expected from passive transfer of maternal IgG antibody, or by isolation of the virus which may be shed from the throat and urine for as long as a year.

2. **Infectious agent**—Rubella virus (family Togaviridae; genus *Rubivirus*).

3. **Occurrence**—Worldwide; universally endemic except in remote and isolated communities, especially certain island groups which have epidemics every 10-15 years. It is prevalent in winter and spring.

Extensive epidemics occurred in the USA in 1935, 1943 and 1964, and in Australia in 1940. Before vaccine was licensed in 1969, peaks of rubella incidence occurred in the USA every 6-9 years. In unvaccinated populations, rubella is primarily a disease of childhood, but it occurs more often in adolescents and adults than does measles or chickenpox. Where children are well immunized, adolescent and young adult infections become more important, with epidemics in institutions, colleges and military populations. Congenital rubella incidence has declined significantly in the USA since 1979.

4. **Reservoir**—Man.

5. **Mode of transmission**—Contact with nasopharyngeal secretions of infected persons. Infection is by droplet spread or direct contact with patients. In closed environments such as among military recruits, all exposed susceptibles may be infected. Infants with congenital rubella shed large quantities of virus in their pharyngeal secretions and in urine, and serve as a source of infection to their contacts.

6. **Incubation period**—Sixteen to 18 days with a range of 14-23 days.

7. **Period of communicability**—For about 1 week before and at least 4 days after onset of rash; highly communicable. Infants with congenital rubella may shed virus for months after birth.

8. **Susceptibility and resistance**—Susceptibility is general after loss of transplacentally acquired maternal antibody. Active immunity is acquired by natural infection or by vaccination; it is usually permanent after natural infection and thought to be long-term, probably lifelong, after vaccination. In the USA, 10-20% of young adults remain susceptible. Infants born to immune mothers are ordinarily protected for 6-9 months, depending on the amount of maternal antibody acquired transplacentally.

9. **Methods of control**—Rubella control is needed primarily to prevent defects in the offspring of women who acquire the disease during pregnancy.

A. *Preventive measures:*

1) Educate the general public on modes of transmission and the need for immunization.
2) A single dose of live, attenuated rubella virus vaccine (Rubella Virus Vaccine, Live) elicits a significant antibody response in approximately 98-99% of susceptibles. The

vaccine is in dried form and after reconstitution must be kept at 2-8°C (35.6-46.4°F) or colder and protected from light to retain potency. Vaccine virus may be recovered from the nasopharynx of some recipients for several weeks but is not communicable. In the USA, immunization of all children 15 months of age or older is recommended as part of a combined vaccine containing measles and mumps vaccine (MMR). The continuing occurrence of rubella among women of childbearing age indicates that emphasis should continue to be placed on vaccinating susceptible adolescent and adult females of childbearing age. Vaccine is recommended for all susceptible premarital and postpartum women, especially for teachers and young adults who congregate at colleges and other types of institutions. Medical personnel likely to come into contact with individuals who have rubella, and also in contact with patients in prenatal clinics, should show proof of immunity by presence of rubella-specific antibodies or written documentation of immunization performed on or after the first birthday.

Vaccine should not be given to anyone with an immunodeficiency or on immunosuppressive therapy. Because of theoretical concerns, women known to be pregnant should not be vaccinated; however, no defects attributable to vaccine virus have been detected in about 200 offspring of susceptible women vaccinated with the RA 27/3 vaccine (which is the one now used in the USA) shortly before conception or during the first trimester of pregnancy.

Reasonable precautions in a rubella immunization program include asking postpubertal females if they are pregnant, excluding those who say they are, and explaining the theoretical risks to the others and emphasizing the need to prevent pregnancy for the next 3 months. The immune status of an individual can be determined reliably only by serologic testing, but this is not necessary before vaccination since vaccine can be given safely to an immune person. In some countries (e.g., Australia) routine immunization is given to girls between 11-13 years with or without prior antibody testing. For greater general detail, see Measles, 9A1.

3) In case of natural infection early in pregnancy, abortion should be considered because of high risk of damage to the fetus. Although vaccine virus has been isolated from products of conception, congenital defects in live-born infants have not been seen; therefore, vaccination of a

woman subsequently discovered to be pregnant need not be considered an indication for abortion, but the potential risks should be explained; the final decision rests with the individual woman and her physician.

4) IG given after exposure early in pregnancy may not prevent infection or viremia, but it may modify or suppress symptoms. It is sometimes given in huge doses (20 ml) to a susceptible pregnant woman exposed to the disease who would not consider abortion under any circumstances, but its value has not been established.

B. Control of patient, contacts and the immediate environment:

1) Report to local health authority: All cases of rubella and of congenital rubella should be reported. In the USA, report is obligatory, Class 3B (see Preface). Early reporting of suspected cases will permit early establishment of control measures.

2) Isolation: In hospitals and institutions, patients suspected of having rubella should be managed under contact isolation precautions and placed in a private room; attempts should be made to prevent exposure of nonimmune pregnant women (see 9B5, below). Exclude children from school and adults from work for 7 days after onset of rash.

3) Concurrent disinfection: None.

4) Quarantine: None.

5) Immunization of contacts: Immunization, while not contraindicated (except during pregnancy), will not necessarily prevent infection or illness. Passive immunization with IG is not indicated (except possibly as in 9A4, above).

6) Investigation of contacts and source of infection: Identify pregnant female contacts, especially those in the first trimester. Such contacts should be tested serologically for susceptibility or early infection (IgM antibody) and advised accordingly.

7) Specific treatment: None.

C. Epidemic measures: An outbreak of rubella in a school or comparable population may justify mass immunization. The medical community and general public should be informed about rubella epidemics in order to identify and protect susceptible pregnant women.

D. Disaster implications: None.

E. International measures: None.

EXANTHEM SUBITUM
(Roseola infantum)

ICD-9 057.8

An acute illness of viral etiology, usually in children under 4 years (most common in 2 year-olds) caused by human herpesvirus-6 (HHV-6) or a virus closely related to HHV-6. A fever, sometimes as high as 41°C (106°F), appears suddenly and lasts 3-5 days. A maculopapular rash on the trunk and later on the rest of the body ordinarily follows lysis of the fever, and the rash usually fades rapidly. Symptoms are generally mild, but febrile seizures have been reported. Incidence is greatest in the spring. The incubation period is about 10 days. Unrecognized infections occur; immunity follows illness.

SALMONELLOSIS

ICD-9 003

1. **Identification**—A bacterial disease commonly manifested by an acute enterocolitis, with sudden onset of headache, abdominal pain, diarrhea, nausea and sometimes vomiting. Dehydration, especially among infants, may be severe. Fever is almost always present. Anorexia and diarrhea often persist for several days. Infection may begin as acute enterocolitis and develop into septicemia or focal infection. The infectious agent may rarely localize in any tissue of the body, producing abscesses and causing arthritis, cholecystitis, endocarditis, meningitis, pericarditis, pneumonia, pyoderma or pyelonephritis. Ordinarily, deaths are uncommon, except in the very young, the very old, and the debilitated. However, morbidity and associated costs of salmonellosis may be high.

In cases of septicemia, *Salmonella* may be isolated on enteric media from feces and from blood during the acute stages of illness. In cases of enterocolitis, fecal excretion usually persists for several days or weeks beyond the acute phase of illness; administration of antibiotics may increase the duration of excretion of organisms. For detection of asymptomatic infections, 3-10 g of fecal material is preferred to rectal swabs; specimens should be collected over several days since excretion of the organisms may be intermittent. Serologic tests are not useful in diagnosis.

2. **Infectious agents**—Numerous serotypes of *Salmonella* are pathogenic for both animals and man (strains of human origin causing typhoid and paratyphoid fevers are presented in a separate chapter). There is much variation in the relative prevalence of the different serotypes from country to country; in most countries which maintain *Salmonella* surveillance, *S. typhimurium* and *S. enteritidis* are the two most commonly

reported. Of approximately 2,000 known serotypes, only about 200 are detected in the USA in any given year. In most areas, a small number of serotypes account for the majority of confirmed cases.

3. **Occurrence**—Worldwide; more extensively reported in N America and Europe; classified as a foodborne disease (see Foodborne disease) because contaminated food is the predominant mode of transmission. Only a small proportion of cases are recognized clinically, and as few as 1% of clinical cases are reported. The incidence rate of infection is highest in infants and young children. Epidemiologically, *Salmonella* enterocolitis may occur in small outbreaks in the general population. Large outbreaks in hospitals, institutions for children, restaurants and nursing homes are common and usually arise from food contaminated at its source, or, less often, during handling by an ill patient or a carrier, but person-to-person spread can occur. There are estimated to be 5 million *Salmonella* infections in the USA annually.

4. **Reservoir**—Domestic and wild animals, including poultry, swine, cattle, rodents and pets such as tortoises, turtles, terrapins, chicks, dogs and cats; also humans, i.e., patients, convalescent carriers and, especially, mild and unrecognized cases. Chronic carriers are rare in humans but prevalent in animals and birds.

5. **Mode of transmission**—By ingestion of the organisms in food derived from infected food animals or contaminated by feces of an infected animal or person. This includes raw and undercooked (inadequate time for a given temperature) eggs and egg products, raw milk and raw milk products, meat and meat products, poultry and poultry products; as well as pet turtles and chicks, and unsterilized pharmaceuticals of animal origin. Infection is transmitted to animals by animal feeds and fertilizers prepared from contaminated meat scraps, tankage, fish meal and bones. Fecal-oral transmission from person to person is important, especially when diarrhea is present; infants and stool-incontinent adults pose a greater risk of transmission than do asymptomatic carriers. The ingestion of only a few organisms can cause infection, but usually $>10^{2\text{-}3}$ organisms are required.

Epidemics of *Salmonella* infection are usually traced to foods such as commercially processed meat products, inadequately cooked poultry and poultry products, raw sausages, uncooked or lightly cooked foods containing eggs and egg products, unpasteurized milk and dairy products, including dried milk, and foods contaminated with feces by an infected foodhandler. They are also traced to foods such as meat and poultry products that have been processed or prepared with contaminated utensils or on work surfaces or tables contaminated in previous use. The organisms can multiply in a variety of foods, especially milk, to attain a very high infectivity level. Hospital epidemics tend to be protracted, with organisms persisting in the environment; they often start with contaminated food and continue by person-to-person transmission via the hands of personnel or contaminated instruments. Maternity units with infection (at times asymptomatic) of the infants are sources of further spread. Fecal contamination of unchlorinated public water supplies has caused some extensive outbreaks.

6. **Incubation period**—Six to 72 hours, usually about 12-36 hours.

7. **Period of communicability**— Throughout the course of infection; extremely variable, usually several days to several weeks. A temporary carrier state occasionally continues for months, especially in infants. About 1% of infected adults and 5% of children under 5 years excrete the organism for >1 year. The administration of antibiotics, even those to which the organisms are sensitive in laboratory tests, can prolong the period of communicability.

8. **Susceptibility and resistance**—Susceptibility is general and usually increased by achlorhydria, antacid therapy, GI surgery, prior or current broad-spectrum antibiotic therapy, neoplastic disease, immuno-suppressive therapy and other debilitating conditions, including malnutrition. Severity of the disease is related to the serotype, the number of organisms ingested and host factors. Patients with AIDS are at risk of recurrent non-typhoidal *Salmonella* septicemia. Septicemia in persons with sickle cell disease increases the risk of focal systemic infection, e.g., osteomyelitis.

9. **Methods of control**—

   A. *Preventive measures:*

   1) Thoroughly cook all foodstuffs derived from animal sources, particularly poultry, pork, egg products and meat dishes. Avoid recontamination within the kitchen after cooking is completed. Avoid consuming raw or incompletely cooked eggs, as in eggnogs or homemade ice cream, and using dirty or cracked eggs. Pasteurized egg products should be used to prepare dishes in which eggs would otherwise be pooled before cooking. All milk, milk products and egg products should be pasteurized. Refrigerate prepared foods in small containers.

   2) Educate foodhandlers and food-preparers on the importance of handwashing before, during and after food preparation; and on the importance of refrigerating food, maintaining a sanitary kitchen, and protecting prepared foods against rodent and insect contamination.

   3) Exclude individuals with diarrhea from foodhandling and from care of hospitalized patients, the elderly and children.

   4) Thoroughly indoctrinate known carriers on the need for

very careful postdefecatory handwashing (and before handling food), and discourage them from handling food for others as long as they shed the organisms.

5) Recognize, control and prevent *Salmonella* infections in domestic animals and pets. Chicks, ducklings and turtles are particularly dangerous pets for small children.

6) Inspect for sanitation and adequately supervise abattoirs, food-processing plants, feed-blending mills, egg-grading stations and butcher shops.

7) Radiation pasteurize poultry products, a procedure approved by the Food and Drug Administration, USPHS and the Food Safety Inspection Service (USDA).

8) Adequately cook or heat-treat, including radiation pasteurization, animal-derived foods prepared for animal consumption (meat meal, bone meal, fish meal, pet food), followed by measures to avoid recontamination.

B. *Control of patient, contacts and the immediate environment:*

1) Report to local health authority: Obligatory case report, Class 2B (see Preface).

2) Isolation: For hospitalized patients, enteric precautions in handling feces and contaminated clothing and bed linen. Exclude symptomatic individuals from foodhandling and from direct care of infants, elderly, immunocompromised and institutionalized patients. Exclusion of asymptomatic infected individuals is indicated for those with questionable hygienic habits and may be required by local or state regulations. When exclusion is mandated, release to return to work as foodhandler or in patient care generally requires 2 consecutive negative stool cultures for *Salmonella* collected not less than 24 hours apart; if antibiotics have been given, the initial culture should be taken at least 48 hours after the last dose. Proper handwashing should be stressed.

3) Concurrent disinfection: Of feces and articles soiled therewith. In communities with a modern and adequate sewage disposal system, feces can be discharged directly into sewers without preliminary disinfection. Terminal cleaning.

4) Quarantine: None.

5) Immunization of contacts: No immunization available.

6) Investigation of contacts and source of infection: Culture stools of any household contacts who are involved in foodhandling, direct patient care, or care of young children or elderly persons in institutional settings.

7) Specific treatment: For uncomplicated enterocolitis, none

generally indicated except rehydration and electrolyte replacement with oral glucose-electrolyte solution (see Cholera, 9B7). Antibiotics may prolong the carrier state and lead to resistant strains. However, in infants under 2 months, the elderly, the debilitated and those with sickle cell disease, or in patients with continued or high fever or manifestations of extra-intestinal infection, antibiotic therapy should be given. Antimicrobial resistance of non-typhoidal Salmonellae is variable. Ampicillin or amoxicillin is usually recommended; co-trimoxazole and chloramphenicol are alternates when antimicrobial-resistant strains are involved.

C. *Epidemic measures:* See Foodborne disease, Staphylococcal food poisoning, 9C1 and 9C2. Search for a history of foodhandling errors, such as use of unsafe raw ingredients, inadequate cooking, time-temperature abuses and cross contamination. In the USA, in *S. enteritidis* outbreaks in which egg-containing dishes are implicated, initiate trace-back to the egg source and report to the US Dept of Agriculture is advised.

D. *Disaster implications:* A danger in a situation with mass feeding and poor sanitation.

E. *International measures:* WHO Collaborating Centres (see Preface).

SCABIES
(Sarcoptic itch, Acariasis)

ICD-9 133.0

1. **Identification**—A parasitic disease of the skin caused by a mite, whose penetration is visible as papules, vesicles, or tiny linear burrows containing the mites and their eggs. Lesions are prominent around finger webs, anterior surfaces of wrists and elbows, anterior axillary folds, belt line, thighs and external genitalia in men; nipples, abdomen, and the lower portion of the buttocks are frequently affected in women. In infants, the head, neck, palms and soles may be involved; these areas are usually spared in older individuals. Itching is intense, especially at night, but complications are limited to lesions secondarily infected from scratching. In immunodeficient individuals and in senile patients, infestation often appears as a generalized dermatitis more widely distributed than the burrows, with extensive scaling, and sometimes vesiculation and crusting ("Norwegian scabies"); the usual severe itching may be reduced or

absent. When scabies is complicated by beta-hemolytic streptococcal infection, risk of acute glomerulonephritis is present.

Diagnosis may be established by recovering the mite from its burrow and identifying it microscopically. Care should be taken to choose lesions for scraping or biopsy which have not been excoriated by repeated scratching. Prior application of mineral oil facilitates collecting the scrapings and examining them under a cover slip. Applying ink to the skin and then washing it off will disclose the burrows.

2. **Etiologic agent**—*Sarcoptes scabiei,* a mite.

3. **Occurrence**—Widespread. Past epidemics were attributed to poverty, poor sanitation, and crowding due to war and economic crises. The recent wave of infestation in the USA and Europe has evolved in the absence of major social disturbances and has affected people of all socioeconomic levels, without regard to age, sex, race, or standards of personal hygiene. It is endemic in many developing countries.

4. **Reservoir**—Man; *Sarcoptes* spp. and other mites of animals can live on man but do not reproduce in the skin.

5. **Mode of transmission**—Transfer of parasites is by direct skin-to-skin contact; can be acquired during sexual contact. Transfer from undergarments and bedclothes occurs only if these have been contaminated by infested persons immediately beforehand. Mites can burrow beneath the skin surface in 2.5 minutes. Norwegian scabies is highly transmissible because of the large number of mites in the exfoliating scales.

6. **Incubation period**—Two to 6 weeks before onset of itching in persons without previous exposure. Persons who have been previously infested develop symptoms 1-4 days after re-exposure.

7. **Period of communicability**—Until mites and eggs are destroyed by treatment, ordinarily after 1 or occasionally 2 courses of treatment, a week apart.

8. **Susceptibility and resistance**—Some resistance is suggested since immunologically compromised persons are susceptible to hyperinfestation; fewer mites succeed in establishing themselves on persons previously infested than on those with no prior exposure.

9. **Methods of control**—

   A. *Preventive measures:* Educate the public and medical community on mode of transmission, early diagnosis and treatment of infested patients and contacts.

B. *Control of patient, contacts and the immediate environment:*

1) Report to local health authority: Official report not ordinarily justifiable, Class 5 (see Preface).

2) Isolation: Exclude infested individuals from school or work until the day after treatment. For hospitalized patients, contact isolation for 24 hours after start of effective treatment.

3) Concurrent disinfection: Laundering underwear, clothing and bed sheets worn or used by the patient in the 48 hours prior to treatment using hot cycles of both washer and dryer has been suggested but is of questionable value.

4) Quarantine: None.

5) Immunization of contacts: None.

6) Investigation of contacts and source of infestation: Search for unreported and unrecognized cases among companions and household members; single infestations in a family are uncommon. Treat persons prophylactically who have had skin-to-skin contact with infested persons (including family members and sexual contacts).

7) Specific treatment: Apply 1% gamma benzene hexachloride (lindane, Kwell®), crotamiton (Eurax®), tetraethylthiuram monosulfide (Tetmosol®) in 5% solution twice daily (not available in the USA), or an emulsion of benzyl benzoate to the whole body except the head and neck; treatment details vary with the drug. On the next day, a cleansing bath is taken and a change made to fresh clothing and bedclothes. Itching may persist for 1-2 weeks, and during this period, should not be regarded as a sign of drug failure or reinfestation; overtreatment is common and should be avoided because of toxicity of some of these agents, especially gamma benzene hexachloride. In about 5% of cases, a second course of treatment may be necessary after an interval of 7-10 days if eggs survived the first treatment. Close supervision of treatment, including bathing, is necessary.

C. *Epidemic measures:*

1) Treatment is undertaken on a coordinated mass basis.

2) Case-finding efforts are extended to screen whole families, military units or institutions, with segregation of infested individuals if possible.

3) Soap and facilities for mass bathing and laundering are essential. Tetmosol soap, where available, helps to prevent infestation.

4) Health education of infested individuals and others at risk, as well as treatment. Cooperation of civilian or military authorities, often both, is needed.

D. **Disaster implications:** A potential nuisance in situations of overcrowding.

E. **International measures:** None.

SCHISTOSOMIASIS   ICD-9 120
(Bilharziasis, Snail fever)

1. **Identification**—A blood fluke (trematode) infection with adult male and female worms living in mesenteric or vesical veins of the host over a life span of many years. Eggs produce minute granulomata and scars in organs where they lodge or are deposited. Symptomatology is related to the number and location of the eggs in the human host: *Schistosoma mansoni* and *S. japonicum* give rise primarily to hepatic and intestinal symptoms, including diarrhea, abdominal pain and hepato-splenomegaly; *S. haematobium* to urinary manifestations, including dysuria, frequency and hematuria at the end of urination.

The most important pathologic effects are the complications that arise from chronic infection: liver fibrosis, portal hypertension, and possibly colorectal malignancy in the intestinal form; obstructive uropathy, superimposed bacterial infection and possibly bladder cancer in the urinary form of schistosomiasis. CNS manifestations may occur during the acute or chronic stages of infection from deposition of eggs in ectopic sites.

The larvae of certain schistosomes of birds and mammals may penetrate the human skin and cause a dermatitis, sometimes known as "swimmer's itch"; these schistosomes do not mature in man. Such infections may be prevalent among bathers in lakes in many parts of the world, including the Great Lakes region of N America and certain California coastal beaches.

Definitive diagnosis depends on the demonstration of eggs in the stool, urine or biopsy specimens. Useful immunologic tests include the circum-oval precipitin test, IFA and ELISA with egg or adult worm antigen, and RIA with purified egg or adult antigens; positive results on serologic tests do not constitute proof of current infection.

2. **Infectious agents**—*Schistosoma mansoni*, *S. haematobium* and *S. japonicum* are the major species causing human disease. *S. mekongi*, *S. malayensis*, *S. mattheei* and *S. intercalatum* are of importance only in limited areas.

3. **Occurrence**—*S. mansoni* is found in Africa (including Madagascar); the Arabian Peninsula; Brazil, Surinam and Venezuela in S America; and in some Caribbean islands. *S. haematobium* is found in Africa (including Madagascar and Mauritius) and the Middle East. *S. japonicum* is found in

China, Japan, the Philippines and Sulawesi (Indonesia). *S. mekongi* is found in the Mekong River area of Laos, Cambodia (Kampuchea) and Thailand. *S. intercalatum* occurs in parts of West Africa, including Cameroon, Central African Republic, Chad, Gabon, São Tomé and Zaire. *S. mattheei* is found in southern Africa. *S. malayensis* is known only from peninsular Malaysia. None of these species is indigenous to N America.

4. **Reservoir**—Man is the principal reservoir of *S. haematobium, S. intercalatum* and *S. mansoni*. Man, dogs, cats, pigs, cattle, water buffalo, horses and wild rodents are potential hosts of *S. japonicum;* their relative epidemiologic importance varies in different regions. *S. malayensis* appears to be a rodent parasite, occasionally infecting man. Persistence of the parasite depends on the presence of an appropriate snail as intermediate host; i.e., species of the genera *Biomphalaria* for *S. mansoni; Bulinus* for *S. haematobium, S. intercalatum,* and *S. mattheei; Oncomelania* for *S. japonicum; Tricula* for *S. mekongi;* and *Robertsiella* for *S. malayensis.*

5. **Mode of transmission**—Infection is acquired from water containing free-swimming larval forms (cercariae) which have developed in snails. The eggs of *S. haematobium* leave the mammalian body mainly in the urine, those of the other species in the feces. The eggs hatch in water and the liberated larvae (miracidia) penetrate into suitable freshwater snail hosts. After several weeks, the cercariae emerge from the snail and penetrate human skin, usually while the person is working, swimming or wading in water; they enter the bloodstream, are carried to blood vessels of the lungs, migrate to the liver, develop to maturity, and then migrate to veins of the abdominal cavity. Adult forms of *S. mansoni, S. japonicum, S. mekongi, S. mattheei* and *S. intercalatum* usually remain in mesenteric veins; those of *S. haematobium* usually migrate through anastomoses into the vesical plexus of the urinary bladder. Eggs are deposited in venules and escape into the lumen of the bowel or urinary bladder, or lodge in other organs, including the liver and the lungs.

6. **Incubation period**—Acute systemic manifestations (Katayama fever) may occur in primary infections 2-6 weeks after exposure, immediately preceding and during initial egg deposition. Acute manifestations are rare with *S. haematobium* infections.

7. **Period of communicability**—Not communicable from person to person, but persons with chronic schistosomiasis may spread the infection by discharging eggs in urine and/or feces into bodies of water for as long as they excrete eggs; it is common for human infections with *S. mansoni* and *S. haematobium* to last in excess of 10 years. Infected snails will release cercariae for as long as they live, a period which may last from several weeks to about 3 months.

8. **Susceptibility and resistance**—Susceptibility is universal; any

resistance developing as a result of infection is variable and poorly defined.

9. **Methods of control—**

   A. *Preventive measures:*

   1) Educate the public in endemic areas regarding mode of transmission and methods of protection.

   2) Dispose of feces and urine so that viable eggs will not reach bodies of fresh water containing intermediate snail hosts. Control of animals infected with *S. japonicum* is desirable but usually not practical.

   3) Improve irrigation and agriculture practices; reduce snail habitats by removing vegetation or by draining and filling.

   4) Treat snail-breeding sites with molluscicides. (Cost may limit use of these agents.)

   5) Prevent exposure to contaminated water (e.g., use rubber boots). To minimize cercarial penetration, towel dry, vigorously and completely, skin surfaces wet with suspected water. Apply 70% alcohol immediately to the skin to kill surface cercariae.

   6) Provide water for drinking, bathing and washing clothes from sources free of cercariae or treated to kill them.

   7) Treat patients in endemic areas to prevent disease progression and to reduce transmission by reducing egg passage.

   B. *Control of patient, contacts and the immediate environment:*

   1) Report to local health authority: In selected endemic areas; in many countries not a reportable disease, Class 3C (see Preface).

   2) Isolation: None.

   3) Concurrent disinfection: Sanitary disposal of feces and urine.

   4) Quarantine: None.

   5) Immunization of contacts: None.

   6) Investigation of contacts and source of infection: Examine contacts for infection from a common source. Search for source is a community effort (see 9C, below).

   7) Specific treatment: Praziquantel (Biltricide®) is the drug of choice against all species. Alternative drugs are oxamniquine for *S. mansoni* and metrifonate for *S. haematobium*.

   C. *Epidemic measures:* Examine for schistosomiasis and treat all who are infected, but especially those with moderate to heavy intensities of egg passage; pay particular attention to children.

Provide clean water, warn people against contact with waters potentially containing cercariae, and prohibit contamination of water. Treat areas which have high snail densities with molluscicides.

D. **Disaster implications:** None.

E. **International measures:** WHO Collaborating Centres (see Preface).

SHIGELLOSIS
ICD-9 004
(Bacillary dysentery)

1. **Identification**—An acute bacterial disease involving the large and distal small intestine, characterized by diarrhea accompanied by fever, nausea and sometimes toxemia, vomiting, cramps and tenesmus. In typical cases the stools contain blood, mucus and pus (dysentery) resulting from the confluent microabscesses caused by the invasive organisms; however, about one-third of cases present with a watery diarrhea. Convulsions may be an important complication in young children. Bacteremia is uncommon. Mild and asymptomatic infections occur. Illness is usually self-limited, lasting several days to weeks, with an average of 4-7 days. The severity of illness and the case fatality rate are functions of the host (age and pre-existing state of nutrition) and the serotype. *Shigella dysenteriae* 1 (Shiga's bacillus) is often associated with serious disease, including toxic megacolon and the hemolytic-uremic syndrome; case fatality rates have been as high as 20% among hospitalized cases even in recent years. In contrast, many infections with *Shigella sonnei* result in a short clinical course and an almost negligible case fatality rate, except in compromised hosts.

Bacteriologic diagnosis is made by isolation of *Shigella* from feces or rectal swabs. Prompt laboratory processing of specimens and use of several media increase the likelihood of *Shigella* isolation. Infection is usually associated with the presence of pus cells in the stool.

2. **Infectious agents**—The genus *Shigella* is comprised of 4 species or subgenera: Group A, *S. dysenteriae;* Group B, *S. flexneri;* Group C, *S. boydii;* and Group D, *S. sonnei.* Groups A, B and C are further divided into some 40 serotypes, designated by arabic numbers. A specific virulence plasmid is necessary for the epithelial cell invasiveness manifested by *Shigellae.*

3. **Occurrence**—Worldwide; two-thirds of the cases, and most of the deaths, are in children under 10 years. Illness in infants under 6 months is unusual. Secondary attack rates in households can be as high as 40%.

Outbreaks commonly occur under conditions of crowding and where personal hygiene is poor, such as in jails, institutions for children, day-care centers, mental hospitals and crowded camps; also in homosexual groups. Shigellosis is endemic in both tropical and temperate climates; reported cases represent only a small proportion of cases, even in developed areas.

More than one serotype is commonly present in a community; mixed infections with other intestinal pathogens also occur. In general, *S. boydii, S. dysenteriae* and *S. flexneri* account for most isolates from developing countries. In contrast, *S. sonnei* is most common and *S. dysenteriae* is uncommon in developed countries. Multi-antibiotic-resistant *Shigella* (including *S. dysenteriae* 1) have appeared in many areas of the world, related to widespread use of antimicrobial agents.

4. **Reservoir**—The only significant reservoir is man. However, outbreaks have occurred in primate colonies.

5. **Mode of transmission**—By direct or indirect fecal-oral transmission from a patient or carrier. Infection may occur after the ingestion of very few (10-100) organisms. Individuals primarily responsible for transmission are those who fail to clean hands and under fingernails thoroughly after defecation. They may then spread infection to others directly by physical contact or indirectly by contaminating food. Water and milk transmission may occur as the result of direct fecal contamination; flies may transfer organisms into a non-refrigerated food item in which they can multiply to an infectious dose. Dogs which have ingested infected human feces may be the source of exposure to susceptible persons, especially children.

6. **Incubation period**—Twelve to 96 hours (usually 1-3 days) up to one week for *S. dysenteriae* 1.

7. **Period of communicability**—During acute infection and until the infectious agent is no longer present in feces, usually within 4 weeks after illness. Asymptomatic carriers may transmit infection; rarely, the carrier state may persist for months, or longer. Appropriate antimicrobial treatment usually reduces duration of carriage to less than a week.

8. **Susceptibility and resistance**—Susceptibility is general, with infection following ingestion of a small number of organisms; the disease is more severe in children than in adults, among whom many infections may be asymptomatic. The elderly, debilitated individuals, and persons of all ages suffering from malnutrition are particularly susceptible to severe disease and death. Studies with experimental serotype-specific live oral vaccines have shown protection of short duration against infection with the homologous serotype.

9. **Methods of control**—Because of the diverse problems which may be involved in shigellosis, local health authorities must be prepared to

evaluate the local situation and take appropriate steps to prevent the spread of infection. It is not possible to provide a specific set of guidelines applicable to all situations. The potentially high case fatality rate in infections with *S. dysenteriae* type 1, coupled with antibiotic resistance, calls for measures comparable to those for typhoid fever, including the need to identify source(s) of infection. In contrast, an infection with *S. sonnei* in a private home would not merit such an approach. Institutional outbreaks, without regard to the infecting species, may require special measures, including separate housing for cases and new admissions, and repeated cultures of patients and attendants. The most difficult epidemics to control are those involving young children (not yet toilet-trained), the mentally disabled, and situations where there is an inadequate supply of water. Closure of affected day-care centers may lead to placement of infected children in other centers, with subsequent transmission in those centers, and is not by itself an effective control measure.

A. **Preventive measures:** Same as those listed under typhoid fever, 9A, 1-10, except that no commercial vaccines are available.

B. **Control of patient, contacts and the immediate environment:**

1) Report to local health authority: Case report is obligatory in most states and countries, Class 2B (see Preface). Recognition and report of epidemics in schools and institutions are especially important.

2) Isolation: During acute illness, enteric precautions. Because of the extremely small infective dose, patients with known *Shigella* infections should not be employed to handle food or to provide child or patient care until 2 successive fecal samples or rectal swabs (collected ≥24 hours apart, but not sooner than 48 hours following discontinuance of antimicrobials) are found to be free of *Shigella*. Patients must be advised of the importance and effectiveness of handwashing with soap and water after defecation as a means of curtailing transmission of *Shigella* to contacts.

3) Concurrent disinfection: Of feces and contaminated articles. In communities with a modern and adequate sewage disposal system, feces can be discharged directly into sewers without preliminary disinfection. Terminal cleaning.

4) Quarantine: None.

5) Management of contacts: Whenever feasible, ill contacts of shigellosis patients should be excluded from foodhandling and the care of children or patients until diarrhea ceases and 2 successive negative stool cultures are ob-

tained. Thorough handwashing after defecation and before handling food or caring for children or patients must be stressed if such contacts are unavoidable.

6) Investigation of contacts and source of infection: The search for unrecognized mild cases and convalescent carriers among contacts may be unproductive in sporadic cases and seldom contributes to the control of an outbreak. Cultures of contacts should generally be confined to foodhandlers, attendants and children in hospitals, and other situations where the spread of infection is particularly likely.

7) Specific treatment: Fluid and electrolyte replacement is important when diarrhea is watery or there are signs of dehydration (see Cholera, 9B7). Antibacterials (cotrimoxazole, ampicillin and quinolones) shorten the duration and severity of illness and the duration of pathogen excretion; they should be used in individual cases if warranted by the severity of the illness or to protect contacts (i.e., in day-care centers or institutions) when epidemiologically indicated. Multi-resistance to antibiotics is common, so the choice of specific agents will depend on the antibiogram of the isolated strain or on local antimicrobial susceptibility patterns. Antimotility agents are contraindicated; they may prolong the illness.

C. *Epidemic measures:*

1) Report at once to the local health authority any group of cases of acute diarrheal disorder, even in the absence of specific identification of the causal agent.

2) Investigate food, water and milk supplies, and use general sanitation measures.

3) Prophylactic administration of antibiotics is not recommended.

4) Publicize the importance of handwashing after defecation; provide soap and individual paper towels if otherwise not available.

D. *Disaster implications:* A potential problem where personal hygiene and environmental sanitation are deficient (see Typhoid fever).

E. *International measures:* WHO Collaborating Centres (see Preface).

SMALLPOX   ICD-9 050

The last naturally acquired case of smallpox in the world occurred in October 1977; global eradication was certified two years later by the WHO and confirmed by the World Health Assembly in May 1980. Thus, the occurrence of even a single case anywhere in the world is an international public health emergency. Because of the imperative need for rapid diagnosis and immediate institution of effective control measures should a case occur (in nature or from a laboratory accident), this disease, although now extinct, warrants this full presentation.

1. **Identification**—A systemic viral disease with an exanthem which is usually characteristic. Onset is sudden, with fever, malaise, headache, severe backache, prostration, and occasionally abdominal pain. After 2-4 days the temperature falls and a rash appears. The rash passes through successive stages of macules, papules, vesicles, pustules and finally scabs which fall off at the end of the third-fourth week; fever frequently rises as the rash progresses to the pustular stage. The lesions, appearing first on the face and subsequently on the body and extremities, are more abundant on the face and extremities than on the trunk (centrifugal distribution), and are abundant over prominences and extensor surfaces. In previously vaccinated persons, the rash may be significantly modified to the extent that systemic symptoms are mild to nil, and only a few highly atypical lesions are seen, which sometimes do not pass through the usual successive stages of rash.

Two principal clinico-epidemiologic varieties of smallpox were recognized: variola minor (alastrim) and variola major (classical smallpox). In variola major, the case fatality rate among the unvaccinated was 15-40%; death occurred as early as the third-fourth day, but more usually during the second week. Approximately 3% of hospitalized variola major cases experienced a fulminating disease characterized by a severe prodrome, prostration, and bleeding into the skin and mucous membranes, uterus and genital tract, especially in pregnant women; such hemorrhagic cases were rapidly fatal. In the highly lethal "flat" variety, observed in about 5% of cases, the focal lesions were slow to develop, and the vesicles containing very little fluid tended to project only slightly above the surrounding skin and were soft and velvety to the touch. In the few patients with this type who survived, the lesions sometimes resolved without the usual pustulation and crusting.

Outbreaks of variola minor were associated with a case fatality rate of <1%. Although the rash was similar to that observed in variola major, the patient generally experienced less severe systemic reactions, and "hemorrhagic" and "flat" types were rarely observed.

Most frequently confused with varicella (chickenpox), smallpox was usually distinguished by the clear-cut prodromal illness, the centrifugal distribution of the rash, the appearance of all lesions more or less simultaneously, the similarity in appearance of all lesions in a given area, and its more deeply seated lesions.

Laboratory confirmation is made by isolation of the virus on chicken embryo chorioallantoic membrane or cell culture from scrapings of lesions, vesicular or pustular fluid or crusts, and by a rise in titer in serologic tests. A rapid provisional diagnosis is often possible by EM or, if not available, by the precipitation-in-gel technique. These procedures cannot distinguish smallpox from vaccinia or monkeypox, in which case differentiation is made by DNA endonuclease digest electrophoresis.

2. Infectious agent—Variola virus, a species of *Orthopoxvirus*.

3. Occurrence—Formerly a worldwide disease, the WHO global program culminated in the eradication of smallpox. The last known case of naturally acquired variola major occurred in Bangladesh on 16 October 1975. Variola minor persisted in the Horn of Africa until 26 October 1977. Since that date, 2 cases of smallpox occurred in 1978 in Birmingham, England, related to escape of the virus from a research laboratory.

4. Reservoir—Prior to eradication, man was the reservoir; now it is held only in stocks of virus in 2 restricted laboratories.

5. Mode of transmission—By close contact with respiratory; discharges and, less frequently, by skin lesions of patients, or material which they had recently contaminated; infrequently airborne spread. Household, hospital and school contacts were especially at risk. Spread to laundry workers by bedding and other linens was observed. Inapparent infections have not been implicated, but unrecognized cases sometimes led to extensive secondary spread.

6. Incubation period—From 7-17 days; commonly 10-12 days to onset of illness and 2-4 days more to onset of rash.

7. Period of communicability—From the time of the development of the earliest lesions to disappearance of all scabs; about 3 weeks. Most communicable during first week.

8. Susceptibility and resistance—Susceptibility is universal; long-term immunity usually followed recovery; second attacks were rare.

9. Methods of control—

    A. Preventive measures:

        1)   Since smallpox has now been eradicated, routine vaccination is no longer justified. International Certificates of Vaccination against smallpox are no longer required of travelers.

        2)   Vaccination is recommended only for those few research workers in laboratories still conducting research on variola virus or related orthopoxviruses; in the USA, vaccine

for this purpose can be obtained from the CDC, Division of Host Factors, Atlanta GA 30333; telephone (404) 639-3356 or (404) 639-2888 after working hours.

3) Military forces in some countries continue to be vaccinated to protect against the remote possibility of biological warfare, even though international convention precludes such warfare. Appropriate measures should be taken by such services to minimize risk to unvaccinated contacts (see 9A4, below).

4) Vaccination, should it ever be required, is accomplished by inserting a live WHO-recommended vaccine strain into the superficial layers of the skin. Freeze-dried vaccine, stockpiled by WHO and many countries, retains adequate potency. The preferred site for vaccination is the outer aspect of the upper arm over the insertion of the deltoid muscle. No cleansing of the skin is needed unless the vaccination site is obviously dirty, in which case it should be gently cleansed with water, and permitted to dry.

Two different vaccination techniques may be used; multiple puncture or jet injection. In the **multiple puncture technique,** a forked (bifurcated) needle is used. The needle is dipped into the vaccine and then, holding the needle perpendicular to the skin, punctures are made in an up-and-down manner within an area about 3 mm (1/8″) in diameter. Five punctures are made for previously unvaccinated and 15 for revaccinations. A trace of blood should be observed at the vaccination site. Any vaccine on the surface should be removed. For **jet injection,** a special bacteria-free vaccine is required.

To minimize risk of infection of unvaccinated contacts, a loose dressing should be applied over any lesion which might develop; the individual should avoid physical contact with others, especially those with a history of eczema. Vaccination is repeated as above at least 1 week later unless a "major reaction" is apparent, indicating that an immunizing vaccinial infection has occurred. A "major reaction" is one which, 1 week after vaccination, presents a vesicular or pustular lesion, or an area of definite induration or erythema surrounding a scab or ulcer remaining at the point of vaccine insertion. All other responses are "equivocal reactions" and the individual should be vaccinated again, using more vigorous application of vaccine. All primary vaccinations should elicit a major reaction; revaccinations, except in highly immune groups, should produce major reactions in 80-90% of subjects. Persons with a high level of cellular immunity may exhibit an allergic reaction in the first 2-3 days after vaccination (even with a vaccine which has lost its infectivity) consisting of erythema and papules or vesicles resulting in a scab which may still be present at the end of 1 week; however, there may be no antibody response.

Major complications of vaccination include (1) encephalitis, very rare with current vaccine strains; (2) progressive vaccinia occurring in individuals with immunologic defects or who are immunocompromised, e.g., by AIDS, drugs, corticosteroids or radiation; and (3) eczema vaccinatum in those with past or present eczema, which may occur in eczematous siblings of vaccinees. Minor complications include generalized vaccinia with multiple vaccinial lesions appearing in 5-10 days on various parts of the body; autoinoculation of mucous membranes or abraded skin; and a benign erythema multiforme-type rash, usually generalized and symmetrical, which may frequently occur at the height of the vaccinia. Vaccinia immune globulin (VIG), 0.3-0.6 ml/kg, is indicated in the treatment of eczema vaccinatum and progressive vaccinia. It may be obtained in the USA on an emergency basis by contacting the CDC, Atlanta (see Preface). Methisazone (Marboran) may be of benefit in treatment of these conditions.

5) Vaccination is contraindicated in those at special risk of experiencing complications. These include persons with eczema, those with impaired immunodeficiency (whether from disease such as AIDS or from treatment programs with steroids or ionizing radiation), and pregnant women. If such an individual should require vaccination, VIG, 0.3 ml/kg, should be given concurrently with vaccination. If there has been possible exposure to a case of smallpox, there are no contraindications to vaccination even if VIG is not available.

6) Initial vaccination should be limited to household and other close contacts when a presumptive diagnosis of smallpox is established on examination by a physician with extensive experience in the clinical and epidemiologic diagnosis of smallpox and on a laboratory report confirming that poxvirus particles have been demonstrated by electron microscopy.

B. *Control of patient, contacts and the immediate environment:*

1) Report to local health authority: AN INTERNATIONAL EPIDEMIOLOGIC EMERGENCY. REPORT

BY TELEPHONE OR TELEGRAPH TO HEALTH AUTHORITIES. All suspected cases should be investigated immediately by clinical and laboratory study by state, national and, appropriately, international authorities. The occurrence of even one laboratory-confirmed case of smallpox would be an international emergency, as it would call into question the status of eradication or indicate that virus had escaped from a research laboratory. Occurrence of cases only clinically suspected to be smallpox constitutes a public health emergency. Class 1 (see Preface).

2) Isolation: Pending instructions from national and international advisers, strict isolation precautions will be established.

3) Concurrent disinfection: All material in contact with the patient should be boiled, autoclaved or burned. Terminal disinfection will be carried out as recommended by advisers.

4), 5), and 6) Quarantine, Immunization of contacts, and Investigation of contacts and source of infection: Appropriate measures would be defined by national and international advisers.

7) Specific treatment: None.

C. *Epidemic measures:* Immediate reporting of a suspected case will prompt assistance from national and international authorities to provide detailed investigation and for implementation of necessary control measures.

D. *Disaster implications:* Introduction of variola virus into a nonimmune population could result in a major disaster unless controlled promptly.

E. *International measures:*

1) Immediate telegraphic notification by governments to WHO and to adjacent countries if any case of smallpox is found or suspected.

2) In December 1979, the Global Commission for the Certification of Smallpox Eradication concluded that: (1) Smallpox eradication had been achieved throughout the world; and (2) that there was no evidence that smallpox would return as an endemic disease.

MONKEYPOX   ICD-9 051.9

Clinically, human monkeypox is almost identical to smallpox. It remains an infrequent, sporadic zoonosis. Between 1970 and 1986, over

400 cases had been reported from tropical rain forested areas of West and Central Africa; Zaire alone accounted for 95% of these cases.

Clinically, the disease is similar to that of ordinary and modified forms of smallpox. Lymphadenopathy is more prominent and occurs in the early stage of the disease. Pleomorphism and "cropping," similar to that in chickenpox, are observed in 20% of patients. The prognosis depends largely on the presence of severe complications. The case fatality rate is 10-15%, comparable to that of smallpox when it was in that area.

Most cases have occurred either singly or in small clusters in small, remote villages close to, or in, the tropical rainforest, where the population usually has multiple contacts with a variety of wild animals. Recent ecologic studies indicate that squirrels (genus *Funisciurus* and *Heliosciurus*), abundant among the oil-palms surrounding the villages, are a significant host and reservoir of the monkeypox virus. The majority of human infections are attributable to contact with affected animals.

The disease affects all age groups, but children under 10 years are at the highest risk. Human-to-human transmission occurs from primary human cases, with a secondary attack rate of about 10%, but very rarely from secondary cases. The longest reported chain of interhuman transmission consisted of only four serial cases.

The virus is a separate species of *Orthopoxvirus,* with biological properties and genome map distinct from variola virus; smallpox vaccination protects against disease. Recent studies have shown that transmission of the virus is uncommon in its enzootic areas, even where smallpox vaccination levels are very low. Cases are expected to continue to occur, but there is no evidence that monkeypox will become a public health problem.

SPOROTRICHOSIS   ICD-9 117.1

1. **Identification**—A fungal disease, usually of the skin, often of an extremity, which begins as a nodule. As the nodule grows, lymphatics draining the area become firm and cordlike and form a series of nodules, which in turn may soften and ulcerate. Arthritis, pneumonitis and other visceral infections are rare. Fatalities are uncommon.

Laboratory confirmation is made by culture of the pus or exudate, preferably aspirated from an unopened lesion; organisms are rarely visualized by direct smear. Biopsied tissue should be examined with fungal stains.

2. **Infectious agent**—*Sporothrix schenckii,* a dimorphic fungus.

3. **Occurrence**—Reported from all parts of the world, in males more

frequently than in females, and in adults more than in children; an occupational disease of farmers, gardeners and horticulturists. The disease is characteristically sporadic, and relatively uncommon. An epidemic among gold miners in South Africa involved some 3,000 persons; fungus was growing on mine timbers. In 1988, 84 cases occurred in 14 states (USA) in persons who handled conifer seedlings packed with sphagnum moss.

4. **Reservoir**—Soil, decaying vegetation, wood, moss and hay.

5. **Mode of transmission**—Introduction of fungus through the skin by pricks of thorns or barbs, the handling of sphagnum moss or by slivers from wood or lumber. Outbreaks have occurred among children playing and adults working with baled hay; a recent outbreak was associated with sphagnum moss wrapped around conifer seedlings. Pulmonary sporotrichosis is assumed to arise by inhalation of conidia.

6. **Incubation period**—The lymphatic form may develop one week to 3 months after injury.

7. **Period of communicability**—Not transmitted from person to person.

8. **Susceptibility and resistance**—People probably are highly susceptible.

9. **Methods of control**—

   A. *Preventive measures:* Treat lumber with fungicides in industries where disease occurs.

   B. *Control of patient, contacts and the immediate environment:*

      1) Report to local health authority: Official report not ordinarily justifiable, Class 5 (see Preface).
      2) Isolation: None.
      3) Concurrent disinfection: Of discharges and dressings. Terminal cleaning.
      4) Quarantine: None.
      5) Immunization of contacts: None.
      6) Investigation of contacts and source of infection: To seek undiagnosed and untreated cases.
      7) Specific treatment: Orally administered iodides are effective in lymphocutaneous infection; in other forms, amphotericin B (Fungizone®) is often effective.

   C. *Epidemic measures:* Determine source to limit future exposures. In the South African epidemic, mine timbers were sprayed with a mixture of zinc sulfate and triolith. This and other sanitary measures controlled the epidemic.

D. *Disaster implications:* None.

E. *International measures:* None.

STAPHYLOCOCCAL DISEASE

Staphylococci produce a variety of syndromes with clinical manifestations ranging from a single pustule to septicemia and death. A lesion or lesions containing pus is the primary clinical finding, abscess formation the typical pathology. Virulence of bacterial strains varies greatly. The most useful index of pathogenicity is the ability to coagulate plasma; almost all pathogenic strains are coagulase-positive.

Staphylococcal disease has distinctly different clinical and epidemiologic patterns in the general community, in newborns, in menstruating women, or among hospitalized patients. Therefore, each will be presented separately. Staphylococcal food poisoning, an intoxication and not an infection, is discussed separately (see Foodborne disease, Staphylococcal).

I. STAPHYLOCOCCAL DISEASE IN THE COMMUNITY
BOILS, CARBUNCLES, FURUNCLES ICD-9 680, 041.1
IMPETIGO ICD-9 684, 041.1
CELLULITIS, ABSCESSES ICD-9 682.9, 041.1
STAPHYLOCOCCAL SEPTICEMIA ICD-9 038.I
STAPHYLOCOCCAL PNEUMONIA ICD-9 482.4
ARTHRITIS, OSTEOMYELITIS ICD-9 730, 041.1
ENDOCARDITIS ICD-9 421.0, 041.1

1. **Identification**—The common skin lesions are impetigo, folliculitis, furuncles, carbuncles, abscesses and infected lacerations. The basic lesion of impetigo is described in II, section 1, below; in addition, a distinctive scalded skin syndrome is associated with certain strains of *Staphylococcus aureus,* most often those of phage group II, which elaborate an exfoliative toxin. The other skin lesions are localized and discrete. Constitutional symptoms are unusual; if lesions extend or are widespread, fever, malaise, headache and anorexia may develop. Usually, lesions are uncomplicated, but seeding of the bloodstream may lead to pneumonia, lung abscess, osteomyelitis, septicemia, endocarditis, pyarthrosis, meningitis or brain abscess. In addition to primary lesions of the skin, staphylococcal

conjunctivitis occurs in newborns and the elderly. Staphylococcal pneumonia is a well recognized complication of influenza. Staphylococcal endocarditis and other complications of staphylococcal bacteremia may result from parenteral use of illicit drugs or be acquired nosocomially through the use of intravenous catheters and other devices. Embolic skin lesions are frequent complications of endocarditis and/or bacteremia.

Coagulase-negative staphylococci may cause septicemia, endocarditis and urinary infections and are increasingly involved in the etiology of disease, usually in connection with prosthetic devices or indwelling catheters.

Diagnosis is confirmed by isolation of the organism.

2. Infectious agent—Various coagulase-positive strains of *Staphylococcus aureus* may be characterized by phage type, antibiotic resistance or serologic agglutination; epidemics are caused by relatively few specific strains. The majority of clinical isolates of *S. aureus*, both community and hospital-acquired, are resistant to penicillin G, and multi-resistant (including methicillin-resistant) strains are increasingly frequent. Coagulase-negative *S. epidermidis* can be pathogenic; *S. saprophyticus* is a common cause of urinary tract infections in young women.

3. Occurrence—Worldwide. Highest incidence is in areas where personal hygiene (especially the use of soap and water) is suboptimal and people are crowded; common among children, especially in warm weather. It occurs sporadically and as small epidemics in families and summer camps, with various members developing recurrent illness due to the same staphylococcal strain.

4. Reservoir—Man, and rarely animals.

5. Mode of transmission—The major site of colonization is the anterior nares; 30-40% of the general population carry coagulase-positive staphylococci there. Auto-infection is responsible for at least one-third of infections. Persons with a draining lesion or any purulent discharge are the most common sources of epidemic spread. Transmission is by contact with a person who either has a purulent lesion or is an asymptomatic (usually nasal) carrier of a pathogenic strain. Some carriers are more effective disseminators of infection than others. The role of contaminated objects has been overstressed; the hands are the most important instrument for transmitting infection. Airborne spread is rare but has been demonstrated in infants with associated viral respiratory disease.

6. Incubation period—Variable and indefinite. Commonly 4-10 days.

7. Period of communicability—As long as purulent lesions continue to drain or the carrier state persists. Auto-infection may continue for the period of nasal colonization or duration of active lesions.

8. Susceptibility and resistance—Immune mechanisms are not well understood. Susceptibility is greatest among the newborn and the chronically ill. Elderly and debilitated persons, drug abusers, and those with diabetes mellitus, cystic fibrosis, chronic renal failure, agammaglobulinemia, agranulocytosis, neoplastic disease and burns are particularly susceptible. Use of steroids and antimetabolites also increases susceptibility.

9. Methods of control—

A. *Preventive measures:*

1) Educate the public in personal hygiene, especially handwashing and the importance of avoiding common use of toilet articles.

2) Treat promptly the initial cases in children and families.

B. *Control of patient, contacts and the immediate environment:*

1) Report to local health authority: Obligatory report of outbreaks in schools, summer camps and other population groups; also any recognized concentration of cases in the community. No individual case report, Class 4 (see Preface).

2) Isolation: Not practical in most communities; infected persons should avoid contact with infants and debilitated persons.

3) Concurrent disinfection: Place dressings from open lesions and discharges in disposable bag and dispose in a practical and safe manner. Terminal cleaning.

4) Quarantine: None.

5) Immunization of contacts: None.

6) Investigation of contacts and source of infection: Search for draining lesions; occasionally, determination of nasal carrier status of the pathogenic strain among family members is useful.

7) Specific treatment: In localized skin infections, systemic antibiotics are not indicated unless infection spreads significantly or complications ensue; local application of an appropriate antibiotic (such as bacitracin, 4 times/day) is adequate. Abscesses should be incised to permit drainage of pus. For severe staphylococcal infections, employ a penicillinase-resistant penicillin or, when hypersensitivity to penicillin is present, use a cephalosporin (unless there is a history of immediate hypersensitivity to penicillin), clindamycin or vancomycin. In severe systemic infections, the selection of antibiotics should be governed by results of susceptibility tests on isolates. Vancomycin is the treatment of choice for severe infections with methicillin-

resistant *S. aureus;* prompt parenteral treatment is important. Staphylococci are generally resistant to sulfonamides unless they are used in combination with trimethoprim (e.g., in co-trimoxazole).

C. *Epidemic measures:*

1) Search for and treat persons with clinical disease, especially those with draining lesions. Institute strict personal hygiene with emphasis on handwashing. Culture for nasal carriers of the epidemic strain, and treat locally (see II, 9C3, below).

2) Investigate any unusual or abrupt increase in prevalence of staphylococcal infections in the community for a possible common source, such as an unrecognized hospital epidemic.

D. *Disaster implications:* None.

E. *International measures:* WHO Collaborating Centres (see Preface).

II. STAPHYLOCOCCAL DISEASE IN HOSPITAL NURSERIES
IMPETIGO   ICD-9 684, 041.1
ABSCESS OF THE BREAST   ICD-9 675.1, 041.1

1. Identification—Impetigo of the newborn (pemphigus neonatorum) and other purulent skin manifestations are the most frequent nursery-acquired staphylococcal diseases. The characteristic skin lesions develop secondary to colonization (with a pathogenic strain) of the nose or umbilicus, conjunctiva, circumcision site or rectum of infants. (Colonization of these sites with nonpathogenic strains of staphylococci is a normal occurrence in infants and does not imply disease.) Lesions most commonly are in diaper and intertriginous areas but may be distributed anywhere on the body; they are initially vesicular, rapidly turning seropurulent, surrounded by an erythematous base. Rupture of pustules favors peripheral spread. Though less common, scalded skin syndrome, or Ritter's disease, may occur with clinical manifestations ranging from diffuse scarlatiniform erythema, to scattered bullous impetigo, to generalized disease. Complications are unusual, although furunculosis, breast abscess, staphylococcal pneumonia, septicemia, meningitis, osteomyelitis, brain abscess and other serious diseases have been reported.

2. Infectious agent—Same as for staphylococcal disease in the community (I, section 2, above).

3. **Occurrence**—Worldwide. Problems occur mainly in hospitals, are promoted by laxity in aseptic techniques and are exaggerated by development of antibiotic-resistant strains of the infectious agent (i.e., hospital strains).

4. **Reservoir**—Same as for staphylococcal disease in the community (I, section 4, above).

5. **Mode of transmission**—Primary mode is spread by hands of hospital personnel; rarely airborne.

6. **Incubation period**—Commonly 4-10 days, but disease may not occur until several months after colonization.

7. **Period of communicability**—Same as for staphylococcal disease in the community (I, section 7, above).

8. **Susceptibility and resistance**—Susceptibility in the newborn appears to be general. Infants remain at risk of disease for duration of colonization with pathogenic strains.

9. **Methods of control**—

    A.   *Preventive measures:*

        1)   Use aseptic techniques when necessary and adequate handwashing before each infant contact in nurseries.

        2)   Use a rotational system ("cohorting") in the nursery, whereby one unit (A) is filled and subsequent babies are admitted to a second nursery (B), while the initial unit (A) discharges infants and is cleaned before new admissions. If facilities are present for rooming-in of baby with mother, this may reduce risk. Colonized or infected infants should be grouped together in another cohort. Assignments of nursing and other ward personnel should be restricted to specific cohorts.

        3)   Surveillance and supervision through an active Hospital Infection Control Committee, including a regular system for investigating, reporting and reviewing all hospital-acquired infections. Illness developing after discharge from hospital should also be investigated and recorded, preferably by active surveillance of all discharged newborns at about one month of age.

        4)   Some advocate routine application of antibacterial substances, such as triple dye (brilliant green, crystal violet, acriflavine), chlorhexidine or bacitracin ointment, to the umbilical cord stump while the baby is in the hospital.

B. *Control of patient, contacts and the immediate environment:*

1) Report to local health authority: Obligatory report of epidemics; no individual case report, Class 4 (see Preface).

2) Isolation: Without delay, place all known or suspected cases in the nursery on contact isolation precautions. Do not permit hospital personnel with minor lesions (pustules, boils, abscesses, paronychia, conjunctivitis, severe acne, otitis externa or infected lacerations) to work in the nursery.

3) Concurrent disinfection: Same as for staphylococcal disease in the community (see I, 9B3, above).

4) Quarantine: None.

5) Immunization of contacts: None.

6) Investigation of contacts and source of infection: See epidemic measures in 9C, below.

7) Specific treatment: For localized impetiginous lesions: remove crusts, cleanse skin, treat with bacitracin ointment or wash with an iodophor solution 4-6 times/day. Systemic antibiotics are not indicated unless disease is progressive with fever, malaise or secondary complications. For serious infections, treat as in I, 9B7, above.

C. *Epidemic measures:*

1) The occurrence of two or more concurrent cases of staphylococcal disease related to a nursery or a maternity ward is presumptive evidence of an epidemic and warrants investigation. Culture all lesions to determine antibiotic resistance pattern of epidemic strain. Clinically important isolates should be kept by the laboratory for 6 months before discarding. This makes possible epidemiologic investigation using antibiotic sensitivity patterns and phage typing.

2) In a nursery outbreak, institute isolation precautions for cases and contacts until all have been discharged. Before admitting new patients, wash cribs, beds, isolettes and other furniture with an approved disinfectant. Autoclave instruments and basins, wipe mattresses and sterilize bedding and diapers.

3) Examine all patient-care personnel, including physicians, nurses, aides and attendants, for draining lesions anywhere on the body. Culture nasal specimens from all persons in contact with infants. Under circumstances of continuing disease, it may become necessary to exclude and treat all carriers of the epidemic strain until cultures are negative. Treatment of asymptomatic carriers is directed at suppression of the nasal carrier state, usually

accomplished by the local application of appropriate antibiotic ointments to the nasal vestibule, sometimes with concurrent rifampin.

4) Investigate adequacy of nursing procedures; emphasize strict handwashing. Personnel assigned to infected or colonized infants should not work with noncolonized newborns.

5) Although prohibited for routine use in the USA because CNS damage may result from systemic absorption, preparations containing 3% hexachlorophene may be employed during an outbreak. Full-term infants may be bathed (in the diaper area only) as soon after birth as possible and daily until they are discharged. After bathing is completed, the hexachlorophene should be washed off thoroughly.

D. *Disaster implications:* None.

E. *International measures:* WHO Collaborating Centres (see Preface).

III. STAPHYLOCOCCAL DISEASE IN MEDICAL AND SURGICAL WARDS OF HOSPITALS   ICD-9 998.5

1. **Identification**—Lesions vary from simple furuncles or stitch abscesses, to extensively infected bedsores or surgical wounds, septic phlebitis, chronic osteomyelitis, fulminating pneumonia, meningitis, endocarditis and septicemia. Postoperative staphylococcal disease is a constant threat to the convalescence of the hospitalized surgical patient. The increasing complexity of surgical operations, with greater organ exposure and more prolonged anesthesia, promotes entry of staphylococci. Increased use of prosthetic devices and indwelling catheters accounts for an increased incidence of nosocomial staphylococcal infections. Frequent and sometimes injudicious use of antibiotic therapy has increased the prevalence of antibiotic-resistant staphylococci. Staphylococcal enteritis is a serious complication which occasionally occurs in antibiotic-treated patients.

Verification depends on isolation of *Staphylococcus aureus,* associated with a clinical illness compatible with the bacteriologic findings.

2. **Infectious agent**—*Staphylococcus aureus;* see I, section 2, above. These are predominantly antibiotic resistant, with 85-90% resistant to penicillin and increasing proportions resistant to semi-synthetic penicillins (e.g., methicillin) and the aminoglycosides (e.g., gentamicin).

3. **Occurrence**—Worldwide. Staphylococcal infection is a major form

of acquired sepsis in the general wards of hospitals. At times, attack rates assume epidemic proportions. Spread to the community may occur when persons infected in the hospital are discharged.

4., 5., 6., and **7. Reservoir, Mode of transmission, Incubation period,** and **Period of communicability:** Same as for staphylococcal disease in the community (I, sections 4, 5, 6, and 7, above).

8. Susceptibility and resistance—Susceptibility is general, but greatest in chronically ill and debilitated patients, those receiving systemic steroid or antimetabolite therapy and those undergoing major and prolonged surgical operation and convalescence. The widespread use of continuous intravenous therapy with in-dwelling plastic catheters and parenteral injections has opened new portals of entry for infectious agents.

9. Methods of control—

   A. *Preventive measures:*

   1) Coordinate through a Hospital Infection Control Committee to enforce strict aseptic technique and to provide programs for monitoring nosocomial infections.
   2) Educate hospital medical staff to use common antibiotics for simple infections and reserve certain antibiotics (e.g., vancomycin, cephalosporins) for penicillin-resistant staphylococcal infections.
   3) Replace all in-dwelling peripheral venous catheters at least every 72 hours; change sites of intravenous infusions every 48 hours.

   B. *Control of patient, contacts and the immediate environment:*

   1) Report to local health authority: Obligatory report of epidemics; no individual case report, Class 4 (see Preface).
   2) Isolation: Whenever a moderate or heavy abundance of staphylococci is known or suspected to be present in draining pus or the sputum of a patient with pneumonia, the patient should be placed on the appropriate isolation precautions promptly. Isolation is not required when wound drainage is scanty, provided that an occlusive dressing is used and care is taken in changing dressings to prevent contamination of the environment.
   3) Concurrent disinfection: As in staphylococcal disease in the community (I, 9B3, above).
   4) Quarantine: None.
   5) Immunization of contacts: None.

6) Investigation of contacts and source of infection: Not practical for sporadic cases (see 9C, below).

7) Specific treatment: Appropriate antibiotics as determined by antibiotic sensitivity tests.

C. *Epidemic measures:*

1) The occurrence of two or more cases with epidemiologic association is sufficient to suspect epidemic spread and to initiate investigation.

2) Same as II, 9C3, above.

3) Review and enforce rigid aseptic techniques.

D. *Disaster implications:* None.

E. *International measures:* WHO Collaborating Centres (see Preface).

TOXIC SHOCK SYNDROME ICD-9 785.59

Toxic Shock Syndrome (TSS) is a severe illness characterized by sudden onset of high fever, vomiting, profuse watery diarrhea and myalgia, followed by hypotension, and in severe cases, shock. An erythematous, "sunburn-like" rash is present during the acute phase; about 10 days after onset, there is desquamation of the skin, especially of palms and soles. Fever is usually higher than 38.9°C (102°F), the systolic blood pressure <90 mm mercury, and three or more organ systems are involved. Those systems involved include the GI; muscular (severe myalgia and/or creatine phosphokinase level greater than twice the normal upper limit); mucous membranes (hyperemia of vaginal, pharyngeal and/or conjunctival); renal (blood urea nitrogen or creatinine more than twice normal and/or sterile pyuria); hepatic (SGOT or SGPT greater than twice normal); hematologic (platelets $<100 \times 10^3$/cu mm); and the CNS (disorientation or alterations in consciousness without focal neurologic signs). Blood, throat and CSF are negative for pathogens on culture, although the recovery of *S. aureus* from any of these sites does not invalidate a case; serologic tests for Rocky Mountain spotted fever, leptospirosis and measles are negative. Although *S. aureus* can rarely be recovered from the vaginas of healthy women, it is regularly found in women with menstrually-associated TSS or in those with TSS who recently underwent gynecologic surgery.

During 1980, almost 900 cases were reported within the USA, 97.1% in women, with a case fatality rate of 5%. Approximately 95% of the reported female cases occurred during the menstrual period. Epidemiologic studies indicated that toxin-producing strains of *S. aureus* were responsible; virtually all isolated strains were penicillin-resistant. Most cases with onset during menstruation have been associated with the use of vaginal tampons. The incidence of severe cases in 1980 was estimated to be 6-16/100,000 women of menstrual age/year. By 1986, the annual incidence had fallen to 1/100,000 women of menstrual age. *S. aureus* has been isolated from focal lesions of the skin, bone and lung in the cases in men and in women not associated with menstruation; 45% of cases now reported are not associated with menstruation. A recent study demonstrated a significantly increased risk of TSS in users of contraceptive diaphragms and vaginal contraceptive sponges.

Menstrual TSS can be almost entirely prevented by avoiding the use of vaginal tampons; the risk may be reduced by using tampons intermittently during each menstrual cycle (that is, not used all day and all night during the period) and by using less absorbent tampons. Instructions for sponge use, indicating that they should not be left in place for more than 30 hours, should be heeded. Women who develop a high fever and vomiting or diarrhea during the menstrual period should discontinue tampon use immediately and consult a physician. It is not known when those who have had an episode of menstrual TSS can safely resume tampon use.

STREPTOCOCCAL DISEASES CAUSED BY GROUP A (BETA-HEMOLYTIC) STREPTOCOCCI
ICD-9 034, 035, 670

(Streptococcal sore throat, Scarlet fever, Impetigo, Erysipelas, Puerperal fever)

1. **Identification**—Group A streptococci cause a variety of diseases. The more frequently encountered conditions are streptococcal sore throat and streptococcal skin infections (impetigo or pyoderma). Other diseases include scarlet fever, puerperal fever, septicemia, erysipelas, cellulitis, mastoiditis, otitis media, pneumonia, peritonsillitis, wound infections, and rarely, toxic shock syndrome. In outbreaks, one form of clinical disease often predominates.

Streptococcal sore throat patients frequently exhibit fever, sore throat, exudative tonsillitis or pharyngitis and tender anterior cervical lymph nodes. The pharynx, the tonsillar pillars and soft palate may be injected and edematous; petechiae may be present against a background of diffuse redness. There may be a minimum of symptoms. Coincident or subsequent otitis media or peritonsillar abscess may occur; acute glomerulonephritis may appear (mean=10 days) or acute rheumatic fever in 1-5 weeks (mean=19 days). In contrast to the other manifestations of rheumatic fever, Sydenham's chorea may occur several months following the streptococcal infection; rheumatic heart disease is a later complication.

Streptococcal skin infection (pyoderma, impetigo) is usually superficial and may proceed through vesicular, pustular and encrusted stages. Scarlatiniform rash is unusual and rheumatic fever is not a sequel; however, glomerulonephritis may occur later, usually three weeks.

Scarlet fever is a form of streptococcal disease characterized by a skin rash; it occurs when the infecting strain of streptococcus produces an erythrogenic toxin, and the patient is sensitized but not immune to the toxin. Clinical characteristics may include all those symptoms associated with a streptococcal sore throat (or it may be associated with a wound, skin or puerperal infection), as well as enanthem, strawberry tongue and exanthem. The rash is usually a fine erythema, commonly punctate, blanching on pressure, often felt (like sandpaper) better than seen and appearing most often on the neck, chest, in folds of the axilla, elbow and groin, and on inner surfaces of the thighs. Typically, the rash does not involve the face, but there is flushing of the cheeks and circumoral pallor. High fever, nausea and vomiting often accompany severe infections. During convalescence, desquamation of the skin occurs at the tips of fingers and toes, less often over wide areas of trunk and limbs, including palms and soles. The case fatality rate in some parts of the world has occasionally been as high as 3%. Scarlet fever may be followed by the same sequelae as streptococcal sore throat.

Erysipelas is an acute cellulitis characterized by fever, constitutional symptoms, leukocytosis and a red, tender, edematous, spreading lesion of the skin, often with a definite raised border. The central point of origin tends to clear as the periphery extends. Face and legs are common sites. Recurrences are frequent. The disease is more common in women and may be especially severe, with bacteremia, in patients suffering from debilitating disease. Case fatality rates vary greatly depending on the part of the body affected and whether there is an associated disease. Erysipelas due to group A streptococci is to be distinguished from erysipeloid, caused by *Erysipelothrix rhusiopathiae*, a localized cutaneous infection seen primarily as an occupational disease of persons handling freshwater fish or shellfish, animals, meat and poultry.

Perianal cellulitis due to group A streptococci has been recognized more frequently in recent years.

Streptococcal puerperal fever is an acute disease, usually febrile, accompanied by local and general symptoms and signs of bacterial invasion of the genital tract and sometimes the bloodstream in the postpartum or postabortion patient. Case fatality rate from streptococcal puerperal fever is low when adequately treated. Puerperal infections may be caused by organisms other than hemolytic streptococci; while clinically similar, they differ bacteriologically and epidemiologically.

Streptococci of other groups can produce human disease. β-hemolytic organisms of group B are frequently found in the human vagina and may cause neonatal sepsis and suppurative meningitis (see Group B Streptococcal Disease of the Newborn, below). Group D organisms (including enterococci), hemolytic or nonhemolytic, are involved in subacute bacterial endocarditis and urinary tract infections. Groups C and G have produced outbreaks of streptococcal tonsillitis, usually foodborne; their role in sporadic cases is less well-defined. Glomerulonephritis has followed group C infections, but only one case has been reported following group G infection; neither group causes rheumatic fever. Alphahemolytic streptococci are also a common cause of subacute bacterial endocarditis.

Provisional laboratory findings which support group A streptococcal disease are based on the identification of group A streptococcal antigen in pharyngeal secretions (the rapid strep test) or on the isolation of organisms from the affected tissues on blood agar or other appropriate media. In cultures, streptococci are identified by the morphology of colonies and production of clear β-hemolysis on blood agar made with sheep's blood; tentative identification is shown by inhibition by special antibiotic discs containing 0.02-0.04 units of bacitracin. Definitive identification depends upon specific sero-grouping procedures; however, rare group A strains produce little or no β-hemolysis (these may be nephritogenic or rheumatogenic). Latex agglutination, IF techniques and coagglutination tests are also available for rapid identification. A rise in serum antibody titer (antistreptolysin O, antihyaluronidase, anti-DNA-ase B) may be demonstrated between acute and convalescent stages of illness. In the USA, the current usual practice is to do a rapid strep test first and, if positive, assume the patient has a group A streptococcal infection. If the results are negative or equivocal, a throat culture should be done to guide management.

2. **Infectious agent**—*Streptococcus pyogenes,* group A streptococci of approximately 80 serologically distinct types which may vary greatly in geographic and time distributions. Group A streptococci producing skin infections are usually of different serologic types from those associated with throat infections. In scarlet fever, 3 immunologically different types of erythrogenic toxin (A, B and C) have been demonstrated. While β-hemolysis is characteristic of group A streptococci, strains of groups B, C and G are often also β-hemolytic.

3. **Occurrence**—Streptococcal sore throat and scarlet fever are common in temperate zones, well recognized in semitropical areas and less frequently recognized in tropical climates. Inapparent infections are at least as common in tropical as in temperate zones. In the USA, streptococcal diseases may be endemic, epidemic or sporadic in character. Group A streptococcal infections due to a limited number of specific types of M protein (M-types), especially types 12, 1, 3, 4 and 25, have frequently been associated with the development of acute glomerulonephritis.

Acute rheumatic fever may occur as a nonsuppurative complication following infection with many group A serotypes which have the capacity to produce clinical infection of the upper respiratory tract. This complication had virtually disappeared from the industrialized countries until several outbreaks appeared in the USA in 1985; increased numbers from many areas of the country are still being reported in 1990. Rheumatic fever remains a great problem in the developing world. Apart from foodborne epidemics, which may occur in any season, the highest incidence is during late winter and spring. The 3-15-year age group is most often affected; no sex or racial differences in incidence have been defined; military and school populations are frequently affected. Together with reappearance of rheumatic fever, more severe streptococcal infections have also been reported, including generalized infections and the toxic shock-like syndrome. A limited number of M-types have been identified in reported cases.

The highest incidence of streptococcal impetigo occurs in young children in late summer and fall in hot climates. Nephritis following skin infections is associated with a limited number of M-types of streptococci (e.g., types 49, 2, 55, 57, 58, 59, 60 and other higher types), which generally differ from those associated with nephritis following infections of the upper respiratory tract.

Geographic and seasonal distributions of erysipelas are similar to those for scarlet fever and streptococcal sore throat; erysipelas is most common in infants and those over 20 years of age. Occurrence is sporadic, even during epidemics of streptococcal infection.

Reliable morbidity data do not exist for puerperal fever. In developed countries, morbidity and mortality have generally declined precipitously since the advent of antibiotics. It is now chiefly a sporadic disease, although epidemics may occur in institutions where aseptic techniques are faulty.

4. **Reservoir**—Man.

5. **Mode of transmission**—Direct or intimate contact with patients or carriers, rarely by indirect contact through objects or hands. Nasal carriers are particularly likely to transmit disease. Casual contact rarely leads to infection. In populations where impetigo is prevalent, group A streptococci may be recovered from the normal skin for 1-2 weeks before skin lesions develop; the same strain may appear in the throat (without clinical evidence of throat infection) usually late in the course of the skin infection. Anal, vaginal, skin and pharyngeal carriers have been responsible for nosocomial outbreaks of wound infections. Dried streptococci reaching the air via contaminated floor dust, lint from bedclothing, handkerchiefs, etc., are viable but apparently noninfectious for mucous membranes and intact skin.

Explosive outbreaks of streptococcal sore throat may follow ingestion of contaminated foods. Milk and milk products have been associated most frequently with foodborne outbreaks; egg salad and deviled hard-boiled eggs have recently been implicated with increasing frequency.

Epidemics of serious streptococcal infections following surgical procedures have been traced to operating room personnel who are carriers of the streptococcal strain causing disease. Identification of the carrier often involves intensive epidemiologic and microbiological investigations. Eradication of the carrier state in these individuals is often difficult and may involve multiple courses of various antibiotics.

6. **Incubation period**—Short, usually 1-3 days, rarely longer.

7. **Period of communicability**—In untreated, uncomplicated cases, 10-21 days; in untreated conditions with purulent discharges, weeks or months. With adequate penicillin therapy, transmissibility generally is terminated within 24-48 hours. Patients with untreated streptococcal pharyngitis may carry the organism in the pharynx for weeks or months, usually in decreasing numbers; the contagiousness of these carriers decreases sharply in 2-3 weeks after onset of infection.

8. **Susceptibility and resistance**—Susceptibility to streptococcal sore throat and scarlet fever is general, although many persons develop either antitoxic or type-specific antibacterial immunity, or both, through inapparent infection. Antibacterial immunity develops only against the specific M-type of group A streptococcus that induced infection and may last for years. Antibiotic therapy may interfere with the development of type-specific immunity. Repeated attacks of sore throat or other streptococcal disease due to different types of streptococci are relatively frequent. Immunity against erythrogenic toxin, and hence to rash, develops within a week after onset of scarlet fever and is usually permanent; second attacks of scarlet fever are rare, but may occur because of the 3 immunologic forms of toxin. Passive immunity to group A streptococcal disease occurs in newborns with transplacental maternal type-specific antibodies.

One attack of erysipelas appears to predispose individuals to subsequent attacks.

9. **Methods of control**—

   A. *Preventive measures:*

   1) Educate the public in modes of transmission, in the relationship of streptococcal infection to acute rheumatic fever, Sydenham's chorea, rheumatic heart disease and glomerulonephritis, and the necessity for completing the full course of antibiotic therapy prescribed for streptococcal infections.

   2) Provide easily accessible laboratory facilities for recognition of group A hemolytic streptococci.

   3) Boil or pasteurize milk and exclude infected persons from handling milk likely to become contaminated.

4) Prepare other foods, such as deviled eggs, just prior to serving or adequately refrigerate in small quantities at ≤5°C (41°F).

5) Exclude those with respiratory illnesses or skin lesions from foodhandling.

6) Strict asepsis in obstetrical procedures, with special attention to avoid contamination from mouths and noses of attendants, as well as by hands and instruments. Protect patients during labor and the postpartum period from attendants, visitors and other patients with respiratory or skin infections.

7) Long-term antimicrobial prophylaxis: Monthly injections of long-acting benzathine penicillin G, or daily penicillin or sulfadiazine orally, for persons to whom recurrent streptococcal infection constitutes a special risk, such as individuals who have had rheumatic fever, chorea, or recurrent erysipelas. Those who do not tolerate penicillin or sulfonamides may be given erythromycin.

B. *Control of patient, contacts and the immediate environment:*

1) Report to local health authority: Obligatory report of epidemics; no individual case report, Class 4 (see Preface).

2) Isolation: Drainage/secretion precautions; may be terminated after 24 hours' treatment with penicillin or other effective antibiotics; therapy should be continued for 10 days to avoid development of rheumatic heart disease.

3) Concurrent disinfection: Of purulent discharges and all articles soiled therewith. Terminal cleaning.

4) Quarantine: None.

5) Immunization of contacts: None.

6) Investigation of contacts and source of infection: Search for and treat carriers in well-documented epidemics of streptococcal infection and in high-risk situations (e.g., evidence of streptococcal infection in families with multiple cases of rheumatic fever, occurrence of cases of rheumatic fever or acute nephritis in a population group such as a school, outbreaks of post-operative wound infections).

7) Specific treatment: Penicillin; several forms are acceptable for treatment: benzathine penicillin G IM (treatment of choice), procaine penicillin G IM, oral penicillin G, or oral penicillin V. Penicillin-resistant strains of streptococci have not occurred. Therapy should provide adequate penicillin levels for 10 days. Such treatment initiated within the first 24-48 hours may ameliorate the acute

illness; however, the bacteria may persist in the pharynx in up to 30% of patients. Therapy will reduce the frequency of suppurative complications and prevent the development of most cases of acute rheumatic fever. Therapy may also reduce the risk of acute glomerulonephritis and prevent further spread of the organism. Erythromycin is the preferred treatment for penicillin-sensitive patients but strains resistant to this antibiotic have been reported. Clindamycin or a cephalosporin can be used when penicillin and erythromycin are contraindicated. Sulfonamides are not effective in eliminating the streptococcus from the throat or in preventing nonsuppurative complications. Many strains are resistant to the tetracyclines.

C. *Epidemic measures:*

1) Determine the source and manner of spread, i.e., person-to-person, by milk or food. Outbreaks can often be traced to an individual with an acute or persistent streptococcal infection or carrier state (nose, throat, skin, vagina or perianal area) through identification of the serologic type of the streptococcus.

2) Investigate promptly any unusual grouping of cases to identify possible common sources, such as contaminated milk or foods.

3) In outbreaks in special groups in which individuals have especially close contact, such as military populations and newborn nurseries, it may be necessary to administer penicillin to the entire group to terminate spread.

D. *Disaster implications:* Patients with thermal burns or wounds are highly susceptible to streptococcal infections of the affected area.

E. *International measures:* WHO Collaborating Centres (see Preface).

GROUP B STREPTOCOCCAL DISEASE OF THE NEWBORN
ICD-9 038.0

Group B streptococci (*S. agalactiae*) of human subtypes produce important diseases of newborn infants. Two distinct forms of illness occur: Early onset disease (1-7 days) is characterized by sepsis, respiratory distress, apnea, shock, pneumonia and meningitis; it has a case fatality rate of about 50%, is acquired in utero or during delivery, and occurs more frequently in low-birth-weight infants. Late onset disease (7 days to several months) is characterized by sepsis and meningitis; it has a case fatality rate of about 25%, is acquired by person-to-person contact, and occurs in full-term infants. Sequelae have been described among survivors of meningitis and include speech, hearing and visual problems, psychomotor retardation and seizure disorders.

While the manner of acquisition is unclear, approximately 10-30% of pregnant women harbor Group B streptococci in the genital tract. Approximately 1% of their offspring develop symptomatic infection; risk of serious disease is greatest in premature infants.

Attempts to eradicate genital tract group B streptococci in women during pregnancy with oral antibiotics have been only partially successful. There are high relapse rates when antibiotics have been discontinued, possibly due to reinfection from rectal carriage of the organism or by possible reacquisition from culture-positive sexual partners.

The administration of intravenous penicillin or ampicillin at the onset and throughout labor to women who are colonized with group B streptococci and who are at high risk of delivering an infected infant (premature gestational age, premature rupture of membranes or intrapartum fever) should be considered. Preliminary studies suggest that this interrupts transmission of group B streptococci to newborn infants and may decrease actual infection and mortality. While group B streptococci are sensitive to penicillin G and ampicillin, penicillin-tolerant strains have been described, suggesting that severe infections should be treated with a penicillin plus an aminoglycoside, preferably gentamicin. A vaccine for pregnant women to stimulate antibody production against invasive disease in newborns is under development.

STRONGYLOIDIASIS ICD-9 127.2

1. **Identification**—A helminthic infection of the duodenum and upper jejunum, often asymptomatic. Clinical manifestations include transient dermatitis when larvae of the parasite penetrate the skin on initial infection; cough, râles and sometimes a demonstrable pneumonitis when they pass through the lungs; or abdominal symptoms caused by the adult female in the mucosa of the intestine. Symptoms of chronic infection may be mild or severe, depending upon intensity of infection. Classic symptoms are abdominal pain (usually epigastric and often suggesting peptic ulcer), diarrhea and urticaria; they may also include nausea, weight loss, vomiting, weakness and constipation. Intensely pruritic dermatitis radiating from the anus may occur; stationary wheals lasting 1-2 days may occur as well as a migrating serpiginous rash moving several cm/hour across the trunk. Rarely, intestinal autoinfection with increasing worm

burden may lead to disseminated strongyloidiasis with wasting, pulmonary involvement and death, particularly, but not exclusively, in the immunocompromised host. In these cases, secondary Gram-negative sepsis is common. Eosinophilia is usually moderate in the chronic stage, but may be absent with dissemination.

Diagnosis is made by identifying larvae in stool specimens (motile in freshly passed feces), in duodenal aspirates or, occasionally, in sputum. Held at room temperature for ≥24 hours, feces may show developing stages of the parasite, including filariform (infective) larvae (which must be distinguished from larvae of hookworm species) and free-living adults.

2. Infectious agents—*Strongyloides stercoralis* and *S. fuelleborni,* nematodes.

3. Occurrence—Throughout tropical and temperate areas; more common in warm, wet regions. Prevalence in endemic areas is not accurately known. May be prevalent in institutions where personal hygiene is poor. *S. fuelleborni* has been reported only in Africa and Papua New Guinea.

4. Reservoir—Man, dogs, cats and non-human primates.

5. Mode of transmission—Infective (filariform) larvae, which develop in feces or moist soil contaminated with feces, penetrate the skin, enter the venous circulation and are carried to the lungs. They penetrate capillary walls, enter the alveoli, ascend the trachea to the epiglottis, and descend into the digestive tract to reach the upper part of the small intestine where development of the adult female is completed. The adult worm, a parthenogenetic female, lives embedded in the mucosal epithelium of the intestine, especially the duodenum, where eggs are deposited. They hatch and liberate rhabditiform (noninfective) larvae which migrate into the lumen of the intestine, leave the host in the feces and develop into either infective filariform larvae (which may infect the same or a new host) or into free-living adults after reaching the soil. The free-living, fertilized females produce eggs that soon hatch, liberating rhabditiform larvae, which may become filariform larvae within 24-36 hours. In some individuals, rhabditiform larvae may develop to the infective stage before leaving the body and penetrate through the intestinal mucosa or perianal skin; the resulting autoinfection can cause massive and persistent infection for many years.

6. Incubation period—From penetration of the skin by filariform larvae until rhabditiform larvae appear in the feces is about 2 weeks; the period until symptoms appear is indefinite and variable.

7. Period of communicability—As long as living worms remain in the intestine; up to 35 years in cases of autoinfection.

8. Susceptibility and resistance—Susceptibility is universal. Acquired immunity has been demonstrated in laboratory animals but not in man. Patients with malignant disease or on immunosuppressive medication may experience dissemination.

9. **Methods of control—**

A. *Preventive measures:*

1) Dispose of human feces in a sanitary manner.
2) Rigid attention to hygienic habits, including use of footwear in endemic areas.
3) Rule out strongyloidiasis before initiating immunosuppressive therapy.
4) Examine and treat infected dogs, cats and monkeys that are in contact with man.

B. *Control of patient, contacts and the immediate environment:*

1) Report to local health authority: Official report not ordinarily justifiable, Class 5 (see Preface).
2) Isolation: None.
3) Concurrent disinfection: Sanitary disposal of feces.
4) Quarantine: None.
5) Immunization of contacts: None.
6) Investigation of contacts and source of infection: Members of the same household or institution should be examined for evidence of infection.
7) Specific treatment: Because of the potential for autoinfection, all infections, regardless of worm burden, should be treated, preferably with thiabendazole (Mintezol®) or alternatively, albendazole (Zentel®). Repeated courses of treatment may be required.

C. *Epidemic measures:* Not applicable; a sporadic disease.

D. *Disaster implications:* None.

E. *International measures:* None.

SYPHILIS
I. VENEREAL SYPHILIS   ICD-9 090-097
(Lues)

1. **Identification**—An acute and chronic treponemal disease characterized clinically by a primary lesion, a secondary eruption involving skin and mucous membranes, long periods of latency, and late lesions of skin, bone, viscera, the CNS and the cardiovascular system. The primary lesion

(chancre) usually appears about three weeks after exposure as an indurated, painless ulcer with a serous exudate at the site of initial invasion. Invasion of the bloodstream precedes the initial lesion, and a firm, nonfluctuant, painless satellite lymph node (bubo) commonly follows. Infection may occur without a clinically evident chancre; i.e., it may be in the rectum or on the cervix. After 4-6 weeks, even without specific treatment, the chancre begins to involute and a generalized secondary eruption may appear, often accompanied by mild constitutional symptoms. This symmetrical maculopapular rash involving the palms and soles, with associated adenopathy, is classic. Secondary manifestations disappear spontaneously within weeks up to 12 months, with subsequent clinical latency of weeks to years. In the early years of latency, there may be recurrence of infectious lesions of the skin and mucous membranes.

CNS disease may occur at any time: as acute syphilitic meningitis in secondary or early latent syphilis, later as meningovascular syphilis, and finally as paresis or tabes dorsalis. Latency sometimes continues through life. In other instances, and unpredictably, late (5-20 years after initial infection), disabling lesions occur in the aorta (cardiovascular syphilis) or gummas may occur in the skin, viscera, bone and/or mucosal surfaces. Death or serious disability rarely occurs during early stages; late manifestations shorten life, impair health and limit occupational efficiency. Concurrent HIV infection may increase the risk of CNS syphilis; neurosyphilis must be considered in the differential diagnosis of an HIV-infected individual with CNS symptoms.

Fetal infection occurs with high frequency in untreated early infections of pregnant women and with lower frequency later in latency. It frequently causes abortion or stillbirth and may cause infant deaths due to preterm delivery of low-birth-weight infants or from generalized systemic disease. Congenital infection may result in late manifestations, occasionally causing such stigmata as Hutchinson's teeth, saddlenose, saber shins, interstitial keratitis and deafness.

The laboratory diagnosis of syphilis is usually made by serologic tests of blood and CSF when indicated. Positive tests with nontreponemal antigens (e.g., RPR, VDRL) should be confirmed by tests employing treponemal antigens (i.e., FA or treponemal hemagglutination) to aid in excluding biological false-positive reactions. Primary and secondary syphilis can be confirmed by darkfield or phase-contrast examination or by FA antibody staining of exudates from lesions or aspirates from lymph nodes (if no antibiotic has been administered). (Serologic tests are negative during the primary and early secondary stages.) A darkfield examination of all genital ulcerative lesions is indicated and is indispensable in suspected early seronegative primary syphilis.

2. **Infectious agent**—*Treponema pallidum,* a spirochete.

3. **Occurrence**—Widespread; involving primarily young people between 20-35 years. Racial differences in incidence are related to social

rather than biological factors. Syphilis is usually more prevalent in urban than rural areas, and, in some cultures, in males than females. The high prevalence among homosexual men seen in the late 1970s and early 1980s has decreased since 1983. In many areas of the USA, reported rates of syphilis have increased beginning in 1986 and continuing into 1990. This increase has occurred primarily in lower socioeconomic classes; risk factors include illicit drug use and prostitution. Early venereal syphilis has also increased significantly throughout much of the world since 1957.

4. **Reservoir**—Man.

5. **Mode of transmission**—By direct contact with infectious exudates from obvious or concealed, moist, early lesions of skin and mucous membranes, body fluids and secretions (saliva, semen, blood, vaginal discharges) of infected persons during sexual contact; rarely by kissing or fondling children with early congenital disease. Transmission can occur through blood transfusion if the donor is in the early stages of disease. Infection by contact with contaminated articles is theoretically possible. Health professionals have developed primary lesions on the hands following clinical examination of infectious lesions. Fetal infection occurs through placental transfer or at delivery.

6. **Incubation period**—Ten days to 3 months, usually 3 weeks.

7. **Period of communicability**—Variable and indefinite; during primary and secondary stages and also in mucocutaneous recurrences which may occur during the first four years of latency. Extent of communicability through sexual activity during this period is not established, although inapparent lesions make this period potentially infectious. Congenital transmission is most probable during early maternal syphilis but can occur throughout the latent period. Adequate penicillin treatment usually ends infectivity within 24-48 hours.

8. **Susceptibility and resistance**—Susceptibility is universal, though only approximately 30% of exposures result in infection. Infection leads to developing immunity against *Treponema pallidum* gradually and, to some extent, against heterologous treponemes; immunity may fail to develop because of early treatment in the primary and secondary stages. Concurrent HIV infection may reduce the normal host response to *T. pallidum*.

9. **Methods of control**—

    A. *Preventive measures:* In general, the following preventive measures are applicable to all sexually transmitted diseases (STD): syphilis, AIDS, chancroid, lymphogranuloma venereum, granuloma inguinale, gonorrhea, herpes simplex type 2 virus infection, genital human papillomavirus infections (genital warts), trichomonal vaginitis, bacterial vaginosis, sexually transmitted hepatitis B, and diseases caused by *Chlamydia* and the genital mycoplasma.

Emphasis on control of patients with transmissible syphilis should not preclude search for persons with latent syphilis to prevent relapse and disability due to late manifestations.

1) General health promotion measures, health and sex education. Syphilis serology should be included in the workup of all cases of STD and as a routine part of prenatal examination. Congenital syphilis is prevented by serologic examination in early pregnancy and again in late pregnancy and at delivery in high-prevalence populations, with treatment of positive reactors.

2) Protect the community by preventing and controlling STD in prostitutes and their clients; by discouraging sexual promiscuity (in cooperation with social agencies); and by teaching methods of personal prophylaxis applicable before, during and after exposure, especially the use of condoms in sexual contacts with persons not known to be free to STD.

3) Provide facilities for early diagnosis and treatment; encourage their use through education of the public about symptoms of STD and modes of spread, and through making these services readily accessible and acceptable, regardless of economic status. Establish intensive case-finding programs, to include interviewing of patients and tracing of contacts; for syphilis, repeated mass serologic examination of special groups with known high incidence of STD.

B. *Control of patient, contacts and the immediate environment:*

1) Report to local health authority: Case report of early infectious syphilis and congenital syphilis is required in all states, and variously in other countries, Class 2A (see Preface); report of positive serology and darkfield examinations by laboratories is required in most states. Privacy of the individual must be safeguarded.

2) Isolation: For hospitalized patients, drainage/secretion precautions; blood/body fluid precautions are appropriate for patients with primary, secondary and early congenital syphilis. Precautions are unnecessary for late latent and tertiary disease. Patients should refrain from sexual intercourse until lesions clear, and thereafter should refrain from sexual intercourse with untreated infected previous partners to avoid reinfection.

3) Concurrent disinfection: None in adequately treated cases; care to avoid contact with discharges from open lesions and articles soiled therewith.

4) Quarantine: None.

5) Immunization of contacts: None available.

6) Investigation of contacts and source of infection: A fundamental feature of programs for syphilis control is the interviewing of patients to identify contacts from whom infection was acquired and those whom the patient may have infected. Trained interviewers obtain best results. The stage of disease determines the criteria for contact-tracing: (1) For primary syphilis, all sexual contacts during the 3 months preceding onset of symptoms; (2) for secondary syphilis, contacts during the preceding 6 months; (3) for early latent syphilis, those of the preceding year, if time of primary and secondary lesions cannot be established; (4) for late and late latent syphilis, marital partners and children of infected mothers; and (5) for congenital syphilis, all members of the immediate family. **All identified sexual contacts of confirmed cases of early syphilis should receive treatment.**

7) Specific treatment: Long-acting penicillin G (benzathine penicillin), 2.4 million units (m.u.) given in a single IM dose on the day of diagnosis of primary, secondary or early latent syphilis, assures effective therapy even if the patient fails to return.

Alternative therapy for penicillin-allergic patients: either oral doxycycline, 100 mg twice daily for 14 days, or oral tetracycline, 500 mg four times/day for 14 days.

Serologic testing is important to insure adequate therapy; tests are repeated at 3 and 6 months after treatment. In HIV-infected patients, testing should be repeated at 1, 2 and 3 months, and at 3-month intervals thereafter. Any fourfold titer rise indicates the need for retreatment.

Increased dosages and longer periods of therapy are indicated for the late stages of syphilis (i.e., benzathine penicillin, 2.4 m.u. IM weekly for 3 weeks). Consideration should be given to analysis of the CSF, especially if increased risk of neurosyphilis exists: those who have failed therapy, those who are infected with HIV, and those with neurologic findings.

For neurosyphilis, aqueous crystalline penicillin G, 12-24 m.u./day, administered 2-4 m.u. every 4 hours IV for 10-14 days. An alternative therapy is aqueous crystalline penicillin G, 2-4 m.u. IM, plus oral probenecid, 500 mg, each four times/day for 10-14 days. Success in therapy should be checked by following serologic titers and appropriate CSF examinations every 6 months until cell count is normal.

Penicillin-sensitive pregnant women should have their allergy confirmed with skin tests to the major and minor penicillin determinants, if the test antigens are available. Patients with a confirmed penicillin allergy can be desensitized and then given the usual dose of penicillin, based on the stage of their syphilis. Erythromycin had been used for penicillin-sensitive pregnant women but is no longer recommended because of high failure rates.

C. *Epidemic measures:* Intensification of measures outlined under 9A and 9B, above.

D. *Disaster implications:* None.

E. *International measures:*

1) Appropriately examine groups of adolescents and young adults moving from areas of high prevalence of treponemal infections.

2) Adhere to agreements among nations (e.g., Brussels' Agreement) as to records, provision of diagnostic and treatment facilities and contact interviews at seaports for foreign merchant seamen.

3) Provide for rapid international exchange of information on contacts.

4) WHO Collaborating Centres (see Preface).

II. NONVENEREAL ENDEMIC SYPHILIS   ICD-9 104.0
(Bejel, Njovera)

1. Identification—An acute disease of limited geographic distribution, characterized clinically by an eruption of skin and mucous membrane, usually without an evident primary sore. Mucous patches of the mouth are often the first lesions, soon followed by moist papules in skin folds and by drier lesions of the trunk and extremities. Other early skin lesions are macular or papular, often hypertrophic, and frequently circinate, resembling those of venereal syphilis. Plantar and palmar hyperkeratoses occur frequently, often with painful fissuring; patchy depigmentation and hyperpigmentation of the skin and alopecia are common. Inflammatory or destructive lesions of skin, long bones and nasopharynx are late manifestations. Unlike venereal syphilis, the nervous and cardiovascular systems are rarely involved. The case fatality rate is low.

Organisms are demonstrable in lesions by darkfield examination during early disease. Serologic tests for syphilis are reactive in the early stages and remain so for many years of latency, gradually tending toward reversal; response to treatment as in venereal syphilis.

2. **Infectious agent**—*Treponema pallidum,* a spirochete indistinguishable from that of syphilis.

3. **Occurrence**—A common disease of childhood in localized areas where poor socioeconomic conditions and primitive sanitary and dwelling arrangements prevail. Present in eastern Mediterranean and Asian countries; numerous foci in Africa, particularly in arid regions.

4. **Reservoir**—Man.

5. **Mode of transmission**—Direct or indirect contact with infectious early lesions of skin and mucous membranes; the latter favored by common use of eating and drinking utensils and generally unsatisfactory hygienic conditions. Congenital transmission does not occur.

6. **Incubation period**—Two weeks to 3 months.

7. **Period of communicability**—Until moist eruptions of skin and mucous patches disappear; sometimes several weeks or months.

8. **Susceptibility and resistance**—Similar to venereal syphilis.

9. **Methods of control**—

A. *Preventive measures:* Those of the nonvenereal treponematoses. See Yaws, 9A.

B. *Control of patient, contacts and the immediate environment:*

1) Report to local health authority: In selected endemic areas; in most countries not a reportable disease, Class 3B (see Preface).
2), 3), 4), 5), 6) and 7): Isolation, Concurrent disinfection, Quarantine, Immunization of contacts, Investigation of contacts and source of infection, and Specific treatment: See Yaws 9B, applicable to all nonvenereal treponematoses.

C. *Epidemic measures:* Intensification of preventive and control activities.

D. *Disaster implications:* None.

E. *International measures:* See Yaws, 9E. WHO Collaborating Centres (see Preface).

TAENIASIS
TAENIASIS DUE TO *TAENIA SOLIUM*   ICD-9 123
INTESTINAL FORM   ICD-9 123.0
(Pork tapeworm)
CYSTICERCOSIS   ICD-9 123.1
(Cysticerciasis, *Taenia solium* cysticercosis)
TAENIASIS DUE TO *TAENIA*   ICD-9 123.2
SAGINATA
(Beef tapeworm)

1. **Identification**—Taeniasis is an intestinal infection with the adult stage of large tapeworms; cysticercosis is a tissue infection with the larval stage of one species, *Taenia solium*. Clinical manifestations of infection with the adult worm, if present, are variable and may include nervousness, insomnia, anorexia, weight loss, abdominal pain and digestive disturbances. Except for the annoyance of having segments of worms emerging from the anus, many infections are asymptomatic. Taeniasis is usually a nonfatal infection, but *T. solium* may cause fatal cysticercosis.

Larval infection of man with the pork tapeworm, cysticercosis, may produce serious somatic disease, usually involving the CNS. When eggs or proglottids of the pork tapeworm are swallowed by man the eggs hatch in the small intestine, and the larvae migrate to the subcutaneous tissues, striated muscles, and other tissues and vital organs of the body where they form cysts (cysticerci). Consequences may be grave when larvae localize in the eye, CNS or heart. In the presence of somatic cysticercosis, epileptiform seizures, signs of intracranial hypertension or psychiatric disturbances strongly suggest cerebral involvement. Neurocysticercosis may cause serious disability with a relatively high case fatality rate.

Infection with an adult tapeworm is diagnosed by identification of proglottids (segments) or eggs of the worm in the feces or on anal swabs. Eggs of *T. solium* and *T. saginata* cannot be differentiated from each other morphologically. Specific diagnosis is based on the morphology of the scolex (head) and/or gravid proglottids. Obtaining the scolex following treatment confirms the identification and assures elimination of the worm (usually only one worm is present). Specific serologic tests should support the clinical diagnosis of cysticercosis. Subcutaneous cysticerci are visible or palpable and may itch; microscopic examination of an excised cysticercus confirms the diagnosis. Neural and visceral cysticercosis may be recognized by ultrasound, CAT scan (especially for uncalcified cysts) or by x-ray when the cysticerci are calcified.

2. **Infectious agents**—*Taenia solium,* the pork tapeworm, causes both intestinal infection with the adult worm and somatic infection with the larvae (cysticerci). *T. saginata,* the beef tapeworm, causes only intestinal infection with the adult worm in man.

3. **Occurrence**—Worldwide; particularly frequent wherever beef or pork is eaten raw or insufficiently cooked and where sanitary conditions permit pigs and cattle to have access to human feces. Prevalence is highest in parts of Latin America, Africa, SE Asia and eastern Europe. Transmission of *T. solium* is rare in the USA and Canada, and exceedingly rare in the UK and Scandinavia, but it is frequently found in immigrants from endemic areas.

4. **Reservoir**—Man is the definitive host of both species of *Taenia;* cattle are the intermediate hosts for *T. saginata,* and pigs for *T. solium.*

5. **Mode of transmission**—Eggs of *T. saginata* passed in the stool of an infected person are infectious only to cattle, in the flesh of which the parasites develop into "cysticercus bovis," the larval stage of *T. saginata.* Infection in man follows ingestion of raw or undercooked beef containing cysticerci; in the intestine, the adult worm develops attached to the jejunal mucosa.

Intestinal infection in man (taeniasis due to *T. solium*) follows ingestion of raw or undercooked infected pork ("measly pork"), with subsequent development of the adult worm in the intestine. However, human cysticercosis may occur by direct transfer of *T. solium* eggs from the feces of persons harboring an adult worm to their own or another's mouth, or indirectly by ingestion of food or water contaminated with eggs. When the eggs of *T. solium* are ingested by either man or pigs, the embryos escape from the shells, penetrate the intestinal wall into lymphatics or blood vessels, and are carried to the various tissues where they develop to produce the human disease of cysticercosis, or "cysticercus cellulosae" in the pig.

6. **Incubation period**—Symptoms of cysticercosis may appear from days to ≥10 years after infection. Eggs appear in the stool 8-12 weeks after infection with the adult *T. solium* tapeworm; 10-14 weeks with *T. saginata.*

7. **Period of communicability**—*T. saginata* is not directly transmitted from person to person, but *T. solium* may be. Eggs of both species are disseminated into the environment as long as the worm remains in the intestine, sometimes more than 30 years; eggs may remain viable in the environment for months.

8. **Susceptibility and resistance**—Susceptibility is general. No apparent resistance follows infection, but more than one tapeworm in a person has rarely been reported.

9. **Methods of control**—

    A. *Preventive measures:*

        1) Educate the public to prevent contamination of soil, water, human and animal food with human feces; to avoid

use of sewage effluents for pasture irrigation; and to cook beef and pork thoroughly.

2) Identification and immediate treatment or institution of enteric precautions for persons harboring adult *T. solium* is essential to prevent human cysticercosis. *T. solium* eggs are infective immediately upon leaving the host and are capable of producing a severe human illness. Appropriate measures to protect patients from themselves and their contacts are necessary.

3) Freezing pork or beef at a temperature below -5°C (23°F) for >4 days kills the cystercerci effectively.

4) Inspection of the carcasses of cattle and swine will detect only a proportion of infected carcasses; these should be condemned or processed.

5) Deny swine access to latrines and human feces.

B. *Control of patient, contacts and the immediate environment:*

1) Report to local health authority: Selectively reportable, Class 3C (see Preface).

2) Isolation: None recommended. Stools of patients with untreated taeniasis due to *T. solium* may be infective (see 9A2, above).

3) Concurrent disinfection: Dispose of feces in a sanitary manner; emphasize rigid sanitation, with handwashing after defecating and before eating, especially for *T. solium*.

4) Quarantine: None.

5) Immunization of contacts: None.

6) Investigation of contacts and source of infection: Evaluate symptomatic contacts.

7) Specific treatment: Niclosamide (Niclocide®, Yomesan®) and praziquantel (Biltricide®) are effective in the treatment of *T. saginata* and *T. solium* intestinal infections. For cysticercosis: surgical intervention may relieve some symptoms. Patients with active CNS cysticercosis should be treated with praziquantel under hospitalization; a short course of corticosteroids is usually given to control cerebral edema from dying cysticerci.

C. *Epidemic measures:* None.

D. *Disaster implications:* None.

E. *International measures:* None.

TETANUS   ICD-9 037
(Lockjaw)

1. **Identification**—An acute disease induced by an exotoxin of the tetanus bacillus, which grows anaerobically at the site of an injury. The disease is characterized by painful muscular contractions, primarily of the masseter and neck muscles, secondarily of trunk muscles. A common first sign suggestive of tetanus is abdominal rigidity, though rigidity is sometimes confined to the region of injury. Generalized spasms occur, frequently induced by sensory stimuli; typical features of the tetanic spasm are the position of opisthotonus and the facial expression known as "risus sardonicus." History of an injury or apparent portal of entry may be lacking. The case fatality rate ranges from 30 to 90%, being highest in infants and the elderly, and varying inversely with the length of the incubation period.

Attempts for laboratory confirmation are of little help. The organism is rarely recovered from the site of infection and usually there is no detectable antibody response.

2. **Infectious agent**—*Clostridium tetani,* the tetanus bacillus.

3. **Occurrence**—Worldwide. Sporadic and relatively uncommon in the USA and most industrial countries. Currently, about 50-90 cases and 20-30 deaths are reported annually in the USA. About 60% occur in persons ≥60 years. More common in agricultural regions and in underdeveloped areas where contact with animal excreta is more likely and immunization is inadequate. An important cause of death in many countries of Asia, Africa and S America, especially in rural and tropical areas where tetanus neonatorum is common (see below). Parenteral use of drugs by addicts, particularly intramuscular or subcutaneous use, can result in individual cases and occasional circumscribed outbreaks.

4. **Reservoir**—Intestine of horses and other animals, including man, in which the organism is a harmless normal inhabitant. Soil or fomites contaminated with animal and human feces.

5. **Mode of transmission**—Tetanus spores introduced into the body, usually through a puncture wound contaminated with soil, street dust or animal or human feces; through lacerations, burns and trivial or unnoticed wounds; or by injected contaminated street drugs. Tetanus occasionally follows surgical procedures. The presence of necrotic tissue and/or foreign bodies favors growth of the anaerobic pathogen. Cases have followed injuries considered too trivial for medical consultation.

6. **Incubation period**—Usually 3-21 days, although it may range from 1 day to several months, depending on the character, extent and location of the wound; average 10 days. Most cases occur within 14 days. In general, shorter incubation periods are associated with more heavily

contaminated wounds, more severe disease and a worse prognosis.

7. **Period of communicability**—Not directly transmitted from person to person.

8. **Susceptibility and resistance**—Susceptibility is general. Active immunity is induced by tetanus toxoid and persists for at least 10 years after full immunization; transient passive immunity follows injection of tetanus immune globulin (TIG) or tetanus antitoxin (equine origin). Infants born from actively immunized mothers acquire passive immunity which protects them from neonatal tetanus. Recovery from tetanus may not result in immunity; second attacks can occur. Primary immunization is indicated after recovery.

9. **Methods of control**—

A. *Preventive measures:*

1) Educate the public on the necessity of complete immunization with tetanus toxoid, the kinds of injury particularly liable to be complicated by tetanus, and the potential need after injury for active and/or passive prophylaxis.

2) Universal active immunization with adsorbed tetanus toxoid, which gives durable protection for at least 10 years; after the initial basic series has been completed, single booster doses elicit high levels of immunity. The toxoid is generally administered together with diphtheria toxoid and pertussis vaccine as a triple (DTP) antigen (or double [DT] antigen for children under 7 years with contraindications to pertussis vaccine), or Td for older persons. In some countries, DTP, DT and T are available combined with inactivated polio vaccine. There is no advantage to nonadsorbed ("plain") preparations, whether for primary immunization or booster shots. Reactions following tetanus toxoid injections are infrequent, but do occur, particularly after excessive numbers of prior doses have been given.

a) The schedule recommended for tetanus immunization is the same as for diphtheria (q.v.).

b) While tetanus toxoid is recommended for universal use regardless of age, it is especially important for workers in contact with soil, sewage and domestic animals, members of the military forces, policemen and others with greater than usual risk of traumatic injury. Vaccine-induced maternal immunity is important in preventing neonatal tetanus.

c) Active protection should be maintained by administering booster doses of Td every 10 years.

    d) Where logistics or costs make the standard schedule impractical, there is evidence that a single dose of some toxoids may immunize 50-90% of children and adults; a second dose given one month or more later usually brings all subjects above the immune threshold. Following a third dose, protection persists for a long time.

3) Prophylaxis in wound management: Tetanus prophylaxis in patients with wounds is based on careful assessment of whether the wound is clean or contaminated, the immune status of the patient, proper use of tetanus toxoid and/or TIG (see table, below), wound cleansing and, where required, surgical debridement and the proper use of antibiotics.

    a) Those who have been completely immunized who sustain minor and uncontaminated wounds require a booster dose of toxoid only if more than 10 years have elapsed since the last dose was given. For major and/or contaminated wounds, a single booster injection of a tetanus toxoid (preferably Td) should be administered promptly on the day of injury if the patient has not received tetanus toxoid within the preceding 5 years.

    b) Persons who have not completed a full primary series of tetanus toxoid require a dose of toxoid as soon as possible following the wound and may require passive immunization with human TIG if it is a major wound and/or it is contaminated. DTP, DT or Td, as determined by the age of the patient and previous immunization history, should be used at the time of the wound, and ultimately, to complete the primary series. Passive immunization with at least 250 IU of TIG IM (or 1,500 to 5,000 IU of antitoxin of animal origin if TIG is not available) is indicated for patients with other than clean, minor wounds and a history of no, unknown, or less than three previous tetanus toxoid doses. When tetanus toxoid and TIG or antitoxin are given concurrently, separate syringes and separate sites must be used. When antitoxin of animal origin is given, it is essential that anaphylaxis be avoided by injecting 0.1 ml (with adrenalin on hand in a syringe), waiting 15 minutes, injecting 0.25 ml and, if there is no reaction after an additional 30 minutes, inject the full dose. Penicillin given for 7 days may kill *C. tetani* in the wound, but this does not obviate the need for prompt treatment of the wound together with appropriate immunization.

B. *Control of patient, contacts and the immediate environment:*

1) Report to local health authority: Case report required in most states (USA) and countries, Class 2B (see Preface).
2) Isolation: None.
3) Concurrent disinfection: None.
4) Quarantine: None.
5) Immunization of contacts: None.
6) Investigation of contacts and source of infection: Case investigation to determine circumstances of injury.
7) Specific treatment: TIG IM (or IV if a preparation safe for intravenous administration is available) in doses of 3,000-6,000 IU. If TIG is not available, tetanus antitoxin (equine origin) in a single large dose should be given intravenously following appropriate testing for hypersensitivity; parenteral penicillin in large doses should be given daily for 10-14 days. Intrathecal administration of TIG 250-500 IU or antitoxin (free of phenolic preservatives) has given promising results. (TIG is not licensed for intrathecal use in the USA.) The wound should be debrided widely and excised if possible. Maintain an adequate airway and employ sedation as indicated; muscle relaxant drugs together with tracheostomy or nasotracheal intubation and mechanically assisted respiration may be life-saving. Active immunization should be initiated concurrently with therapy.

C. *Epidemic measures:* In the rare outbreak, search for contaminated street drugs.

D. *Disaster implications:* Social upheavals (wars, riots) and natural disasters (floods, hurricanes, earthquakes) which cause many traumatic injuries in unimmunized populations will result in an increased need for TIG or tetanus antitoxin and toxoid for injured patients.

E. *International measures:* Up-to-date immunization against tetanus is advised for international travelers.

Summary guide to tetanus prophylaxis in routine wound management.[1]

History of teta-nus immunization (doses)	Clean, minor wounds		All other wounds	
	Td*	TIG	Td*	TIG
Uncertain or < 3	Yes	No	Yes	Yes
3 or more	No[2]	No	No[3]	No

[1]Important details in the text.
*For children <7 yrs old, DTP (DT, if pertussis vaccine is contraindicated) is preferred to tetanus toxoid alone. For persons ≥7 yrs, Td is preferred to tetanus toxoid alone.
[2]Yes, if >10 years since last dose.
[3]Yes, if >5 years since last dose. (More frequent boosters are not needed and can accentuate side effects.)

TETANUS NEONATORUM   ICD-9 771.3

Tetanus neonatorum is a serious health problem in many developing countries where maternity care services are limited and immunization against tetanus is inadequate. The mortality rates due to tetanus neonatorum range from 2 to 60/1000 live births in the developing world. WHO estimates that up to one million cases of neonatal tetanus occur annually in the developing world (1% of all births) with about 800,000 deaths. Most newborn infants with tetanus have been delivered outside a hospital to unimmunized mothers delivered by a traditional birth attendant.

The disease usually occurs through introduction via the umbilical cord of tetanus spores during delivery by cutting the cord with an unclean instrument, or after delivery by "dressing" the umbilical stump with substances heavily contaminated with tetanus spores, frequently as part of natal rituals.

Tetanus neonatorum is typified by a newborn infant who sucks and cries well for the first few days after birth and subsequently develops progressive difficulty and then inability to feed because of trismus, generalized stiffness with spasms or convulsions and opisthotonus. The average incubation period is about 6 days, with a range from 3 to 28 days. Overall, neonatal tetanus case fatality rates are very high; among cases with short incubation periods, these exceed 80%.

Prevention of tetanus neonatorum can be achieved by a combination of two approaches: by improving maternity care with emphasis on increasing the proportion of deliveries attended by trained attendants, and by increasing the immunization coverage of women of childbearing age, especially pregnant women, with tetanus toxoid.

Important control measures include licensing of midwives; providing professional supervision and education as to methods, equipment and techniques of asepsis in childbirth; and educating mothers, relatives and attendants in the practice of strict asepsis of the umbilical stump of newborn infants. The latter is especially important in many less developed areas where strips of bamboo are used to sever the umbilical cord and where ashes, cow dung poultices or other contaminated substances are traditionally applied to the umbilicus. In those areas, any woman of childbearing age visiting a health facility should be screened and offered immunization, no matter what the reason for the visit.

Unimmunized women in circumstances where risk of neonatal tetanus exists should receive at least five doses of tetanus toxoid according to the foliowing schedule: the first at first contact or as early as possible during pregnancy, the second 4 weeks after the first and preferably at least 2 weeks before delivery. The third dose should be given 6 to 12 months after the second, or during her next pregnancy. The remaining two doses should be given at least at annual intervals when the mother is in contact with the health service or during her subsequent pregnancies. This total of five doses protects her through her entire child-bearing period.

TOXOCARIASIS ICD-9 128.0
(Visceral larva migrans [VLM], Larva migrans visceralis, Ocular larva migrans, *Toxocara [canis] [cati]* infection)

1. **Identification**—A chronic and usually mild disease, predominantly of young children, but increasingly recognized in adults, due to migration of certain nematode larvae in the organs and tissues. It is characterized by eosinophilia of variable duration, hepatomegaly, hyperglobulinemia, pulmonary symptoms and fever. With heavy infestation, the WBC count may reach $\geq 100,000$/cu mm, with 80-90% eosinophils. Symptoms may persist for a year or longer. Pneumonitis, chronic abdominal pain, a generalized rash and focal neurologic disturbances may occur. Endophthalmitis (caused by larvae entering the eye) may occur, usually in children older than those with visceral larva migrans (VLM), with loss of vision in the affected eye. Retinal lesions may resemble retinoblastoma, which may lead to unnecessary enucleation of the eye. The disease is rarely fatal.

ELISA testing with larval stage antigens, after absorbing the serum with *Ascaris suum* (not necessary with *Toxocara* ES antigens), is 75-90% sensitive in VLM and in ocular infections. Demonstration of larvae of *Toxocara* by liver biopsy confirms the clinical diagnosis, but the diagnostic yield is low, and biopsy is rarely justified.

2. **Infectious agents**—*Toxocara canis* and *T. cati,* predominantly the former.

3. **Occurrence**—Probably worldwide. The disease has had most attention in the USA and the UK, but prevalence is probably no greater in these countries than in many others. The severe form occurs sporadically as isolated cases in a family, affecting mainly children 14-40 months, but it also occurs at older ages. The next older or younger sibling often shows eosinophilia or other evidence of light or residual infection. Serologic studies in asymptomatic children using the ELISA test have shown a mean seroprevalence of 3%, reaching 23% in some USA subpopulations. Adults are less frequently infected.

4. **Reservoir**—Dogs and cats, for *T. canis* and *T. cati,* respectively. Nearly all puppies are infected by transplacental and transmammary migration of larvae. Puppies start to pass eggs in their stools by the time they are 4 weeks old.

5. **Mode of transmission**—By direct or indirect transmission of infective *Toxocara* eggs from contaminated soil to the mouth; directly by pica (dirt-eating) by young children, indirectly by eating unwashed raw vegetables. Eggs reach the soil in feces of infected dogs and cats; up to 24% of soil samples from certain parks in the USA and the UK contained eggs. The eggs require 1-3 weeks incubation to become infective, but remain viable and infective in soil for many months; they are adversely affected by desiccation. After ingestion, embryonated eggs hatch in the intestine, larvae penetrate the wall and migrate to the liver and lungs by the lymphatic and circulatory systems. From the lungs, larvae spread to other tissues, particularly to the abdominal organs (visceral larva migrans) or the eyes (ocular larva migrans), causing damage by migration and induction of granulomatous lesions. Since the organisms cannot replicate in the human host, disease persists until the immune response (or medication) has killed all nematodes.

6. **Incubation period**—Weeks or months, depending upon intensity of infection, reinfection and sensitivity of the patient. Ocular manifestations may occur as late as 4-10 years after initial infection.

7. **Period of communicability**—Not directly transmitted from person to person.

8. **Susceptibility and resistance**—The lower incidence in older children and adults relates mainly to less exposure. Reinfection can occur. Dogs usually acquire infection as puppies; infection in the female dog may end or become dormant with sexual maturity; with pregnancy, however, *T. canis* larvae become active and infect the fetuses, and the newborn pups through the milk. Sex and age differences are less marked for cats; older animals are somewhat less susceptible than young.

9. **Methods of control—**

A. *Preventive measures:*

1) Educate the public and especially pet owners concerning sources and origin of the infection, particularly the danger of pica and of exposure to areas contaminated with the feces of untreated puppies. Parents of toddlers should consider carefully the hazard of pets in the household.
2) Prevent contamination of soil by dog and cat feces in areas immediately adjacent to houses and children's play areas, especially in urban areas and multiple housing projects.
3) Require removal of canine and feline feces passed in play areas. Children's sandboxes offer an attractive site for defecating cats; cover when not in use.
4) Deworm dogs and cats beginning at 3 weeks of age, repeated at 2-week intervals for 3 treatments, and every 6 months thereafter. Also treat lactating bitches. Dispose of feces passed as a result of treatment, as well as other stools, in a sanitary manner.
5) Always wash hands after handling soil and before eating.
6) Prevent pica in children.

B. *Control of patient, contacts and the immediate environment:*

1) Report to local health authority: Official report not ordinarily justifiable, Class 5 (see Preface).
2) Isolation: None.
3) Concurrent disinfection: None.
4) Quarantine: None.
5) Immunization of contacts: None.
6) Investigation of contacts and source of infection: Search for site of infection of index case; identify others exposed. Intensify preventive measures (see 9A, above). Treatment of asymptomatic, ELISA-positive individuals is not indicated.
7) Specific treatment: Diethylcarbamazine (DEC, Banocide®, Hetrazan®, Notezine®) and thiabendazole have been used; effectiveness is questionable at best.

C. *Epidemic measures:* Not applicable.

D. *Disaster implications:* None.

E. *International measures:* None.

GNATHOSTOMIASIS   ICD-9 128.1

Another visceral larva migrans, common in Thailand and elsewhere in SE Asia, is caused by *Gnathostoma spinigerum,* a nematode parasite of dogs and cats. Following ingestion of undercooked fish and poultry containing third-stage larvae, the parasites migrate through the tissues of man or animals, forming transient inflammatory lesions or abscesses in various parts of the body. Larvae may invade the brain, producing focal cerebral lesions associated with eosinophilic pleocytosis.

CUTANEOUS LARVA MIGRANS   ICD-9 126
DUE TO *ANCYLOSTOMA*   ICD-9 126.2
BRAZILIENSE
DUE TO *ANCYLOSTOMA CANINUM*   ICD-9 126.8
(Creeping eruption)

Infective larvae of dog and cat hookworm, *Ancylostoma braziliense* and *Ancylostoma caninum,* cause a dermatitis in man called "creeping eruption." This is a disease of utility men, gardeners, children, seabathers and others who come in contact with damp sandy soil contaminated with dog and cat feces; in the USA, most prevalent in the southeast. The larvae enter the skin and migrate intracutaneously for long periods; eventually they penetrate to deeper tissues. Each larva causes a serpiginous track, advancing several millimeters to a few centimeters a day, with intense itching more marked at night. The disease is self-limited, with spontaneous cure after several weeks or months. Individual larvae can be killed by freezing the area with ethyl chloride spray; thiabendazole is effective systemically and as a topical ointment.

TOXOPLASMOSIS   ICD-9 130
CONGENITAL TOXOPLASMOSIS   ICD-9 771.2

1. **Identification**—A systemic protozoan disease; infections are frequently asymptomatic or present as an acute disease resembling infectious mononucleosis, with fever, lymphadenopathy and lymphocytosis persisting for days or weeks. With development of antibodies the parasitemia decreases, but *Toxoplasma* cysts remaining in the tissues contain viable organisms. Among immunodeficient individuals, primary infection may include cerebral signs, pneumonia, generalized skeletal muscle involvement, myocarditis, a maculopapular rash and death. The dormant organisms from an earlier infection can reactivate as in AIDS patients, among whom cerebral toxoplasmosis occurs. A primary infection during early pregnancy may lead to fetal infection with death of the fetus or chorioretinitis, brain damage with intracerebral calcification, hydrocephaly, microcephaly, fever, jaundice, rash, hepatosplenomegaly,

xanthochromic CSF and convulsions evident at birth or shortly thereafter. Later in pregnancy, maternal infection results in mild or subclinical fetal disease with delayed manifestations, especially recurrent or chronic chorioretinitis.

Diagnosis is based on clinical signs and supportive serologic results, demonstration of the agent in body tissues or fluids by biopsy or necropsy, or isolation in animals or cell culture. Rising antibody levels are corroborative of active infection; specific IgM and titer rises in sequential sera of infants are conclusive evidence of congenital infection. High antibody levels may persist for years without relation to active disease.

2. Infectious agent—*Toxoplasma gondii,* an intracellular coccidian protozoan of cats, belonging to the family Sarcocystidae, grouped with the Sporozoa.

3. Occurrence—Worldwide in mammals and birds. Infection in man is common.

4. Reservoir—The definitive hosts of *T. gondii* are cats and other felines, which acquire infection mainly from eating infected mammals (especially rodents) or birds and rarely as a feces-borne infection from other cats. Only felines harbor the parasite in the intestinal tract where the sexual stage of the life cycle takes place, with excretion of the oocysts in feces for 10-20 days or, rarely, longer.

The intermediate hosts of these 2-host coccidia are sheep, goats, rodents, swine, cattle, chickens and birds; all may carry an infective stage (cystozoite or bradyzoite) of *T. gondii* encysted in tissue, especially muscle and brain. Tissue cysts remain viable for long periods, perhaps the life of the animal.

5. Mode of transmission—Transplacental infection in humans occurs only when a pregnant woman has a primary infection with the rapidly dividing tachyzoites circulating in the bloodstream. Children are at risk by ingesting infective oocysts from dirt in sandboxes, playgrounds and yards in which cats have defecated. Infections may be acquired by eating raw or undercooked infected meat (pork or mutton, more rarely beef) containing tissue cysts, or by the ingestion of infective oocysts in food or water contaminated with feline feces. Inhalation of sporulated oocysts was associated with one outbreak. Milk of infected goats and cattle may contain tachyzoites; one outbreak was associated epidemiologically with consumption of raw goat's milk. Infection may rarely be acquired by blood transfusion or organ transplantation from an infected donor.

6. Incubation period—Ten to 23 days in one common-source outbreak from ingestion of undercooked meat; 5-20 days in an outbreak associated with cats.

7. Period of communicability—Not directly transmitted from person to person except in utero. The oocysts shed by cats sporulate and become infective 1-5 days later and may remain infective in water or moist soil for about a year. Cysts in the flesh of an infected animal remain infective as long as the meat is edible and uncooked.

8. Susceptibility and resistance—Susceptibility to infection is general, but immunity is readily acquired, and most infections are asymptomatic. Duration and degree of immunity are unknown but assumed to be long-lasting or permanent; antibodies persist for years, probably for life. Patients undergoing cytotoxic or immunosuppressive therapy are highly susceptible, and usually display reactivated infection; a complication of AIDS.

9. Methods of control—

A. *Preventive measures:*

1) Cook meats thoroughly (until color changes). Freezing meat reduces infectivity but does not eliminate it.

2) Feed cats dry, canned or boiled food, and discourage hunting (i.e., keep them as indoor pets only).

3) Dispose of cat feces and litter daily (before sporocysts become infective). Feces can be flushed down the toilet, burned or deeply buried. Disinfect litter pans daily by scalding; wear gloves when handling potentially infective material. Dried litter should be disposed of without shaking, to avoid dispersal of oocysts in the air.

4) Unless they are known to have antibodies to *T. gondii,* pregnant women should avoid cleaning litter pans or contact with cats of unknown feeding history. Wear gloves during gardening, and wash hands thoroughly after work and before eating.

5) Wash hands thoroughly after handling raw meat or contact with soil possibly contaminated with cat feces, and before eating.

6) Educate pregnant women about these preventive measures.

7) Control stray cats and prevent them from gaining access to sandboxes and sand piles used by children for play. Sandboxes should be covered when not in use.

8) Patients with AIDS should receive prophylactic treatment throughout life with pyrimethamine (50 mg/week) plus sulfadoxine (1 g/week); or Fansidar (2 tablets weekly).

B. *Control of patient, contacts and the immediate environment:*

1) Report to local health authority: Not ordinarily required, but desirable to facilitate further understanding of the epidemiology of the disease, Class 3C (see Preface).

2) Isolation: None.

3) Concurrent disinfection: None.
4) Quarantine: None.
5) Immunization of contacts: None.
6) Investigation of contacts and source of infection: In congenital cases, determine antibodies in mother and members of the household; in acquired cases, determine contact with infected animals and common exposure to cat feces, soil or raw meat.
7) Specific treatment: Treatment is not routinely indicated for a healthy immunocompetent host, except in an initial infection during pregnancy or the presence of chorioretinitis, myocarditis or other organ involvement. Pyrimethamine (Daraprim®) combined with sulfadiazine and folinic acid (to avoid bone marrow depression) for 4 weeks is the preferred treatment for those with severe symptomatic disease. Treatment of pregnant women is problematic. Spiramycin is commonly used; the addition of pyrimethamine and sulfadiazine should be considered when fetal infection is documented. Congenitally infected, asymptomatic children should be treated prophylactically with pyrimethamine-sulfadiazine-folinic acid during their first year of life to prevent chorioretinitis and other sequelae.

C. *Epidemic measures:* None.

D. *Disaster implications:* None.

E. *International measures:* None.

TRACHOMA   ICD-9 076

1. **Identification**—A chlamydial conjunctivitis of insidious or abrupt onset; the infection may persist for a few years if untreated, but the characteristic lifetime duration of active disease in hyperendemic areas is the result of frequent reinfection. It is characterized by the presence of lymphoid follicles and diffuse conjunctival inflammation (papillary hypertrophy), particularly on the tarsal conjunctiva lining the upper eyelid. The inflammation produces superficial vascularization of the cornea (pannus) and scarring of the conjunctiva. This scarring increases with the severity and duration of the inflammatory disease. Marked conjunctival scarring causes in-turned eye lashes and lid deformities (entropion and trichiasis) which cause chronic abrasion of the cornea with visual impairment and

blindness later in adult life. Associated bacterial infections are common in populations with endemic trachoma and contribute to the communicability and severity of the disease.

Early stages of infection may be indistinguishable from that of chlamydial conjunctivitis (q.v.), which occurs as sporadic cases in sexually active adults, while early trachoma is an endemic childhood disease in families or communities in some developing countries.

Other forms of chronic follicular conjunctivitis, occasionally with scarring and corneal pannus, include molluscum contagiosum nodules of the eyelids, toxic reactions to chronically administered eye drops and chronic staphylococcal lid margin infection. An allergic reaction to contact lens wear (giant papillary conjunctivitis) may produce a trachoma-like syndrome with tarsal nodules (giant papillae), conjunctival scarring and corneal pannus.

Laboratory diagnosis is made by detection of intracytoplasmic chlamydial elementary bodies in epithelial cells of conjunctival scrapings by Giemsa-stained smears, or by IF after methanol fixation of the smear, by detection of chlamydial antigen by EIA, or by isolation of the agent in special cell culture.

2. **Infectious agent**—*Chlamydia trachomatis* of serovars A, B, Ba, and C. Some strains are indistinguishable from those of chlamydial conjunctivitis (q.v.).

3. **Occurrence**—Worldwide, occurring as an endemic disease most often in the poorer rural communities in developing countries. In endemic areas, trachoma presents in childhood, then subsides in adolescence, leaving varying degrees of potential disabling scarring. Blinding trachoma is still widespread in the Middle East, northern and sub-Saharan Africa, parts of the Indian subcontinent and in SE Asia. Pockets of blinding trachoma occur in Latin America, Australia (among aborigenes) and the Pacific Islands. In the USA, it is rarely present, occurring among population groups with poor hygiene, poverty, and crowded living conditions, particularly in dry, dusty regions such as some Indian reservations in the Southwest. The late complications of trachoma (in-turned lids and corneal scarring) occur in older persons who had infectious trachoma in childhood; these people are rarely infectious.

4. **Reservoir**—Man.

5. **Mode of transmission**—By direct contact with ocular discharges on fingers and clothes, and nasopharyngeal discharges from infected persons and materials soiled therewith. Flies contribute to spread of the disease, especially *Musca sorbens* in Africa and the Middle East and *Hippelates* species in the southern USA, but transmission occurs in the absence of flies. In children with active trachoma, *Chlamydia* can be recovered from the nasopharynx and rectum, but the trachoma serovars do not appear to have a genital reservoir in endemic communities.

6. **Incubation period**—Five to 12 days (based on volunteer studies).

7. **Period of communicability**—As long as active lesions are present in the conjunctivae and adnexal mucous membranes; this may last a few years. Concentration of the agent in the tissues is greatly reduced with cicatrization, but increases again with reactivation and recurrence of infective discharges. Infectivity is terminated within 2-3 days of antibiotic treatment, long before the clinical disease improves.

8. **Susceptibility and resistance**—Susceptibility is general; there is no evidence that infection confers immunity, or that experimental vaccines are useful in preventing infection or in reducing the severity of established cases. In endemic areas, children have active disease more frequently than adults. The severity of disease often is related to living conditions, particulary poor hygiene. Exposure to dry winds, dust and fine sand may contribute to the severity of the disease.

9. **Methods of control**—

   A. *Preventive measures:*

      1) Educate the public on the need for personal hygiene, especially the risk in common use of toilet articles.
      2) Improve basic sanitation, including availability and use of soap and water; avoid common-use towels.
      3) Provide adequate case-finding and treatment facilities, with emphasis on preschool children.
      4) Conduct epidemiologic investigations to determine important factors in the occurrence of the disease in each specific situation.

   B. *Control of patient, contacts and the immediate environment:*

      1) Report to local health authority: Case report required in some states (USA) and countries of low endemicity, Class 2B (see Preface).
      2) Isolation: Not practical in most areas where the disease occurs. For hospitalized patients, drainage/secretion precautions.
      3) Concurrent disinfection: Of eye and nasal discharges and contaminated articles.
      4) Quarantine: None.
      5) Immunization of contacts: None.
      6) Investigation of contacts and source of infection: Members of family, playmates and schoolmates.
      7) Specific treatment: In areas where the disease is severe and highly prevalent, mass treatment of the whole population, especially the children, with topical tetracycline or erythromycin ointments is used with varying schedules,

such as twice daily for 5 consecutive days, once monthly for 6 months. Oral tetracyclines and erythromycin are also effective in the active stages of the disease.

C. *Epidemic measures:* In regions of hyperendemic prevalence, mass treatment campaigns have been successful in reducing severity and frequency when associated with education of the people in personal hygiene and improvement of the sanitary environment, particularly a good water supply.

D. *Disaster implications:* None.

E. *International measures:* WHO Collaborating Centres (see Preface).

TRENCH FEVER
(Wolhynian fever, Quintana fever)

ICD-9 083.1

1. **Identification**—A nonfatal, febrile, bacterial disease varying in manifestations and severity. It is characterized by headache, malaise, pain and tenderness, especially on the shins; onset is either sudden or slow, with a fever which may be relapsing, typhoid-like, or limited to a single febrile episode lasting for several days. Splenomegaly is common, and a transient macular rash may occur. Symptoms may continue to recur many years after the primary infection, which may be subclinical with organisms circulating in the blood for months, with or without repeated recurrence of symptoms.

Laboratory diagnosis is made by culture of patient's blood on blood agar under 5% CO_2 tension in air. Microcolonies are visible after 2 weeks incubation at 37°C (98.6°F). Infection evokes specific antibodies detectable by serologic tests; ELISA tests are highly sensitive.

2. **Infectious agent**—*Rochalimaea quintana (Rickettsia quintana).*

3. **Occurrence**—Epidemics occurred in Europe during World Wars I and II among troops and prisoners-of-war living under crowded, unhygienic conditions. Sporadic cases in endemic foci probably are not recognized.

The organism probably can be found wherever the human body louse exists. Endemic foci of infection have been detected in Poland, the USSR, Mexico, Bolivia, Burundi, Ethiopia and North Africa.

4. **Reservoir**—Man. The intermediate host is the body louse, *Pediculus humanus.* The organism multiplies extracellularly in the gut lumen for the duration of the insect's life, which is approximately 5 weeks after

hatching. No transovarian transmission occurs.

5. **Mode of transmission**—Not directly transmitted from person to person. Man is infected by inoculation of the organism in louse feces through a break in the skin, either from the bite of the louse or other means. Infected lice begin to excrete infectious feces 5-12 days after ingesting infective blood and continue for the rest of their lifespan. Nymphal stages may become infected. The disease spreads when lice leave abnormally hot (febrile) or cold (dead) bodies in search of a normothermic clothed body.

6. **Incubation period**—Generally 7-30 days.

7. **Period of communicability**—Organisms may circulate in the blood (by which lice are infected) for weeks, months or years and may recur with or without symptoms. A history of trench fever is a permanent contraindication to blood donation.

8. **Susceptibility and resistance**—Susceptibility is general. After infection, the degree of protective immunity to either infection or disease is unknown.

9. **Methods of control**—

A. *Preventive measures:* Delousing procedures will destroy the vector and prevent transmission to man. Dust clothing and body with an effective insecticide.

B. *Control of patient, contacts and the immediate environment:*

1) Report to local health authority: Cases should be reported so that an evaluation of louse infestation in the population may be made and appropriate measures taken, since lice also transmit epidemic typhus and relapsing fever, Class 3B (see Preface).

2) Isolation: None after delousing.

3) Concurrent disinfection: Louse-infested clothing should be treated to kill the lice.

4) Quarantine: None.

5) Immunization of contacts: None.

6) Investigation of contacts and source of infection: Search the bodies and clothing of people at risk for the presence of lice; delouse if indicated.

7) Specific treatment: Tetracyclines and chloramphenicol are probably effective, but have not yet been adequately tested in clinical cases.

C. *Epidemic measures:* Systematic application of residual insecticide to the clothing of all persons in the affected population (see 9A, above).

D. **Disaster implications:** Risk is increased when louse-infested people are forced to live in crowded, unhygienic shelters (see 9B1, above).

E. **International measures:** WHO Collaborating Centres (see Preface).

TRICHINELLOSIS   ICD-9 124
(Trichiniasis, Trichinosis)

1. **Identification**—A disease caused by an intestinal roundworm whose larvae (trichinae) migrate to and become encapsulated in the muscles. Clinical disease in man is highly variable and can range from inapparent infection to a fulminating, fatal disease, depending on the number of larvae ingested. Sudden appearance of muscle soreness and pain, together with edema of upper eyelids are common early and characteristic signs. These are sometimes followed by subconjunctival, subungual and retinal hemorrhages, pain and photophobia. Thirst, profuse sweating, chills, weakness, prostration and rapidly increasing eosinophilia may follow shortly after the ocular signs. Gastrointestinal symptoms, such as diarrhea, due to the intraintestinal activity of the adult worms, may precede the ocular manifestations. Remittent fever is usual, sometimes as high as 40°C (104°F); the fever terminates after 1-6 weeks, depending on intensity of infection. Cardiac and neurologic complications may appear in the third to sixth week; death due to myocardial failure may occur in either the first to second week or between the fourth and eighth weeks.

Serologic tests and marked eosinophilia may aid in diagnosis. Biopsy of skeletal muscle, not earlier than about 10 days after exposure to infection, frequently provides conclusive evidence of infection by demonstrating the uncalcified parasite cyst.

2. **Infectious agent**—*Trichinella spiralis,* an intestinal nematode. Separate taxonomic designations have been proposed for isolates found in the Arctic *(T. spiralis nativa)* and in Africa *(T. s. nelsoni).*

3. **Occurrence**—Worldwide, but variable in incidence, depending in part on practices of eating and preparing pork or wild animal meat, and the extent to which the disease is recognized and reported. Necropsy surveys in the mid-20th century revealed a prevalence of 16.7% in the USA; the age-adjusted rate is now 2% or less. Cases usually are sporadic and outbreaks localized, in several instances resulting from eating home-made sausage and other meat products using pork or shared meat from

Arctic mammals. Outbreaks due to infected horse meat have recently been reported.

4. Reservoir—Swine, dogs, cats, rats and many wild animals, including fox, wolf, bear, polar bear, wild boar and marine mammals in the Arctic, and hyena, jackal, lion and leopard in the tropics.

5. Mode of transmission—By eating raw or insufficiently cooked flesh of animals containing viable encysted larvae, chiefly pork and pork products, and "beef products," such as hamburger adulterated either intentionally or inadvertently with raw pork. In the epithelium of the small intestine, larvae develop into adults. Gravid female worms then produce larvae, which penetrate the lymphatics or venules and are disseminated via the bloodstream throughout the body. The larvae become encapsulated in skeletal muscle.

6. Incubation period—Systemic symptoms usually appear about 8-15 days after ingestion of infected meat; varies between 5 and 45 days depending on the number of worms involved. Gastrointestinal symptoms may appear within a few days.

7. Period of communicability—Not transmitted directly from person to person. Animal hosts remain infective for months, and meat from such animals stays infected for appreciable periods unless cooked or frozen to kill the larvae (see 9A1 and 9A6, below).

8. Susceptibility and resistance—Susceptibility is universal. Infection results in partial immunity.

9. Methods of control—

A. *Preventive measures:*

1) Educate the public on the need to cook all fresh pork and pork products and meat from wild animals at a temperature and for a time sufficient to allow all parts to reach at least 77°C (171°F), or until meat changes from pink to gray, which allows a sufficient margin of safety. This should be done unless it has been established that these meat products have been processed either by heating, curing or freezing adequate to kill trichinae.

2) Grind pork in a separate grinder or clean the grinder thoroughly before and after processing other meats.

3) Adopt regulations to assure adequate commercial processing of pork products. Testing carcasses for infection with a digestion technique is useful. Immunodiagnosis with the ELISA test is also adequate.

4) Adopt laws and regulations to require and enforce the cooking of garbage and offal before feeding to swine.

5) Educate hunters to cook thoroughly the meat of walrus,

seal, wild boar, bear and other wild animals.

6) Freezing temperatures maintained throughout the mass of the infected meat are effective in killing trichinae; i.e., holding pieces of pork up to 15 cm thick at a temperature of -15°C (+5°F) for 30 days or -25°C (-13°F) or lower for 10 days will effectively destroy all common types of *Trichinella* cysts. Hold thicker pieces at the lower temperature for at least 20 days. These temperatures will not kill the cold-resistant Arctic strains (*T. s. nativa*) found in walrus and bear meat, and rarely in swine.

7) Exposure of pork cuts or carcasses to low level gamma irradiation effectively kills trichina larvae.

B. *Control of patient, contacts and the immediate environment:*

1) Report to local health authority: Case report required in most states (USA) and countries, Class 2B (see Preface).
2) Isolation: None.
3) Concurrent disinfection: None.
4) Quarantine: None.
5) Immunization of contacts: None.
6) Investigation of contacts and source of infection: Check other family members and persons who have eaten suspected meat for evidence of infection. Confiscate any remaining suspected food.
7) Specific treatment: Thiabendazole may be effective in the intestinal stage; mebendazole (Vermox®) is used in the muscular stage. Corticosteroids are indicated only in severe cases since they delay elimination of the adult worms from the intestine.

C. *Epidemic measures:* Institute epidemiologic study to determine the common food involved. Confiscate remainder of suspected food and correct faulty practices.

D. *Disaster implications:* None.

E. *International measures:* WHO Collaborating Centres (see Preface).

TRICHOMONIASIS   ICD-9 131

1. Identification—A common, persistent, protozoan disease of the genitourinary tract, characterized in women by vaginitis, with small

petechial or sometimes punctate hemorrhagic lesions and a profuse, thin, foamy, yellowish discharge with foul odor; frequently asymptomatic. In men, the infectious agent invades and persists in the prostate, urethra, or seminal vesicles, but rarely produces symptoms or demonstrable lesions; it is thought to cause about 3% of nongonococcal urethritis, and is associated with prostatitis in these cases.

Diagnosis is made through identification of the motile parasite, either by microscopic examination of discharges or by culture, which is more sensitive.

2. **Infectious agent**—*Trichomonas vaginalis*, a flagellate protozoan.

3. **Occurrence**—Widespread; a frequent disease of all continents and all races, primarily of adults, with the highest incidence among females 16-35 years. In sampled areas of the USA, the prevalence of infection among patients in gynecology clinics has been as high as 50%.

4. **Reservoir**—People.

5. **Mode of transmission**—By contact with vaginal and urethral discharges of infected persons during sexual intercourse and presumably by contact with contaminated articles.

6. **Incubation period**—Four to 20 days, average 7 days.

7. **Period of communicability**—For the duration of the persistent infection, which may last for years.

8. **Susceptibility and resistance**—Susceptibility to infection is general but clinical disease is mainly in females.

9. **Methods of control**—

    A.   *Preventive measures:* Educate the public as to the symptoms and mode of transmission; encourage women with symptoms to seek immediate treatment and to avoid sexual intercourse until treatment is completed.

    B.   *Control of patient, contacts and the immediate environment:*

        1)   Report to local health authority: Official report not ordinarily justifiable, Class 5 (see Preface).

        2)   Isolation: None; avoid sexual relations during period of infection and treatment.

        3)   Concurrent disinfection: None; the organism cannot withstand drying.

        4)   Quarantine: None.

        5)   Immunization of contacts: None.

        6)   Investigation of contacts and source of infection: Sexual partners should be treated concurrently.

        7)   Specific treatment: Metronidazole (Flagyl®) by mouth is

effective in both male and female patients. It is contraindicated during the first trimester of pregnancy. Concurrent treatment of sexual partner(s) to prevent reinfection. Metronidazole resistance is uncommon but has been reported.

C. *Epidemic measures:* None.

D. *Disaster implications:* None.

E. *International measures:* None.

TRICHURIASIS
(Trichocephaliasis, Whipworm disease)

ICD-9 127.3

1. **Identification**—A nematode infection of the large intestine, usually asymptomatic. Heavy infections may cause bloody, mucoid stools and diarrhea. Rectal prolapse may occur in heavily infected children.

Diagnosis is made by demonstration of eggs in feces or by sigmoidoscopic observation of worms attached to the wall of the lower colon in heavy infections. Eggs must be differentiated from those of *Capillaria* species.

2. **Infectious agent**—*Trichuris trichiura (Trichocephalus trichiurus),* a nematode; the human whipworm.

3. **Occurrence**—Worldwide, especially in warm, moist regions.

4. **Reservoir**—Man.

5. **Mode of transmission**—Indirect; not immediately transmissible from person to person. Eggs passed in feces require a minimum of 10-14 days in warm moist soil to become infective. Ingestion of infective eggs from contaminated soil is followed by hatching of the larvae, their attachment to the mucosa of the cecum and proximal colon, and development into mature worms. Eggs appear in the feces about 90 days after ingestion of the embryonated eggs; symptoms may appear much earlier.

6. **Incubation period**—Indefinite.

7. **Period of communicability**—Several years in untreated carriers.

8. **Susceptibility and resistance**—Susceptibility is universal.

9. **Methods of control**—

A. *Preventive measures:*

1) Provide adequate facilities for feces disposal.

2) Educate all members of the family, particularly children, in the use of toilet facilities.
3) Encourage satisfactory hygienic habits, especially hand-washing before foodhandling; avoid ingestion of soil by washing thoroughly vegetables and other soil-contaminated foods.

B. **Control of patient, contacts and the immediate environment:**

1) Report to local health authority: Official report not ordinarily justifiable, Class 5 (see Preface). Advise school health authorities of unusual frequency in school populations.
2) Isolation: None.
3) Concurrent disinfection: None; sanitary disposal of feces.
4) Quarantine: None.
5) Immunization of contacts: None.
6) Investigation of contacts and source of infection: Examine feces of all symptomatic members of the family group, especially children and playmates.
7) Specific treatment: Mebendazole (Vermox®) or albendazole (Zentel®) is the drug of choice; both are contraindicated in pregnancy. Oxantel is an alternative drug (not available in the USA).

C. **Epidemic measures:** Not applicable.

D. **Disaster implications:** None.

E. **International measures:** None.

TRYPANOSOMIASIS
I. AFRICAN TRYPANOSOMIASIS
(Sleeping sickness)

ICD-9 086
ICD-9 086.5

1. **Identification**—A systemic protozoan disease. In the early stages, a painful chancre may be found at the primary tsetse fly bite site; also there may be fever, intense headache, insomnia, painless enlarged lymph nodes, anemia, local edema and rash. In the late stage, there is body wasting, somnolence and signs referable to the CNS. The gambiense disease (ICD-9 086.3) may run a protracted course of several years; the rhodesiense disease (ICD-9 086.4) in East Africa is lethal within weeks or

a few months without treatment. Both forms of the disease are always fatal without treatment.

Diagnosis is made by finding trypanosomes in blood, lymph or CSF. Parasite concentration may be required particularly in the gambiense disease. Inoculation of laboratory rats or mice is sometimes useful in rhodesiense disease. Lymph node aspirates may help in diagnosing the gambiense disease. Specific antibodies may be demonstrated by ELISA, IFA and agglutination tests; high levels of immunoglobulins, especially IgM, are common in African trypanosomiasis.

2. **Infectious agents**—*Trypanosoma brucei gambiense* and *T. b. rhodesiense*, hemoflagellates. Criteria for species differentiation are not absolute; isolates from cases of virulent, rapidly progressive disease are considered to be *T. b. rhodesiense*, especially if contracted in East Africa; West and Central African cases are usually more chronic and considered to be due to *T. b. gambiense*.

3. **Occurrence**—The disease is confined to tropical Africa between 15°N and 20°S latitude, corresponding to the distribution of the tsetse fly. In endemic regions, infection has been found in 0.1-2% of the population. Outbreaks can occur when, for any reason, man-fly contact is intensified, or when virulent strains of trypanosomes are introduced into a tsetse-infested area by movement of infected flies or reservoir hosts. Where flies of the *Glossina palpalis* group are the principal vectors, as in West and Central Africa, infection occurs mainly along streams. In East Africa and around Lake Victoria, where the main vectors are of the Morsitans group, disease occurs over the broader dry savannas. *G. fuscipes*, which belongs to the Palpalis group, has been responsible for outbreaks of rhodesiense sleeping sickness in Kenya and is the vector transmitting the disease in a large epidemic in peridomestic situations in Uganda since 1976.

4. **Reservoir**—In *T. b. gambiense*, man is the major reservoir; however, the role of domestic and wild animals is not clear. Wild animals, especially bushbuck and antelopes, and domestic cattle are the chief animal reservoirs of *T. b. rhodesiense*.

5. **Mode of transmission**—By the bite of an infective *Glossina*, the tsetse fly. Six species are the principal vectors in nature: *Glossina palpalis*, *G. tachinoides*, *G. morsitans*, *G. pallidipes*, *G. swynnertoni* and *G. fuscipes*. The tsetse fly is infected by ingesting blood of a man or animal that carries trypanosomes. The parasite multiplies in the fly for 12-30 days, depending on temperature and other factors, until infective forms develop in the salivary glands. Once infected, a tsetse fly remains infective for life (up to 3 months); infection is not passed from generation to generation in flies. Congenital transmission can occur in man. Direct mechanical transmission is possible by blood on the proboscis of *Glossina* and other man-biting insects, such as horseflies, or in laboratory accidents.

6. **Incubation period**—In *T. b. rhodesiense* infection, usually 3 days to 3 weeks; in *T. b. gambiense* infection, there is a variable patent period which may last several months, or even years.

7. **Period of communicability**—Communicable to the tsetse fly as long as the parasite is present in the blood of the infected person or animal. Parasitemia occurs in waves of varying intensity in untreated cases and occurs in all stages of the disease. In one study of rhodesiense disease, parasitemia was detected in only 60% of infected cases.

8. **Susceptibility and resistance**—Susceptibility is general. Occasional inapparent infections have been documented with both *T. b. gambiense* and *T. b. rhodesiense*. Spontaneous recovery in cases with the gambiense form without CNS involvement has been claimed but this has not been confirmed.

9. **Methods of control**—

    A. *Preventive measures:* Selection of appropriate methods of prevention must be based on knowledge of the local ecology of the vectors and infectious agents. Thus, in a given geographic area, priority must be given to one or more of the following:

        1) Educate the public on personal measures to protect against tsetse fly bites.

        2) Reduce the parasite population by survey of the human population for infection; treat those infected.

        3) Destroy vector tsetse fly habitats. If cleared areas can be reclaimed for agricultural use, a permanent solution to the vector problem may result.

        4) Reduce the fly population by appropriate use of traps impregnated with decamethrin and by local use of residual insecticides (synthetic pyrethroids, 5% DDT and 3% dieldrin are effective); in emergency situations, use aerosol insecticides sprayed by helicopter and fixed-wing aircraft.

        5) Prohibit blood donation from those who have visited or lived in endemic areas in Africa.

    B. *Control of patient, contacts and the immediate environment:*

        1) Report to local health authority: In selected endemic areas, establish records of prevalence and encourage control measures; not a reportable disease in most countries, Class 3B (see Preface).

        2) Isolation: Not practicable. Prevent tsetse flies from feeding on patients with trypanosomes in their blood. In some countries, legal restrictions are placed on the movement of untreated patients.

3) Concurrent disinfection: None.
4) Quarantine: None.
5) Immunization of contacts: None.
6) Investigation of contacts and source of infection: None.
7) Specific treatment: If the CNS shows no changes in cellular or protein content, suramin is the drug of choice for *T. b. rhodesiense* infections, and pentamidine for *T. b. gambiense* infections. Melarsoprol (Mel-B®) has been used effectively for treatment of patients with abnormal CSF with either parasite, but severe adverse side effects may occur in 5-10% of patients. Suramin and melarsoprol are available from CDC Drug Service, Atlanta, on an investigational basis (see Preface). Recent studies have shown that eflornithine (DFMO) may be preferable treatment for gambiense CNS disease; it is available as Ornidyl through compassionate protocol from Marion Merrell Dow, Cincinnati OH 45242, USA. All treated patients should be checked at 3, 6, 12, and 24 months after treatment for possible relapsed infections.

C. *Epidemic measures:* Mass surveys, treatment for identified infections and tsetse fly control are urgent. If epidemics recur in an area despite control measures, it may be necessary to move whole villages to safer districts; other measures as in 9A, above.

D. *Disaster implications:* None.

E. *International measures:* Promote cooperative efforts of governments in endemic areas. Disseminate information and increase the availability of simple diagnostic tests for screening and simple means of vector control. Develop systems for effective distribution of reagents and drugs. Stimulate training at national and international levels. WHO Collaborating Centres (see Preface).

II. AMERICAN TRYPANOSOMIASIS ICD-9 086.2
(Chagas disease)

1. Identification—Acute disease generally occurs in children, while chronic manifestations generally appear later in life. Many infected people have no clinical manifestations. The acute disease is characterized by variable fever, malaise, lymphadenopathy and hepatosplenomegaly. An inflammatory response at the site of infection (chagoma) may last up to 8 weeks. Unilateral bipalpebral edema (Romaña's sign) occurs in a significant percentage of acute cases. Life-threatening or fatal manifestations include myocarditis and meningoencephalitis. Chronic sequelae

include myocardial damage with cardiac dilatation, arrhythmias and major conduction abnormalities, and intestinal tract involvement with megaesophagus and megacolon. Late manifestations are relatively rare in Panamanian infections, and megaviscera do not occur.

Infection with *Trypanosoma rangeli* occurs in focal areas of endemic Chagas disease, extending from Central America to Peru and Venezuela; a prolonged parasitemia occurs, sometimes coexisting with *T. cruzi* flagellates (with which it shares reservoir hosts), but no clinical manifestations attributable to this infection have been noted.

Diagnosis of Chagas disease in the acute phase is established by demonstration of the organism in blood (rarely, in a lymph node or skeletal muscle) by direct examination or after hemoconcentration, culture, intracerebral inoculation of suckling mice, or xenodiagnosis (feeding uninfected triatomid bugs on the patient and finding the parasite in the bug's feces several weeks later). Parasitemia is most intense during febrile episodes early in the course of infection. In the chronic phase, xenodiagnosis and blood culture on diphasic media may be positive, but other methods rarely reveal parasites. Parasites are differentiated from those of *T. rangeli* by their shorter length (20μm v. 36μm). Serologic tests are valuable for individual diagnosis as well as for screening purposes.

2. Infectious agent—*Trypanosoma cruzi (Schizotrypanum cruzi)*, a protozoan that occurs in man as a hemoflagellate and as an intracellular parasite without an external flagellum.

3. Occurrence—The disease is confined to the Western Hemisphere, with wide geographic distribution in rural Mexico and Central and S America; highly endemic in some areas. Three acute vector-borne human infections acquired within the USA have been reported (2 in Texas, 1 in California); three additional infections were acquired by blood transfusion. Serologic studies suggest the possible occurrence of other asymptomatic cases. *T. cruzi* has been found in small mammals in Alabama, Arizona, Arkansas, California, Florida, Georgia, Louisiana, Maryland, New Mexico, Texas and Utah. Recent studies found infection in 4.9% of migrants from Central America living in the Washington DC, area.

4. Reservoir—Man, and over 150 species of domestic and wild animals, including dogs, cats, rats, mice, and other domestic animals; plus marsupials, edentates, rodents, chiropters, carnivores and primates.

5. Mode of transmission—Infected vectors, i.e., blood-sucking species of *Reduviidae* (cone-nosed bugs), especially from the genera *Triatoma, Rhodnius* and *Panstrongylus* spp. have the trypanosomes in their feces. Defecation occurs during feeding; infection of humans and other mammals occurs when the freshly excreted bug feces contaminates conjunctiva, mucous membranes, abrasions or skin wounds (including the bite wound). The bugs become infected when they feed on a parasitemic animal; the organisms multiply in the gut. Transmission may also occur by blood transfusion, with the increasing rate of infected donors in cities due to migrants from rural areas. Organisms may also cross the placenta to cause congenital infection; transmission through lactation seems highly unlikely, so there is currently no reason to restrict lactation by chagasic mothers. Accidental laboratory infections occur occasionally; transplantation of organs from chagasic donors presents a growing risk of *T. cruzi* transmission.

6. **Incubation period**—About 5-14 days after bite of the insect vector; 30-40 days if infected through blood transfusion.

7. **Period of communicability**—Organisms are present regularly in the blood during the acute period and may persist in very small numbers throughout life in symptomatic and asymptomatic people. The vector becomes infective in 10-30 days after biting an infected host, and the gut infection in the bug persists for life (as long as 2 years).

8. **Susceptibility and resistance**—All ages are susceptible, but the disease is usually more severe in younger people.

9. **Methods of control**—

    A. *Preventive measures:*

        1) Educate the public on the mode of spread and methods of prevention.

        2) Systematically attack vectors infesting poorly constructed houses by use of effective insecticides with residual action, by spraying, or by use of insecticidal paints or fumigant canisters.

        3) Construct or repair living areas to eliminate lodging places for the insect vector and shelter for domestic and wild reservoir animals.

        4) Use bed nets in houses infested by the vector.

        5) Screen blood donors living in or coming from endemic areas by appropriate serologic tests to prevent infection by transfusion. Addition of gentian violet (25 ml of 0.5% solution/500 ml of blood 24 hours before use) may prevent transmission.

    B. *Control of patient, contacts and the immediate environment:*

        1) Report to local health authority: In selected endemic areas; not a reportable disease in most countries, Class 3B (see Preface).

        2) Isolation: Not generally practical. Blood/body fluid precautions for hospitalized patients.

        3) Concurrent disinfection: None.

        4) Quarantine: None.

5) Immunization of contacts: None.
6) Investigation of contacts and source of infection: Search thatched roofs, bedding and rooms for the vector. All members of the family of a case should be examined. Perform serologic tests and blood examinations on all blood donors implicated as possible sources of transfusion-acquired infection.
7) Specific treatment: Nifurtimox, a nitrofurfurylidene derivative, is most useful in treatment of acute cases and is available from the CDC Drug Service, Atlanta, on an investigational basis (see Preface) and from major hospitals in the endemic area. Benznidazole, a 2-nitroimidazole derivative, has also proven to be effective in acute cases.

C. *Epidemic measures:* In areas of high incidence, field survey to determine distribution and density of vectors and animal hosts.

D. *Disaster implications:* None.

E. *International measures:* None.

TUBERCULOSIS (TB)

ICD-9 010-018

1. **Identification**—A mycobacterial disease important as a cause of disability and death in many parts of the world. The initial infection usually goes unnoticed; tuberculin sensitivity appears within a few weeks. Lesions commonly heal, leaving no residual changes except occasional pulmonary or tracheobronchial lymph node calcifications. Approximately 95% of those initially infected enter this latent phase from which there is lifelong risk of reactivation. In approximately 5%, the initial infection may progress directly to pulmonary tuberculosis or, by lymphohematogenous dissemination of bacilli, to pulmonary, miliary, meningeal or other extrapulmonary involvement. Serious outcome of the initial infection is more frequent in infants, adolescents and young adults.

Extrapulmonary tuberculosis is much less common than pulmonary. It may affect any organ or tissue and includes tuberculous meningitis, acute hematogenous (miliary) tuberculosis, and involvement of lymph nodes, pleura, pericardium, kidneys, bones and joints, larynx, skin, intestines, peritoneum and eyes.

Progressive pulmonary tuberculosis arises from exogenous reinfection or endogenous reactivation of a latent focus remaining from the initial infection. If untreated, about half the patients will die within a two-year period. Appropriate chemotherapy nearly always results in a cure. Clinical status is based mainly on the presence or absence of tubercle bacilli in the sputum and also on the nature of changes seen on chest radiographs. Abnormal x-ray densities indicative of pulmonary infiltration, cavitation and fibrosis can occur before clinical manifestations. Fatigue, fever and weight loss may occur early, while localizing symptoms of cough, chest pain, hemoptysis and hoarseness become prominent in advanced stages.

People who are or have been infected with Mycobacterium tuberculosis, M. africanum and M. bovis will almost always react to a low dose tuberculin skin test, i.e., bio-equivalent to 5 International Units (IU) of the International Standard of Purified Protein Derivative-Standard (PPD-S). The reaction may be suppressed in critically ill tuberculosis patients; during certain acute infectious diseases, notably measles; by vaccination with live attenuated viruses; and in persons who are immunosuppressed by disease or drugs. Reactions caused by other mycobacteria, including BCG, tend to be smaller; their relative frequency varies with the prevalence of these other mycobacteria in the environment. When non-specific sensitivity is prevalent, a positive reaction is usually defined as one with a diameter of ≥10 mm of induration; this must be recognized as an arbitrary cut-point and not suitable for all situations and age groups.

The cut-point for true positive reactions will vary and may be as high as an induration of 15 mm in diameter for adults living in areas with little tuberculosis but a high frequency of other mycobacteria; on the other hand, among household contacts of infectious tuberculosis cases and persons with HIV infection, as little as 5 mm of induration should be considered indicative of tuberculous infection. When repeated tuberculin testing of adults is done, a subsequent reaction with an increase in size to a diameter which meets the criteria for a positive reaction in the population being tested, is considered conversion, indicative of a recent tuberculous infection. This definition is also arbitrary; the larger the increase in reaction size and the absolute size of the reaction, the greater the likelihood of recent tuberculous infection. Tuberculous infection may also be inferred when a single test presents ≥10 mm of induration.

In developed countries, a presumptive diagnosis of current active disease is made by demonstration of acid-fast bacilli in stained smears from sputum or other body fluids; a positive smear justifies initiation of antituberculosis therapy. The diagnosis is confirmed by isolation of tubercle bacilli on culture; this also permits determination of the drug susceptibility of the infecting organism. In the absence of bacteriologic confirmation, current disease can be presumed if there is strong clinical evidence of an ongoing disease process with histologic, biochemical or radiologic confirmation.

2. **Infectious agents**—*Mycobacterium tuberculosis* and *M. africanum* primarily from humans, and *M. bovis* primarily from cattle. Other

mycobacteria occasionally produce disease clinically indistinguishable from tuberculosis; the etiologic agents can be identified only by culture of the organisms.

3. Occurrence—Worldwide; developed countries had shown downward trends of mortality and morbidity for many years, but in the 1980s, morbidity plateaued or increased in areas and population groups with a high prevalence of HIV infection. Mortality and morbidity rates increase with age, and in older persons, they are higher in males than females. They are much higher among the poor than the rich, and usually higher in cities than in rural areas. In 1989, the reported incidence of clinical disease in the USA was 9.5/100,000 population. In low incidence areas, such as the USA, most tuberculosis is endogenous, i.e., it results from a reactivation from latent foci remaining from the initial infection. Although tuberculosis ranks low among communicable diseases in infectiousness per unit of time of exposure, the long exposure of some contacts, notably household associates, may lead to a 30% risk of becoming infected, and a 1-5% chance of the infection progressing to disease within a year. For infected infants, the lifetime risk of developing disease may approach 10%. For persons co-infected with HIV, the annual risk has been estimated as 7%. Epidemics have been reported among persons congregated in enclosed spaces, such as nursing homes, shelters for the homeless, hospitals, schools, prisons, and office buildings.

Prevalence of infection detected by tuberculin testing increases with age. The incidence of infection in developed countries has declined rapidly in recent decades; in the USA, the annual risk of new infection is estimated to average about 20/100,000 persons or less. In areas where human infection with mycobacteria other than tubercle bacilli is prevalent, cross reactions complicate interpretation of the tuberculin reaction.

Infection with the bovine tubercle bacillus in man is rare in the USA, but is still a problem in areas where the disease in cattle has not been controlled and milk is consumed raw.

4. Reservoir—Primarily man. In some areas, diseased cattle; rarely primates, badgers or other mammals.

5. Mode of transmission—Exposure to bacilli in airborne droplet nuclei produced by persons with pulmonary or laryngeal tuberculosis during expiratory efforts, such as coughing, singing or sneezing. Laryngeal tuberculosis is highly contagious. Prolonged close exposure to an infectious case may lead to infection of contacts. Direct invasion through mucous membranes or breaks in the skin may occur, but is extremely rare. Bovine tuberculosis results from exposure to tuberculous cattle, usually by ingestion of unpasteurized milk or dairy products, and sometimes by airborne spread to farmers and animal handlers. Extrapulmonary tuberculosis, other than laryngeal, is generally not communicable, even if there is a draining sinus.

6. **Incubation period**—From infection to demonstrable primary lesion or significant tuberculin reaction, about 4-12 weeks. While the subsequent risk of progressive pulmonary or extrapulmonary tuberculosis is greatest within the first year or two after infection, it may persist for a lifetime as a latent infection.

7. **Period of communicability**—Theoretically, as long as viable tubercle bacilli are being discharged in the sputum. Some untreated or inadequately treated patients may be sputum-positive intermittently for years. The degree of communicability depends on the number of bacilli discharged, the virulence of the bacilli, adequacy of ventilation, exposure of the bacilli to sun or UV light and opportunities for their aerosolization by coughing, sneezing, talking or singing. Effective antimicrobial chemotherapy usually reduces communicability to insignificant levels within days to a few weeks. Children with primary tuberculosis are generally not infectious.

8. **Susceptibility and resistance**—The most hazardous period for development of clinical disease is the first 6-12 months after infection. The risk of developing disease is highest in children under 3 years old, lowest in later childhood and high again among adolescents, young adults and the very old. Reactivations of long latent infections account for a large proportion of cases of clinical disease in older persons. For those infected, susceptibility to disease is markedly increased in those with HIV infection and other forms of immunosuppression, and also increased among underweight and undernourished persons, persons with silicosis, diabetes or gastrectomies, and among substance abusers.

9. **Methods of control**—

   A. *Preventive measures:*

   1) Educate the public in mode of spread and methods of control and the importance of early diagnosis.
   2) Improve those social conditions which increase the risk of becoming infected, such as overcrowding.
   3) Make available medical, laboratory and x-ray facilities for examination of patients, contacts and suspects, and facilities for early treatment of cases and persons at high risk of infection; and beds for those needing hospitalization.
   4) Provide public health nursing and outreach services for home supervision of patients to supervise therapy directly, and to arrange for examination and preventive treatment of contacts.
   5) Use preventive treatment with isoniazid, which has been shown to be effective in preventing the progression of latent infection to clinical disease in a high proportion of individuals. It is routinely indicated for infected persons

under 35 years of age. Because of the increased risk of isoniazid-associated hepatitis among older persons, isoniazid is not routinely advised for infected persons over 35 years of age unless one or more of the following is present: recent infection, close or household association with a current case, an abnormal chest radiograph consistent with old, healed tuberculosis, diabetes, silicosis, prolonged therapy with corticosteroids or immunosuppressants, and immunosuppressive disease such as HIV infection.

Persons started on preventive treatment should be informed of possible adverse effects, such as hepatitis, drug fever or severe rash, and advised to discontinue treatment and seek medical advice if any suggestive symptoms develop. Baseline liver function tests should be obtained on those ≥35 years of age. No more than one month's supply of medication should be given at any time. Patients should be queried at each monthly return visit about adverse effects. Biochemical monitoring for hepatitis need not be done routinely, but is mandatory if symptoms or signs of hepatitis occur.

Isoniazid therapy is contraindicated where there is a history of a previous severe adverse reaction to the drug or when there is acute liver disease of any etiology except tuberculosis. During pregnancy, it may be wise to postpone preventive treatment until after delivery. Isoniazid should be given with added caution to persons who use alcohol regularly.

A policy of preventive treatment, even of special risk groups, is unrealistic and unsuitable for mass application in a community health program unless the treatment program for patients suffering from infectious tuberculosis is widespread and well organized, achieving a high rate of cure.

6) BCG vaccination of uninfected (tuberculin-negative) persons can induce tuberculin sensitivity in >90% of vaccinees. The protection conferred has varied markedly in different field trials, perhaps related to some special characteristics of the population, the quality of the vaccine, or the strain of BCG employed. Some controlled trials have provided evidence that protection may persist for as long as 20 years in high incidence situations, while others have shown no protection at all. Recent case-control and contact studies have consistently demonstrated protection against tuberculous meningitis and disseminated disease in children less than 5 years old.

Because the risk of infection is very low in the USA, BCG is not routinely used. It may be considered for children with negative tuberculin tests who cannot be placed on isoniazid preventive therapy but have continuous exposure to persons with active disease, or who have continuous exposure to patients infected by organisms resistant to isoniazid or rifampin, or who belong to groups with annual rates of new infection greater than 1% per year. BCG is contraindicated for persons with immunodeficiency diseases such as symptomatic HIV infection; asymptomatic persons may be given BCG.

7) Eliminate tuberculosis among dairy cattle by tuberculin testing and slaughter of reactors; pasteurize or boil milk.

8) Take measures to prevent silicosis in industrial plants and mines.

9) In high-incidence areas, examination of sputum by direct microscopy (by culture when possible) of persons who present themselves to health services because of chest symptoms, may give a high yield of infectious tuberculosis. In many situations, direct microscopy may be the most cost-effective method of case finding and is the first priority in developing countries.

10) In the USA and other developed areas where BCG vaccination is not routinely carried out, selective tuberculin testing may be done on groups at high risk of tuberculous and/or HIV infection as a case-finding measure; e.g., immigrants from areas where tuberculosis is prevalent, and groups at high risk for HIV infections such as intravenous drug users. In population groups where disease still occurs, systematic tuberculin testing surveys may be used to monitor trends in the incidence of infection. X-ray examination is especially indicated whenever persistent chest symptoms are noted and bacteriologic tests are negative.

11) Persons infected with HIV should be skin tested with Purified Protein Derivative (PPD) at the time of identification of their HIV infection and started on prophylactic treatment if positive. Conversely, testing for HIV infection should be considered in all persons with evidence of tuberculosis or tuberculous infection.

B. *Control of patient, contacts and the immediate environment:*

1) Report to local health authority: Obligatory case report in most states (USA) and countries, Class 2B (see Preface). Case report should indicate if it is bacteriologically positive or based on positive tuberculin reaction and clinical

and/or x-ray findings. Health departments should maintain a current register of cases requiring treatment.

2) Isolation: For pulmonary tuberculosis, control of infectivity is best achieved by prompt specific drug therapy, which usually produces sputum conversion within a few weeks. Hospital treatment is necessary only for patients with severe illness and for those whose medical or social circumstances make treatment at home impossible. Patients with sputum-positive pulmonary tuberculosis need to be placed in a private room with special ventilation. Patients should be taught to cover the mouth and nose when coughing or sneezing. Persons entering the room should wear masks if the patient is coughing and does not reliably cover his mouth. Patients with primary tuberculosis and those whose sputa are bacteriologically negative, who do not cough, and who are known to be on adequate chemotherapy need not be isolated. The need to adhere to the prescribed chemotherapeutic regimen must be re-emphasized repeatedly to all patients.

3) Concurrent disinfection: Handwashing and good housekeeping practices should be maintained according to routine policy. There are no special precautions necessary for handling fomites (dishes, laundry, bedding, clothes and personal effects). Decontamination of air may be achieved by ventilation and sunlight; this may be supplemented by ultraviolet light.

4) Quarantine: None.

5) Immunization of contacts: Preventive treatment is indicated (see 9A5, above) for close contacts. BCG vaccination of tuberculin-negative household contacts, especially infants and children, may be warranted under special circumstances such as continuing exposure to untreated or ineffectively treated patients with sputum-positive pulmonary tuberculosis (see 9A6, above).

6) Investigation of contacts and source of infection: Tuberculin testing of all members of the household and close extra-household contacts. If negative, a repeat skin test should be performed 2-3 months after exposure has ended. Chest radiographs should be made of positive reactors at either time. Preventive treatment is indicated (see 9A5, above) for contacts who are positive reactors and for initially negative reactors, especially young close contacts, until the repeat skin test is shown to remain negative.

7) Specific treatment: Most initial infections heal without treatment; when they are recognized, preventive antimi-

crobial therapy with isoniazid is indicated to reduce the risk of progressive disease or later reactivation.

Patients with tuberculosis should be given prompt treatment with an appropriate combination of antimicrobial drugs. Regimens currently accepted in the USA include isoniazid (INH) combined with rifampin (RIF), with or without pyrazinamide (PZA). INH, RIF, plus PZA is the combination of choice for initial intensive treatment; regimens including these 3 drugs may be given for a period as short as 6 months. Regimens including only INH and RIF should be continued for 9 months. If INH resistance is suspected, ethambutol (EMB) (or streptomycin) should be added to the regimens above until drug susceptibility studies are available. Since a high proportion of organisms from cases in foreign-born Latin Americans, Africans and Asians have been resistant to INH, it is prudent to include EMB in their therapy and continue this until tests indicate that the organisms are susceptible to the other drugs included in the regimen. If HIV infection is present, a longer duration of therapy may be required.

If sputum fails to become negative after 3-4 months of regular therapy or reverts to positive after a series of negatives, or if clinical response is poor, examination for drug-taking compliance and development of drug resistance is indicated. Treatment failure is usually the result of irregularity in taking drugs, and does not necessitate a change in regimen. If drug resistance is observed, at least 2 drugs to which the organisms are susceptible should be included in the regimen; a single new drug should never be added to a failing regimen. If both INH and RIF cannot be included in the regimen, the minimum duration of therapy is 18 months.

Regimens used in developing countries with low financial resources are usually of a year's duration, consisting of 1-2 months of daily INH plus one or two additional drugs, followed by daily or twice-weekly INH plus another drug for the remainder of the year. The two most commonly used companion drugs with INH are streptomycin and thiacetazone. In some countries, RIF and PZA have been introduced only in the initial phase to strengthen the regimen without increasing the cost excessively; this also permits shortening the regimen and may thus improve compliance.

Children are treated with the same regimens as adults, although many experts advise prolonging therapy for 3-6 months for those with life-threatening extrapulmonary disease such as TB meningitis or miliary tuberculosis. EMB is not used until color vision can be checked; PZA has not been approved by the FDA for use in children.

All drugs occasionally cause adverse reactions. Thoracic surgery is rarely indicated.

C. *Epidemic measures:* Alertness to recognize and treat aggregations of new infections resulting from contact with an unrecognized infectious case, and intensive search for and treatment of the source of infection.

D. *Disaster implications:* None.

E. *International measures:* X-ray screening of individuals from high prevalence countries upon immigration. WHO Collaborating Centres (see Preface).

MYCOBACTERIOSES   ICD-9 031

Mycobacteria, other than *M. tuberculosis, M. africanum, M. bovis* and *M. leprae,* are ubiquitous in nature and may produce disease in man. These acid-fast bacilli in the past have been variously termed atypical, unclassified mycobacteria, or mycobacteria other than tuberculosis (MOTT). Of the numerous identified species only about 15 are recognized as being pathogenic to man.

Clinical syndromes associated with the pathogenic species of mycobacteria can be classified broadly as follows:

(1) systemic bloodborne disease (in the presence of severe immunodeficiency as in AIDS)—mycobacteria of the *M. avium* complex;

(2) pulmonary disease resembling tuberculosis—*M. kansasii, M. avium* complex, *M. fortuitum, M. xenopi;*

(3) lymphadenitis (primarily cervical)—*M. scrofulaceum, M. avium* complex, *M. kansasii;*

(4) skin ulcers—*M. ulcerans* (Buruli ulcer), *M. marinum* (balnei);

(5) injury or injection abscesses—*M. avium, M. fortuitum, M. chelonei;* and

(6) wound infections (sternal following cardiac surgery, mammoplasty wounds and peritonitis)—*M. fortuitum, M. chelonei. M. paratuberculosis* has been suggested as the causative agent in some cases of regional enteritis (Crohn's disease).

The epidemiology of the diseases attributable to these organisms has not been well delineated, but the organisms have been found in soil, milk and water; other factors, such as host tissue damage and immunodeficiency, may predispose to infection. With the exception of organisms causing skin lesions, there is no evidence of person-to-person transmission. A single isolation of these bacilli from sputum, gastric or other specimen is not diagnostic without compatible clinical findings. In general, the diagnosis of disease requiring treatment is based on repeated isolations of many colonies from symptomatic patients with progressive illness. Where human infections with nontuberculosis mycobacteria are prevalent, cross reactions may interfere with the interpretation of the skin test for *M. tuberculosis* infection. Chemotherapy is relatively effective in treating *M. kansasii* disease, but traditional antituberculosis drugs (especially EMB and PZA) may not be effective for the other mycobacterioses. For selection of an efficient drug combination, drug susceptibility tests should be performed on the isolated organisms. Surgery should be given more serious consideration than in tuberculosis, especially when the disease is limited, as in localized pulmonary disease, cervical lymphadenitis or a subcutaneous abscess; surgical excision rather than drug therapy is the treatment of choice in most of these situations.

TULAREMIA   ICD-9 021
(Rabbit fever, Deerfly fever, Ohara disease)

1. **Identification**—A zoonotic, bacterial disease with a variety of clinical manifestations related to the route of introduction and the virulence of the strain. Most often it presents as an indolent ulcer, often on the hand, accompanied by swelling of the regional lymph nodes (ulceroglandular type). There may be no apparent primary ulcer, but only one or more enlarged and painful lymph nodes which may suppurate. Inhalation of infectious material may be followed by a pneumonic disease or a primary systemic (typhoidal) syndrome. Ingestion of organisms may produce a pharyngitis (with or without ulceration), abdominal pain, diarrhea and vomiting. The conjunctival sac is a rare route of introduction (oculoglandular type). Jellison type A strains of organisms, common in rabbits (cottontail, jack and snowshoe), restricted to N America and frequently of tick origin, are more virulent, with a case fatality rate of 5-10%, mainly from typhoidal or pulmonary disease. With appropriate treatment, the case fatality rate is negligible. Jellison type B strains from sources other than rabbits in N America, and strains from all other parts of the Northern Hemisphere from muskrats and water rats, and from rabbits in Japan, are less virulent and, even without treatment, produce few fatalities. Clinically, tularemia may be confused with plague.

Diagnosis is most commonly made by a rise in specific antibodies in the patient's serum; cross agglutinations occur with *Brucella, Proteus* and heterophile antibody. Examination of ulcer exudate, lymph node aspirates and other clinical specimens by FA test may provide rapid diagnosis. The infectious organism can be identified by culture on special media or by inoculation of laboratory animals with material from lesions, blood or sputum; however, this introduces a highly infectious laboratory hazard that requires the exercise of extreme care.

2. **Infectious agent**—*Francisella tularensis (Pasteurella tularensis)*. All isolates seem to be antigenically homogeneous but are differentiated epidemiologically and biochemically into Jellison type A (*F. tularensis* biovar *tularensis*) and type B strains (*F. tularensis* biovar *palaearctica*).

3. **Occurrence**—Throughout N America and in many parts of continental Europe, the USSR, China and Japan. Occurs in the USA all months of the year; incidence may be higher in adults in early winter during rabbit-hunting season and in children during the summer when ticks and deerflies are abundant.

4. **Reservoir**—Numerous wild animals, especially rabbits, hares, muskrats, beavers and some domestic animals; also various hard ticks. In general, *F. t.* biovar *tularensis* is maintained in a rabbit-tick cycle; *F. t.* biovar *palaearctica*, in a rodent-mosquito cycle.

5. **Mode of transmission**—Inoculation of skin, conjunctival sac or oropharyngeal mucosa with blood or tissue while handling infected animals, as in skinning, dressing, or performing necropsies; by fluids of infected flies, ticks or other animals; through the bite of arthropods, including the deerfly *Chrysops discalis* and, in Sweden, the mosquito *Aedes cinereus;* by bite of wood ticks, *Dermacentor andersoni;* dog ticks, *D. variabilis;* and Lone Star ticks, *Amblyomma americanum;* by handling or ingestion of insufficiently cooked rabbit or hare meat; by drinking contaminated water; by inhalation of dust from contaminated soil, grain or hay; rarely, from bites of coyote, squirrel, skunk, hog, cat and dog whose mouth presumably was contaminated from eating an infected rabbit; and also from contaminated pelts and paws of animals. Laboratory infections occur and frequently present as a primary pneumonia or typhoidal tularemia.

6. **Incubation period**—Related to virulence of infecting strain and to size of inoculum; 2-10 days, usually 3 days.

7. **Period of communicability**—Not directly transmitted from person to person. Unless treated, the infectious agent may be found in the blood during the first 2 weeks of disease, and in lesions for a month from onset, sometimes longer. Flies are infective for 14 days and ticks throughout their lifetime (about 2 years). Rabbit meat constantly frozen at -15°C (5°F) has remained infective longer than 3 years.

8. **Susceptibility and resistance**—All ages are susceptible and long-term immunity follows recovery; however, reinfection has been reported.

9. Methods of control—

A. *Preventive measures:*

1) Educate the public to avoid bites of flies, mosquitoes and ticks or handling such arthropods when working in endemic areas, and to avoid drinking, bathing, swimming or working in untreated water where infection prevails among wild animals.

2) Use impervious gloves when skinning or handling animals, especially rabbits. Cook the meat of wild rabbits and rodents thoroughly.

3) Prohibit interstate or interarea shipment of infected animals or their carcasses.

4) Live attenuated vaccines applied intradermally by the multiple-puncture method are used extensively in the USSR, and to a limited extent for occupational risk groups in the USA. An investigational live-attenuated vaccine for laboratory personnel working with the organism is available from U.S. Army Medical Materiel Activity, ATTN: SGRD-UMB, Fort Detrick, Frederick MD 21701-5009, USA.

5) Wear face masks, gowns and impervious gloves when working with cultures of *F. tularensis*.

B. *Control of patient, contacts and the immediate environment:*

1) Report to local health authority: In selected endemic areas (USA); in many countries, not a reportable disease, Class 3B (see Preface).

2) Isolation: Drainage/secretion precautions for open lesions.

3) Concurrent disinfection: Of discharges from ulcers, lymph nodes or conjunctival sac.

4) Quarantine: None.

5) Immunization of contacts: Not indicated.

6) Investigation of contacts and source of infection: Important in each case, with search for the origin of infection.

7) Specific treatment: Streptomycin is the drug of choice; gentamicin and tobramycin have been reported to be effective; the tetracyclines and chloramphenicol are effective when continued until temperature is normal for 4-5 days, but relapses are reported to occur more often than with streptomycin. Fully virulent streptomycin-resistant organisms have been described.

C. *Epidemic measures:* Search for sources of infection related to arthropods, animal hosts, water, soil and crops. Control measures as indicated in 9A, above.

D. *Disaster implications:* None.

E. *International measures:* None.

TYPHOID FEVER
PARATYPHOID FEVER
ICD-9 002.0
ICD-9 002.1-002.3

(Enteric fever, Typhus abdominalis)

1. **Identification**—Systemic bacterial diseases characterized by insidious onset of sustained fever, headache, malaise, anorexia, a relative bradycardia, splenomegaly, rose spots on the trunk, nonproductive cough, constipation more commonly than diarrhea (in adults) and involvement of the lymphoid tissues. Many mild and atypical infections occur.

In typhoid fever, ulceration of Peyer's patches in the ileum can produce intestinal hemorrhage or perforation (about 1% of cases), especially late in untreated cases. Nonsweating fever, mental dullness, slight deafness and parotitis may occur. The usual case fatality rate of 10% can be reduced to ≤1% with prompt antibiotic therapy. Relapses occur in 5-10% of untreated cases and may be more common (15-20%) following antibiotic therapy. Mild and inapparent illnesses occur, especially in endemic areas.

Paratyphoid fever presents a similar clinical picture, but tends to be milder, and the case fatality rate is much lower. Relapses may occur in approximately 3-4% of cases. When the salmonella infections are not systemic, and are manifested only by a gastroenteritis, see Salmonellosis.

The etiologic organisms can be isolated from the blood early in the disease and from urine and feces after the first week; in patients who have already received antibiotics, isolations from bone marrow may still be possible. A fourfold rise in agglutination titer in paired sera appears during the second week in less than 70% of cases of typhoid fever; when it occurs, it supports the diagnosis, provided vaccine had not been given recently. Because of its limited sensitivity, serology is of little diagnostic value.

2. **Infectious agents**—For typhoid fever, *Salmonella typhi,* the typhoid bacillus. Presently 106 types can be distinguished by phage typing, which is of value in epidemiologic studies.

For paratyphoid fever, three serotypes are recognized: (1) *Salmonella paratyphi A;* (2) *S. paratyphi B (S. schottmülleri);* and (3) *S. paratyphi C (S. hirschfeldii).* A number of phage types can be distinguished.

3. **Occurrence**—Worldwide. The number of sporadic cases of typhoid

fever has remained relatively constant in the USA with fewer than 500 cases annually for several years (compared to 2,484 reported in 1950) and, with development of sanitary facilities, has been virtually eliminated from many areas; most cases now are imported from endemic areas. Strains resistant to recommended antibiotics have appeared in several areas of the world. Multi-resistant strains have been reported from Asia, the Middle East and Latin America.

Paratyphoid fever occurs sporadically or in limited outbreaks, probably more frequently than reports suggest. In the USA and Canada, paratyphoid fever is infrequently identified. Of the 3 serotypes, paratyphoid B is most common, A less frequent, and C extremely rare.

4. **Reservoir**—Man for both typhoid and paratyphoid; rarely, domestic animals for paratyphoid. Family contacts may be transient carriers. In most parts of the world, fecal carriers are more common than urinary carriers. The carrier state may follow acute illness or mild or even subclinical infections. The chronic carrier state is most common among persons infected during middle age, especially females; carriers frequently have gall bladder pathology. The chronic urinary carrier state is seen in those with *Schistosoma haematobium* infection. In one outbreak of paratyphoid fever in England, dairy cows excreted *S. paratyphi B* organisms in milk and feces.

5. **Mode of transmission**—By food and water contaminated by feces and urine of patients and carriers. Important vehicles in some parts of the world include shellfish taken from sewage-contaminated beds, raw fruits, vegetables fertilized by nightsoil, contaminated milk and milk products (usually by hands of carriers) and missed cases. Flies may infect foods in which the organisms then multiply to achieve an infective dose.

6. **Incubation period**—The incubation period depends on the size of the infecting dose; usual range is 1-3 weeks. For paratyphoidal gastroenteritis, 1-10 days.

7. **Period of communicability**—As long as the bacilli appear in excreta, usually from the first week throughout convalescence; variable thereafter (commonly 1-2 weeks for paratyphoid). About 10% of untreated typhoid fever patients will discharge bacilli for three months after onset of symptoms, and 2-5% become permanent carriers; some persons infected with paratyphoid organisms may become permanent gall bladder carriers.

8. **Susceptibility and resistance**—Susceptibility is general and is increased in individuals with gastric achlorhydria. Relative specific immunity follows recovery from clinical disease, inapparent infection and active immunization, but is inadequate to protect against subsequent ingestion of large numbers of organisms. In endemic areas, typhoid fever is most common in preschool and school-age children.

9. **Methods of control—**

A. *Preventive measures:*

1) Educate the public about the importance of handwashing. Provide suitable handwashing facilities; this is particularly important for foodhandlers and attendants involved in the care of patients and children.

2) Dispose of human feces in a sanitary manner and maintain fly-proof latrines. Stress use of sufficient toilet paper to minimize finger contamination. Under field conditions, dispose of feces by burial at a site distant and downstream from the source of drinking water.

3) Protect, purify and chlorinate public water supplies; provide safe private supplies; and avoid possible back-flow connections between water and sewer systems. For individual and small-group protection, and while traveling or in the field, treat water chemically or by boiling.

4) Control flies by screening, spraying with insecticides, and using insecticidal baits and traps. Control fly breeding by frequent collection and disposal of garbage, and fly control measures in latrine construction and maintenance.

5) Use scrupulous cleanliness in food preparation and handling; refrigerate as appropriate. Particular attention should be directed to the proper storage of salads and other foods served cold. These provisions apply equally to home and public eating places. If uncertain about sanitary practices, select foods that are cooked and served hot, and fruits peeled by the consumer.

6) Pasteurize or boil all milk and dairy products. Supervise the sanitary aspects of commercial milk production, storage and delivery.

7) Enforce suitable quality-control procedures in all plants preparing food and drink for human consumption. Use chlorinated water for cooling during canned food processing.

8) Encourage breastfeeding throughout infancy; boil all milk and water used for infant feeding.

9) Limit the collection and marketing of shellfish to supplies from approved sources. Boil or steam (for at least 10 minutes) before serving.

10) Instruct patients, convalescents and carriers in personal hygiene. Emphasize handwashing as a routine practice after defecation and before preparing and serving food.

11) Exclude carriers from handling food and from providing patient care. Identify and supervise typhoid carriers; culture of sewage may help in locating carriers. Chronic

carriers should not be released from supervision and restriction of occupation until local or state regulations are met, often not until 3 consecutive negative cultures are obtained from authenticated fecal (and urine in schistosomiasis endemic areas) specimens taken at least 1 month apart and at least 48 hours after antibiotic therapy has stopped. Fresh stool specimens are preferred to rectal swabs; at least 1 of the 3 consecutive negative stool specimens should be obtained by purging. In long-term carriers, gallstones frequently are present or there is x-ray evidence of biliary dysfunction.

Prolonged administration of ampicillin or amoxicillin plus probenecid, or co-trimoxazole, possibly concomitantly, may be effective in the treatment of the carrier, even when biliary disease exists. In preliminary studies, quinolones have produced excellent results.

12) Typhoid fever: Immunization is not routinely recommended in the USA or for travel to developed areas. Current practice is to vaccinate persons subject to unusual exposure to typhoid from occupation or travel to endemic areas, those living in areas of high endemicity and household members of known carriers. The inactivated vaccines are given in a primary series of 2 injections several weeks apart. Periodic, single reinforcing injections are desirable, usually at 3-year intervals, for those at continuing risk of infection. An oral, live vaccine using *S. typhi* strain Ty21a (requiring at least 3 doses) and a parenteral vaccine containing the polysaccharide Vi antigen (single dose required) are available; these vaccines are much less reactogenic than the whole-bacteria vaccine and are at least as protective. However, vaccination may not prevent disease after exposure to large numbers of organisms.

Paratyphoid fever: There is no vaccine against paratyphoid fever; killed whole-cell vaccines were not effective and markedly increased the adverse reactions. The TAB vaccine, which contained killed paratyphoid A and B organisms, was not protective against paratyphoid fever and was significantly more reactogenic.

B. *Control of patient, contacts and the immediate environment:*

1) Report to local health authority: Obligatory case report in most states (USA) and countries, Class 2A (see Preface).

2) Isolation: Enteric precautions while ill; hospital care is desirable during acute illness. Release from supervision by local health authority should be based on not less than

3 consecutive negative cultures of feces (*and* urine in patients with schistosomiasis) taken at least 24 hours apart and at least 48 hours after any antibiotic, and not earlier than 1 month after onset; if any one of these is positive, repeat cultures at intervals of 1 month during the 12-month period following onset until at least 3 consecutive negative cultures are obtained.

3) Concurrent disinfection: Of feces and urine and articles soiled therewith. In communities with modern and adequate sewage disposal systems, feces and urine can be disposed of directly into sewers without preliminary disinfection. Terminal cleaning.

4) Quarantine: None.

5) Immunization of contacts: Routine administration of typhoid vaccine is of doubtful value for family, household and nursing contacts who have been or may be exposed to cases; it could be considered for those who may be exposed to carriers. There is no effective immunization for paratyphoid fever.

6) Investigation of contacts and source of infection: The actual or probable source of infection of every case should be determined by search for unreported cases, carriers, or contaminated food, water, milk or shellfish. All members of travel groups in which a case has been identified should be followed up.

The presence of elevated titers of antibody to purified Vi polysaccharide is highly suggestive of the typhoidal carrier state. Identification of the same phage type in the organisms isolated from patients and a carrier suggests a possible chain of transmission.

Household and close contacts should not be employed in sensitive occupations (e.g., as foodhandlers) until at least 2 negative feces and urine cultures, taken at least 24 hours apart, are obtained.

7) Specific treatment: For enteric fever, chloramphenicol, amoxicillin or co-trimoxazole is the drug of choice for acute infections, with comparably high efficacy. Quinolone derivatives and third-generation cephalosporins are also effective. All isolates should be checked for drug resistance; some strains that are chloramphenicol-, ampicillin- and amoxicillin-resistant are sensitive to co-trimoxazole . Steroids have been effective in some critically ill patients. (See 9A11, above, for treatment of the carrier state.)

C. **Epidemic measures:**

1) Search intensively for the case or carrier who is the source of infection and for the vehicle (water or food) by which infection was transmitted.
2) Exclude suspected food.
3) Pasteurize or boil milk, or exclude milk supplies and other foods suspected on epidemiologic evidence, until safety is assured.
4) Chlorinate suspected water supplies adequately under competent supervision or do not use them. All drinking water must be chlorinated, treated with iodine or boiled before use.
5) Routine use of vaccine is not recommended.

D. **Disaster implications:** With disruption of usual water supply and sewage disposal, and of controls on food and water, transmission of typhoid fever may occur if there are active cases or carriers in a displaced population. Efforts to restore safe drinking water supplies and excreta disposal facilities are more appropriate than mass typhoid vaccination. Vaccination of such populations is generally not recommended.

E. **International measures:**

1) For typhoid fever: Immunization is advised for international travelers to endemic areas, especially if travel will likely involve exposure to unsafe food and water, or close contact with rural areas and indigenous populations. Not a legal requirement for entry into any country.
2) For both typhoid and paratyphoid fevers, WHO Collaborating Centres (see Preface).

TYPHUS FEVER
I. EPIDEMIC LOUSE-BORNE TYPHUS FEVER ICD-9 080
(Louse-borne typhus, Typhus exanthematicus, Classic typhus fever)

1. **Identification**—A rickettsial disease with variable onset; often sudden and marked by headache, chills, prostration, fever and general pains. A macular eruption appears on the 5th-6th day, initially on the upper trunk, followed by spread to the entire body, but usually not to the face, palms or soles. Toxemia is usually pronounced, and the disease terminates by rapid lysis after about two weeks of fever. In the absence of specific therapy, the case fatality rate increases with age and varies from

10 to 40%. Mild infections may occur without eruption, especially in children and persons partially protected by prior immunization. The disease may recrudesce years after the primary attack (Brill-Zinsser disease, ICD-9 081.1); this is milder, has fewer complications, need not be associated with lice, and has a lower case fatality rate.

The IFA test is most commonly used, but it may not discriminate between louse-borne and murine typhus unless the sera are differentially absorbed with the respective rickettsial antigen prior to testing. Other diagnostic methods are CF with group-specific or washed type-specific rickettsial antigens, toxin-neutralization test, and Weil-Felix reaction with *Proteus* OX-19. Antibody tests usually become positive in the second week. In Brill-Zinsser disease, the initial antibody is IgG and the Weil-Felix test may not be positive.

2. Infectious agent—*Rickettsia prowazekii.*

3. Occurrence—In colder areas where people may live under unhygienic conditions and are louse-infested; historically a concomitant of war and famine. Endemic foci exist in mountainous regions of Mexico, Central and S America, in central Africa and numerous countries of Asia. In the USA, the last outbreak of louse-borne typhus occurred in 1921. In the USA, this rickettsia exists as a zoonosis of flying squirrels (*Glaucomys volans);* there is serologic evidence that at least 33 humans have been infected from this source, possibly by the squirrel flea. Most of these have been in the East Coast states, but two cases were reported from Indiana, and one each from California, Illinois, Ohio, Tennessee and W Virginia.

4. Reservoir—Man is the reservoir and is responsible for maintaining the infection during interepidemic periods. The importance of the flying squirrel as a reservoir has not been determined.

5. Mode of transmission—The body louse, *Pediculus humanus,* is infected by feeding on the blood of a patient with acute typhus fever. Patients with recrudescent typhus (Brill-Zinsser disease) can infect lice and may serve as foci for new outbreaks in louse-infested communities. Infected lice excrete rickettsiae in their feces and usually defecate at the time of feeding. Man is infected by rubbing feces or crushed lice into the bite or into superficial abrasions. Inhalation of infective louse feces as dust may account for some infections. Transmission from the flying squirrel is presumed to be by the bite of the squirrel flea, but this has not been documented.

6. Incubation period—From 1 to 2 weeks, commonly 12 days.

7. Period of communicability—The disease is not directly transmitted from person to person. Patients are infective for lice during the febrile illness and possibly for 2-3 days after the temperature returns to normal. The louse is infective by passing rickettsiae in its feces within 2-6 days after the infected blood meal; it is infective earlier if crushed. The

louse invariably dies within two weeks after infection; rickettsiae may remain viable in the dead louse for weeks.

8. Susceptibility and resistance—Susceptibility is general. One attack usually confers long-lasting immunity.

9. Methods of control—

A. *Preventive measures:*

1) Apply an effective residual insecticide powder at appropriate intervals by hand or power blower to clothes and persons of populations living under conditions favoring lousiness. A lousicide should be used which has been shown to be effective on local lice.

2) Improve living conditions with provisions for bathing and washing clothes.

3) Treat prophylactically people who are subject to unusual risk, by application of residual insecticide to clothing by dusting or impregnation.

4) Immunize susceptible persons or groups of persons entering typhus areas, particularly military or labor forces. However, no commercially prepared vaccine is now available in the USA or Canada. A live vaccine prepared from the attenuated strain E of *R. prowazekii* has shown promise.

B. *Control of patient, contacts and the immediate environment:*

1) Report to local health authority: Report of louse-borne typhus fever required as a Disease under Surveillance by WHO, Class 1A (see Preface).

2) Isolation: Not required after proper delousing of patient, clothing, living quarters and household contacts.

3) Concurrent disinfection: Appropriate insecticide powder applied to clothing and bedding of patient and contacts; launder clothing and bedclothes; treat hair for louse eggs (nits) with effective chemical agents. Lice tend to leave abnormally hot or cold bodies in search of a normothermic, clothed body (see 9A1, above). If death from louse-borne typhus occurs before delousing, delouse the body and clothing by thorough application of an insecticide.

4) Quarantine: Louse-infested susceptibles exposed to typhus fever ordinarily should be quarantined for 15 days after application of an insecticide with residual effect.

5) Management of contacts: All immediate contacts should be kept under surveillance for 2 weeks.

6) Investigation of contacts and source of infection: Every effort should be made to trace the infection to the immediate source.

7) Specific treatment: Tetracyclines or chloramphenicol orally in a loading dose of 2-3 g, followed by daily doses of 1-2 g/day in 4 divided doses until the patient becomes afebrile (usually 2 days) plus 1 day. A single dose of doxycycline (5 mg/kg) is also curative. When faced with a seriously ill patient with possible typhus, suitable therapy should be started without waiting for laboratory confirmation.

C. *Epidemic measures:* The imperative measure for rapid control of typhus is application to all contacts of an insecticide with residual effect. Where infestation is known to be widespread, systematic application of residual insecticide to all persons in the community is indicated. If a vaccine is available (see 9A4, above), it should be administered.

D. *Disaster implications:* Typhus can be expected to be a significant problem in endemic areas if social upheavals and crowding occur in louse-infested populations.

E. *International measures:*

1) Telegraphic notification by governments to WHO and to adjacent countries of the occurrence of a case or an outbreak of louse-borne typhus fever in an area previously free of the disease.

2) International travelers: No country currently requires immunization against typhus for entry.

3) Louse-borne typhus is a Disease under Surveillance by WHO. WHO Collaborating Centres (see Preface).

II. MURINE TYPHUS FEVER ICD-9 081.0
(Flea-borne typhus, Endemic typhus fever, Shop typhus)

1. **Identification**—A rickettsial disease whose course resembles that of louse-borne typhus, but is milder. The case fatality rate for all ages is less than 1%; it increases with age.

Absence of louse infestation, seasonal distribution and sporadic occurrence of the disease help to differentiate it from louse-borne typhus. For laboratory diagnosis, see I, section 1, above.

2. **Infectious agent**—*Rickettsia typhi (Rickettsia mooseri).*

3. **Occurrence**—Worldwide. Found in areas where people and rats occupy the same buildings and where large numbers of mice live. In the USA, fewer than 80 cases are reported annually. Seasonal peak is in late

summer and autumn; cases tend to be scattered, but with a high proportion reported from Texas.

4. Reservoir—Rats, mice and possibly other small mammals. Infection is maintained in nature by a rat-flea-rat cycle where rats are the reservoir (commonly *Rattus rattus* and *R. norvegicus*) but infection is inapparent.

5. Mode of transmission—Infective rat fleas (usually *Xenopsylla cheopis*) defecate rickettsiae while sucking blood, contaminating the bite site and other fresh skin wounds. An occasional case may follow inhalation of dried infective flea feces. Infection occurs in opossums, cats and other wild and domestic animals; this is self-limited, but these animals may transport infective fleas to humans. The cat flea, *Ctenocephalides felis,* is a possible vector.

6. Incubation period—From 1 to 2 weeks, commonly 12 days.

7. Period of communicability—Not directly transmitted from person to person. Once infected, fleas remain so for life (up to 1 year).

8. Susceptibility and resistance—Susceptibility is general. One attack confers immunity.

9. Methods of control—

A. *Preventive measures:*

1) Apply insecticide powders with residual action to rat runs, burrows and harborages.
2) To avoid increased exposure of humans, wait until flea populations have first been reduced by insecticides before instituting rodent control measures (see Plague, 9A2-3, 9B6).

B. *Control of patient, contacts and the immediate environment:*

1) Report to local health authority: Case report obligatory in most states (USA) and countries, Class 2B (see Preface).
2) Isolation: None.
3) Concurrent disinfection: None.
4) Quarantine: None.
5) Immunization of contacts: None.
6) Investigation of contacts and source of infection: Search for rodents around premises or home of patient.
7) Specific treatment: As for louse-borne typhus (see I, 9B7, above).

C. **Epidemic measures:** In endemic areas with numerous cases, use of a residual insecticide effective against rat fleas will reduce the flea index of rats and the incidence of infection in rats and man.

D. **Disaster implications:** Cases can be expected when man, rats and fleas are forced to co-exist, but murine typhus has not been a major contributor to disease rates in such situations.

E. **International measures:** WHO Collaborating Centres (see Preface).

III. SCRUB TYPHUS   ICD-9 081.2
(Tsutsugamushi disease, Mite-borne typhus fever)

1. **Identification**—A rickettsial disease often characterized by a primary "punched out" skin ulcer (eschar) corresponding to the site of attachment of an infected mite. The acute febrile onset follows within several days, along with headache, profuse sweating, conjunctival injection and lymphadenopathy. Late in the first week of fever, a dull red, maculopapular eruption appears on the trunk, extends to the extremities and disappears in a few days. Cough and x-ray evidence of pneumonitis are common. Without antibiotic therapy, fever lasts for about 14 days. The case fatality rate in untreated cases varies from 1 to 60%, according to area, strain of rickettsia and previous exposure to disease; it is consistently higher among older persons.

Diagnosis is made by isolation of the infectious agent by inoculating the patient's blood into mice. Serologic tests are complicated by the antigenic differences of various strains of the causal rickettsia; the IFA test is the preferred technique. Many cases develop a positive Weil-Felix reaction with the *Proteus* OXK strain.

2. **Infectious agent**—*Rickettsia tsutsugamushi (Rickettsia orientalis),* with multiple, serologically distinct strains.

3. **Occurrence**—Central, eastern and SE Asia; from southeastern Siberia and northern Japan to northern Australia and the New Hebrides, as far west as Pakistan, and to as high as 10,000 feet above sea level in the Himalayan Mountains. Acquired by man in one of innumerable small, sharply delimited "typhus islands," some covering an area of only a few square feet, where rickettsiae, vectors and suitable rodents exist simultaneously. Occupation greatly influences the sex distribution; restricted mainly to adult workers who frequent scrub-overgrown terrain or other mite-infested areas, such as forest clearings, reforested areas, new settlements, or even newly irrigated desert regions. Epidemics occur when susceptibles are brought into endemic areas, especially in military operations in which 20-50% of men have been infected within weeks or months.

4. **Reservoir**—Infected larval stages of trombiculid mites; *Leptotrombidium akamushi, L. deliensis* and related species (varying with area) are the most common vectors to man. Infection is maintained by transovarian passage in mites.

5. **Mode of transmission**—By the bite of infected larval mites; nymphs and adults do not feed on vertebrate hosts.

6. **Incubation period**—Usually 10-12 days; varies from 6 to 21 days.

7. **Period of communicability**—Not directly transmitted from person to person.

8. **Susceptibility and resistance**—Susceptibility is general. An attack confers prolonged immunity against the homologous strain of *R. tsutsugamushi* but only transient immunity against heterologous strains. Heterologous infection within a few months results in mild disease, but after a year produces the typical illness. Second and even third attacks of naturally acquired scrub typhus (usually benign or inapparent) occur among persons who spend their lives in endemic areas. No experimental vaccine has been effective.

9. **Methods of control**—

   A. *Preventive measures:*

      1) Prevent contact with infected mites by personal prophylaxis against the mite vector, achieved by impregnating clothes and blankets with miticidal chemicals (permethrin and benzyl benzoate) and application of mite repellents (diethyltoluamide, Deet®) to exposed skin surfaces.
      2) Eliminate mites from the specific sites by application of chlorinated hydrocarbons, such as lindane, dieldrin or chlordane to ground and vegetation in environs of camps, mine buildings and other populated zones in endemic areas.
      3) In a small group of volunteers in Malaysia, the administration of 7 weekly doses of doxycycline (200 mg/week in a single dose) was an effective prophylactic regime.

   B. *Control of patient, contacts and the immediate environment:*

      1) Report to local health authority: In selected endemic areas (clearly differentiated from murine and louse-borne typhus). In many countries, not a reportable disease, Class 3A (see Preface).
      2) Isolation: None.
      3) Concurrent disinfection: None.
      4) Quarantine: None.
      5) Immunization of contacts: None.

6) Investigation of contacts and source of infection: None (see 9C, below).

7) Specific treatment: One of the tetracyclines orally in a loading dose, followed by divided doses daily until patient is afebrile (average 30 hours). (See louse-borne typhus, 9B7, above.) If treatment is started within the first 3 days of illness, recrudescence is likely unless a second course of antibiotic is given after an interval of 6 days. In Malaysia, a single dose of doxycycline (5 mg/kg) was effective when given on the seventh day, and in the Pescadores (Taiwan area) when given on the fifth day; earlier administration was associated with some relapses.

C. *Epidemic measures:* Rigorously employ procedures described in III, 9A1-2, above, in the affected area; daily observation of all persons at risk for fever and appearance of primary lesions; institute treatment upon first indication of illness.

D. *Disaster implications:* Only if refugee centers are sited in or near a "typhus island."

E. *International measures:* WHO Collaborating Centres (see Preface).

WARTS, VIRAL   ICD-9 078.1
(Verruca vulgaris, Common wart, Condyloma acuminatum, Papilloma venereum)

1. Identification—A viral disease manifested by a variety of skin and mucous membrane lesions. These include the common wart, a circumscribed, hyperkeratotic, rough-textured, painless papule, varying in size from a pinhead to large masses; filiform warts, elongated, pointed, delicate lesions which may reach 1 cm in length; laryngeal papillomas on vocal cords and the epiglottis in children; flat warts, smooth, slightly elevated, usually multiple lesions varying in size from 1 mm-1 cm; venereal warts (condylomata acuminata), cauliflower-like, fleshy growths, most often seen in moist areas in and around the genitalia, around the anus and within the anal canal, which must be differentiated from condyloma lata of secondary syphilis; flat papillomas of the cervix; and plantar warts, flat, hyperkeratotic lesions of the plantar surface of the feet, which are frequently painful. Both laryngeal papillomas and genital warts have occasionally become malignant. Genital warts have been associated with higher rates of HIV infection.

The diagnosis is usually based on the typical lesion. If there is doubt, it should be excised and examined histologically.

2. **Infectious agent**—Human papillomavirus (HPV) of the papovavirus group of DNA viruses (the human wart viruses). At least 50 human papillomavirus types have been identified with probable specific manifestations; HPV types 16 and 18 have been associated with cervical neoplasia, and types 6 and 11 with genital warts and laryngeal papillomata.

3. **Occurrence**—Worldwide.

4. **Reservoir**—Man.

5. **Mode of transmission**—Usually by direct contact. Warts may be autoinoculated, such as by razors in shaving; contaminated floors are frequently incriminated as the source of infection. Condylomata acuminatum is usually sexually transmitted; laryngeal papillomata are probably transmitted during passage of the infant through the birth canal. The viral types in the genital and respiratory tracts are the same.

6. **Incubation period**—About 2-3 months; range is 1-20 months.

7. **Period of communicability**—Unknown, but probably at least as long as visible lesions persist.

8. **Susceptibility and resistance**—Common and flat warts are most frequently seen in young children, genital warts in sexually active young adults, and plantar warts in school-age children and teenagers. The incidence of warts is increased in immunosuppressed patients.

9. **Methods of control**—

    A. *Preventive measures:* Avoid direct contact with lesions. Use of a condom probably reduces the transmission of venereal warts.

    B. *Control of patient, contacts and the immediate environment:* Treatment of the affected individual will decrease the amount of wart virus available for transmission.

        1) Report to local health authority: None, Class 5 (see Preface).

        2) Isolation: None.

        3) Concurrent disinfection: None.

        4) Quarantine: None.

        5) Immunization of contacts: None.

        6) Investigation of contacts and source of infection: Sexual contacts of patients with venereal warts should be examined and treated if indicated.

        7) Specific treatment: Verrucae usually regress spontaneously within months to years. If treatment is indicated,

freezing with liquid nitrogen for lesions on most of the body surface; salicylic acid plasters and curettage for plantar warts; 10-25% podophyllin in tincture of benzoin for readily accessible genital warts except in pregnant females. Intralesional recombinant interferon alpha-2b (Intron A®, Schering) has been shown to be effective in treatment of condyloma acuminata and is approved for this use. Surgical removal or laser therapy is required for laryngeal papillomata. Cesarean section should be considered if there is extensive papillomatosis in the genital tract.

C. *Epidemic measures:* Usually a sporadic disease.

D. *Disaster implications:* None.

E. *International measures:* None

YAWS
(Frambesia tropica)

ICD-9 102

1. **Identification**—A chronic, relapsing, nonvenereal treponematosis, characterized by contagious, early, cutaneous lesions; and noncontagious, late, destructive lesions. Typical initial lesion (mother yaw) is a papilloma on the face or extremities which persists for several weeks or months. It proliferates slowly and may form a frambesial (raspberry) lesion, or undergo ulceration (ulceropapilloma). Secondary disseminated or satellite papillomata appear before or shortly after the initial lesion heals; these lesions occur in successive crops and are often accompanied by periostitis of the long bones, dactylitis and mild constitutional symptoms. Papillomata and hyperkeratoses on palms and soles may appear in both early and late stages; these lesions are very painful and usually disabling. Lesions heal spontaneously, but relapses may occur at other sites during early and late phases.

The late stage, characterized by destructive lesions of skin and bone, occurs in about 10% of untreated patients, often some years after the early lesions. Unlike syphilis, the brain, eyes, heart, aorta and abdominal organs are not involved. Congenital transmission does not occur and the infection is rarely, if ever, fatal, but can be very disfiguring and disabling.

Diagnosis is confirmed by darkfield or direct FA microscopic examination of exudates from lesions. Non-treponemal serologic tests for syphilis (VDRL, RPR, etc.) become reactive during the initial stage, remain reactive during the early infection and tend to become nonreactive after many years of latency, even without specific therapy; in some, they remain reactive at low titer for life. Treponemal serologic tests (FTA-ABS, MHA-TP, etc.) usually remain reactive for life.

2. **Infectious agent**—*Treponema pallidum,* subspecies *pertenue,* a spirochete.

3. **Occurrence**—Predominantly a disease of children living in rural, warm, humid, tropical areas; more frequent in males. Worldwide prevalence was dramatically decreased by mass penicillin treatment campaigns in the 1950s-1960s, but early yaws has resurged in parts of equatorial and West Africa, with scattered foci of infection persisting in Latin America, the Caribbean islands, SE Asia and the S Pacific islands.

4. **Reservoir**—Man and possibly higher primates.

5. **Mode of transmission**—Principally by direct contact with exudates of early skin lesions of infected persons. Indirect transmission by contamination from scratching, skin-piercing articles and by flies on open wounds is probable but of undetermined importance. Climate influences the morphology, distribution and infectiousness of the early lesions.

6. **Incubation period**—From 2 weeks to 3 months.

7. **Period of communicability**—Variable; may extend intermittently over several years while moist lesions are present. The infectious agent is not usually found in late ulcerative lesions.

8. **Susceptibility and resistance**—No evidence of natural or racial resistance. Infection results in immunity to homologous and heterologous strains; heterologous immunity develops slowly and probably is not complete until after one year.

9. **Methods of control**—

   A. *Preventive measures:* The following are applicable to yaws and other nonvenereal treponematoses. By present techniques, the infectious agents are not differentiable, but it is unlikely the differences in clinical syndromes result only from epidemiologic or environmental factors.

      1) General health promotion measures: health education of the public about treponematosis; better sanitation, including liberal use of soap and water; improvement of social and economic conditions over a period of years to reduce incidence.

      2) Organize intensive control activities on a community level suitable to the local problem; examine entire populations, and treat patients with active or latent disease. Treatment of even asymptomatic contacts is justified, and there may be need to treat the entire population within

defined areas. Periodic clinical resurveys and continuous surveillance are essential for success.

3) Serologically survey for latent cases, particularly in children, to prevent relapses and development of infective lesions that maintain the disease in the community.

4) Provide facilities for early diagnosis and treatment as part of a plan in which the mass control campaign (9A2, above) is eventually consolidated into permanent local health services.

5) Treat disfiguring and incapacitating late manifestations.

B. *Control of patient, contacts and the immediate environment:*

1) Report to local health authority: In selected endemic areas; in many countries not a reportable disease, Class 3B (see Preface). Differentiation of venereal and nonvenereal treponematoses, with proper reporting of each, has particular importance in evaluation of mass campaigns and the consolidation period thereafter.

2) Isolation: None; avoid intimate contact and contamination of the environment until lesions are healed.

3) Concurrent disinfection: Care in disposal of discharges and articles contaminated therewith.

4) Quarantine: None.

5) Immunization of contacts: None.

6) Investigation of contacts and source of infection: All familial contacts should be treated; those with no active disease should be regarded as latent cases. In areas of low prevalence, treat all active cases, all children, and close contacts of infectious cases.

7) Specific treatment: Penicillin. For patients ≥10 years with active disease and contacts, a single injection of benzathine penicillin G (Bicillin), 1.2 million units IM; for patients under 10 years, 0.6 million units.

C. *Epidemic measures:* Active mass treatment programs in areas of high prevalence. Essential features of these programs are: (1) a high percentage of the population examined through field surveys; (2) treatment of active cases extended to the family and community contacts based on the demonstrated prevalence of active yaws; and (3) periodic surveys made at yearly intervals for 1-3 years, as part of the activities of the established rural public health activities of the country.

D. *Disaster implications:* None.

E. *International measures:* To protect countries against risk of reinfection where active mass treatment programs are in progress, adjacent countries in the endemic area should institute suitable measures against yaws. Movement of infected persons across frontiers may need supervision (see Syphilis, 9E). WHO Collaborating Centres (see Preface).

YELLOW FEVER   ICD-9 060

1. **Identification**—An acute infectious viral disease of short duration and varying severity. The mildest cases are clinically indeterminate; typical attacks are characterized by a dengue-like illness, i.e., sudden onset, fever, chills, headache, backache, generalized muscle pain, prostration, nausea and vomiting. As the disease progresses, the pulse slows and weakens, even though the temperature may be elevated (Faget's sign); albuminuria (sometimes pronounced) and anuria may occur. A saddle-back fever curve is common. Leukopenia appears early and is most pronounced about the fifth day. Common hemorrhagic symptoms include epistaxis, buccal bleeding, hematemesis (coffee-ground or black), and melena. Jaundice is moderate early in the disease and is intensified later. The case fatality rate among indigenous populations of endemic regions is <5%, but may exceed 50% among nonindigenous groups and in epidemics.

Laboratory diagnosis is made by isolation of virus from blood by inoculation of suckling mice, mosquitoes or cell cultures (especially those of mosquito cells); by demonstration of viral antigen in the blood or liver tissue by ELISA or FA and in tissues by use of labeled specific antibodies; and by demonstration of viral genome in liver tissue by hybridization probes. Serologic diagnosis is made by demonstrating specific IgM in early sera or a rise in titer of specific antibodies in paired acute-phase and convalescent sera. Serologic cross-reactions occur with other flaviviruses and vaccine-derived antibodies cannot be distinguished from natural immunity. The diagnosis is suggested but not proven by demonstration of typical lesions in the liver.

2. **Infectious agent**—The virus of yellow fever, a flavivirus.

3. **Occurrence**—Except for a few cases in Trinidad in 1954, no outbreak of urban yellow fever has been transmitted by *Aedes aegypti* in the Americas since 1942. Urban yellow fever, when first introduced into the Americas, attacked both sexes and all ages and races. Urban and intermediate yellow fever outbreaks are reported from Africa, arising from enzootic and endemic transmission in the emergent zones of moist and dry savanna during the rainy season, especially in areas contiguous to rain forests where jungle or sylvan yellow fever is enzootic, such as in

Burkina Faso (Upper Volta), with 286 reported deaths in 1983. In 1986, 1987 and 1988, epidemiologically linked outbreaks in Nigeria affected over 30,000 people, causing over 10,000 deaths.

Sylvan yellow fever of tropical America now occurs predominantly among adult males, 20-40 years old, who are exposed in the forest. Approximately 100-200 cases occur each year in northern S America and the Amazon Basin, including the Colombian llanos and eastern regions of Peru and Bolivia. Eighteen cases occurred in Trinidad in 1979 in persons with forest exposure. It has occurred from time to time in all mainland American countries from Mexico to Argentina, with the exception of El Salvador, Uruguay and Chile. In Africa, the endemic zone includes the area between 15°N and 10°S latitude, extending from the Sahara desert south through northern Angola, Zaire, and into Zambia, Tanzania, Uganda, Kenya, Ethiopia, the Somali Republic and southern Sudan. There is no evidence that yellow fever has ever been present in Asia or on the easternmost coast of Africa.

4. **Reservoir**—In urban areas, man and *Aedes aegypti* mosquitoes; in forest areas, vertebrates other than man, mainly monkeys and possibly marsupials, and forest mosquitoes. Transovarian transmission in mosquitoes may contribute to maintenance of infection. Man has no essential role in transmission of jungle yellow fever or in maintaining the virus.

5. **Mode of transmission**—In urban and certain rural areas, by the bite of infective *Aedes aegypti* mosquitoes. In forests of S America, by the bite of several species of forest mosquitoes of the genus *Haemagogus*. In East Africa, *Ae. africanus* is the vector in the monkey population, while semidomestic *Ae. bromeliae* and *Ae. simpsoni,* and probably other *Aedes* species, transmit the virus from monkey to man. In large epidemics in Ethiopia, good epidemiologic evidence incriminated *Ae. simpsoni* as a person-to-person vector. In West Africa, *Ae. furcifer-taylori, Ae. luteocephalus* and other species are responsible for spread between monkey and man. *Ae. albopictus* has been introduced into Brazil and the USA from Asia and has the potential for bridging the sylvatic and urban cycles of yellow fever in the Western Hemisphere. However, no instance of involvement of this species in transmission of yellow fever has been documented.

6. **Incubation period**—Three to 6 days.

7. **Period of communicability**—Blood of patients is infective for mosquitoes shortly before onset of fever and for the first 3-5 days of illness. The disease is highly communicable where many susceptible persons and abundant vector mosquitoes coexist; not communicable by contact or common vehicles. The extrinsic incubation period in *Ae. aegypti* is commonly 9-12 days at the usual tropical temperatures. Once infected, mosquitoes remain so for life.

8. Susceptibility and resistance—Recovery from yellow fever is followed by lasting immunity; second attacks are unknown. Mild inapparent infections are common in endemic areas. Transient passive immunity in infants born to immune mothers may persist for up to 6 months. In natural infections, antibodies appear in the blood within the first week.

9. Methods of control—

A. *Preventive measures:*

1) Institute a program for active immunization of all persons over 9 months of age necessarily exposed to infection because of residence, occupation or travel. A single subcutaneous injection of a vaccine containing viable attenuated yellow fever 17D strain virus, cultivated in chick embryo, is effective in almost 99% of recipients. Antibodies appear from 7 to 10 days after vaccination and may persist for at least 30-35 years, probably much longer, though vaccination or revaccination within 10 years is still required by the International Health Regulations for travel from endemic areas.

   Given the severity of yellow fever and its unpredictability, the vaccine should be considered for incorporation in routine childhood immunization programs in any country falling in the endemic-epidemic belt. The vaccine can be given any time after six months of age and can be administered with other antigens such as measles vaccine.

   The vaccine is contraindicated in the first few months of life and should be considered for those in the 4-6 month age range only if the risk of exposure is judged to exceed the risk of vaccine-associated encephalitis, the principal complication in this age group. The vaccine is also not recommended in circumstances where live vaccines are contraindicated, nor in the first trimester of pregnancy, unless the risk of disease is believed to be higher than the theoretical risk to the pregnancy.

2) Urban yellow fever: By eradication or control of *Ae. aegypti* mosquitoes; vaccination when indicated.

3) Sylvan or jungle yellow fever, transmitted by *Haemagogus* and forest species of *Aedes,* is best controlled by immunization, which is recommended for all persons in rural communities whose occupation brings them into forests in yellow fever areas, and for persons who intend to visit those areas. Protective clothing, bed nets and repellents are advised for persons not immunized.

B. *Control of patient, contacts and the immediate environment:*

1) Report to local health authority: Case report universally required by International Health Regulations (1969), Third Annotated Edition, 1983, WHO, Geneva; Class 1 (see Preface).

2) Isolation: Blood and body fluid precautions. Prevent access of mosquitoes to patient for at least 5 days after onset by screening the sickroom, by spraying quarters with residual insecticide, and by using a bed net.

3) Concurrent disinfection: None; the home of patients and all houses in the vicinity should be sprayed promptly with an effective insecticide.

4) Quarantine: None.

5) Immunization of contacts: Family and other contacts and neighbors not previously immunized should be vaccinated promptly.

6) Investigation of contacts and source of infection: Inquire about all places, including forested areas, visited by patient 3-6 days before onset, to locate focus of yellow fever; observe all persons visiting that focus. Search premises, and places of the patient's work or visits over the preceding several days for mosquitoes capable of transmitting infection; eradicate them with effective insecticide. Investigate mild febrile illnesses and unexplained deaths suggesting yellow fever.

7) Specific treatment: None.

C. *Epidemic measures:*

1) Urban or *Ae. aegypti*-transmitted yellow fever:
   a) Mass vaccination, beginning with persons most exposed and those living in *Ae. aegypti*-infected areas.
   b) Spraying the inside of all houses in the community with insecticides has shown promise for controlling urban epidemics.
   c) Eliminate or apply larvicide to all actual and potential breeding places of *Ae. aegypti*.

2) Jungle or sylvan yellow fever:
   a) Immediate vaccination of all persons living in or near forested areas or entering such areas.
   b) Avoidance by unvaccinated individuals of those tracts of forest where infection has been localized, and by vaccinated persons for the first week after vaccination.
   c) Aerial spraying has shown promise in control of sylvatic vectors.

3) In regions where yellow fever may occur, a diagnostic

viscerotomy service should be organized to collect small specimens of liver post mortem from fatal febrile illnesses of 10 days duration or less; facilities for viral isolation or serologic confirmation are necessary to establish the diagnosis when histopathologic changes in the liver are not pathognomonic of yellow fever.

4) In Central and S America, confirmed deaths of howler and spider monkeys in the forest are presumptive evidence of the presence of yellow fever. Confirmation by the histopathologic examination of livers of moribund or recently dead monkeys or by virus isolation is highly desirable.

5) Immunity surveys by neutralization tests of wild primates captured in forested areas are useful in defining enzootic areas. Serologic surveys of human populations are almost useless where yellow fever vaccine has been widely used.

D. Disaster implications: None.

E. International measures:

1) Telegraphic notification by governments to WHO and to adjacent countries of the first imported, first transferred, or first nonimported case of yellow fever in an area previously free of the disease; and of newly discovered or reactivated foci of yellow fever infection among vertebrates other than man.

2) Measures applicable to ships, aircraft and land transport arriving from yellow fever areas are specified in the International Health Regulations (1969), Third Annotated Edition, 1983, WHO, Geneva.

3) Animal quarantine: Quarantine of monkeys and other wild primates arriving from yellow fever areas may be required until 7 days have elapsed after leaving such areas.

4) International travel: A valid international certificate of vaccination against yellow fever is required by many countries for entry of travelers coming from or through recognized yellow fever zones of Africa and S America; otherwise, quarantine measures are applicable for up to six days. The International Certificate of Vaccination is valid from 10 days after date of vaccination for 10 years; if revaccinated within that period, valid from date of revaccination for 10 years.

YERSINIOSIS   ICD-9 027.8
(Pseudotuberculosis, Enterocolitis)

1. **Identification**—An acute bacterial enteric disease manifested by acute watery diarrhea (especially in young children), enterocolitis, acute mesenteric lymphadenitis mimicking appendicitis (especially in older children), fever, headache, pharyngitis, anorexia, vomiting, erythema nodosum (in about 10% of adults, particularly women), post-infectious arthritis, iritis, cutaneous ulceration, hepatosplenic abscesses, osteomyelitis and septicemia caused by either of two agents, *Yersinia enterocolitica* or *Y. pseudotuberculosis*. *Y. enterocolitica* infections present more commonly with a gastroenterocolitis syndrome, and *Y. pseudotuberculosis* with abdominal pain.

Diagnosis is usually by stool culture. With precautions to prevent overgrowth of fecal flora, the organisms can be recovered on usual enteric media. Cold enrichment in buffered saline at 4°C (39°F) for 2-3 weeks selects for some strains of these organisms, especially from carriers, and may be needed; CIN medium is highly selective, permitting recovery in 24 hours at 32°C (89.6°F) without cold adaptation. In generalized infections, blood cultures are usually positive. Serologic diagnosis can be made by an agglutination test or by ELISA; circulating antibodies appear 1-2 weeks after onset, peak at 3-4 weeks, and gradually disappear in 2-6 months.

2. **Infectious agents**—*Yersinia pseudotuberculosis* comprises 6 serotypes with 4 subtypes; >90% of the infections in man and animals are O-group I strains. *Y. enterocolitica* comprises over 50 serotypes and 5 biotypes, many of which are non-pathogenic. Strains pathogenic for man are generally pyrazinamidase-negative; this includes strains in serotypes O3, O8, O9, and O5,27, and biotypes 1, 2, 3 and 4. Serotypes causing disease may vary in different geographic areas; types O3, O9 and O5,27 account for most of the cases in Europe. Type O8 strains have been responsible for most outbreaks in the USA; however, type O3 now appears to be the most common serotype in New York. Virulence of both *Y. pseudotuberculosis* and *Y. enterocolitica* is mediated by a plasmid that is approximately 70kb in size.

3. **Occurrence**—Worldwide. *Y. pseudotuberculosis* is primarily a zoonotic disease of wild and domesticated birds and mammals, with man as an incidental host. *Y. enterocolitica* has been recovered from a wide variety of animals without signs of disease. The most important source of infection may be pork, as the pharynx of pigs may be heavily colonized by *Y. enterocolitica*. Since the 1960s, *Yersiniae* have been recognized as etiologic agents of gastroenteritis (as high as 1-3% of acute enteritis in some areas) and mesenteric lymphadenitis. Approximately two-thirds of *Y. enterocolitica* cases occur among infants and children; three-fourths of *Y. pseudotuberculosis* cases involve 5-to-20-year-olds. Human cases have been reported in association with disease in household pets, particularly sick

puppies and kittens. Only a small number of human cases are recognized; recognition is dependent largely on the skill and experience of the microbiologist. The highest isolation rates have been reported during the cold season in temperate climates, especially Scandinavia and N America. Epidemics caused by *Y. enterocolitica* have usually been caused by contaminated vehicles such as chocolate milk, soybean cake (tofu) and pork chitterlings. Studies in Europe suggest that many cases are related to ingestion of raw or undercooked pork. Since 20% of infections in older children and adolescents can mimic acute appendicitis, outbreaks can be recognized by local increases in appendectomies.

4. **Reservoir**—Animals are the principal reservoirs for *Yersinia*. The pig is the principal reservoir for pathogenic *Y. enterocolitica;* asymptomatic pharyngeal carriage is common in swine. *Y. pseudotuberculosis* is widespread among many species of avian and mammalian hosts, and particularly among rodents and other small mammals.

5. **Mode of transmission**—Fecal-oral transmission takes place by eating and drinking contaminated food and water or by contact with infected persons or animals. *Y. enterocolitica* has been isolated from a variety of foods; however, pathogenic strains are most commonly isolated from raw pork or pork products. Because of its ability to multiply under refrigeration and microaerophilic conditions, there is an increased risk of infection by *Y. enterocolitica* if uncured meat stored in evacuated plastic bags (usually boxed beef) is undercooked. It has been recovered from natural bodies of water in the absence of *Escherichia coli* organisms. Nosocomial transmission has been reported, as has transmission by transfusion of stored blood from donors who were asymptomatic or had GI illness within 2 weeks.

6. **Incubation period**—Probably 3-7 days, generally under 10 days.

7. **Period of communicability**—There is fecal shedding at least as long as symptoms exist, usually for 2-3 weeks. Untreated cases may excrete the organism for 2-3 months.

8. **Susceptibility and resistance**—Gastroentercolitis (diarrhea) is more severe in children, whereas post-infectious arthritis is more severe in adolescents and older adults. *Y. pseudotuberculosis* exhibits a predilection for male adolescents, while *Y. enterocolitica* attacks both sexes equally. Reactive arthritis has a predilection for persons with the HLA-B27 genetic type; the septicemic form occurs among persons with iron overload (e.g., hemochromatosis) or those who have underlying immunosuppressive illness or therapy.

9. Methods of control—

   A. *Preventive measures:*

      1) Wash hands prior to foodhandling and eating, after handling raw pork and after animal contact.

2) Prepare meat and other foods in a sanitary manner, especially that to be eaten raw; pasteurize milk.

3) Protect water supplies from animal and human feces; purify appropriately.

4) Control rodents and birds (for *Y. pseudotuberculosis*).

5) Dispose of human, dog and cat feces in a sanitary manner.

6) After slaughtering pigs, the head and neck should be removed from the body to avoid contaminating other parts from the heavily colonized pharynx.

B. *Control of patient, contacts and the immediate environment:*

1) Report to local health authority: Case reporting obligatory in many states (USA) and countries; Class 2B (see Preface).

2) Isolation: Enteric precautions for patients in hospitals. Remove those with diarrhea from foodhandling, patient care, and occupations involving care of young children.

3) Concurrent disinfection: Of feces. In communities with modern and adequate sewage disposal systems, feces can be discharged directly into sewers without preliminary disinfection.

4) Quarantine: None.

5) Immunization of contacts: None.

6) Investigation of contacts and source of infection: Search for unrecognized cases and convalescent carriers among contacts is indicated only when a common-source exposure is suspected.

7) Specific treatment: Organisms are sensitive to many antibiotics, but are generally resistant to penicillin and its semisynthetic derivatives. Therapy may be helpful for GI symptoms; definitely indicated for septicemia and other invasive disease. Agents of choice against *Y. enterocolitica* are the aminoglycosides (for septicemia only) and co-trimoxazole. New quinolones such as ciprofloxacin are also effective. Both *Y. enterocolitica* and *Y. pseudotuberculosis* are usually sensitive to the tetracyclines

C. *Epidemic measures:*

1) Any group of cases of acute gastroenteritis or appendicitis syndrome should be reported at once to the local health authority, even in the absence of specific identification of the etiology.

2) Investigate general sanitation and search for common-source vehicle; attention to close contacts with animals, especially pet dogs, cats and other domestic animals.

D. *Disaster implications:* None.

E. *International measures:* None.

ZYGOMYCOSIS   ICD-9 117.7
(Phycomycosis)

Zygomycosis designates all infections caused by fungi of the class Zygomycetes. These include mucormycosis and entomophthoramycosis due to either *Conidiobolus* or *Basidiobolus* species.

MUCORMYCOSIS

1. **Identification**—A group of mycoses usually caused by fungi of the family Mucoraceae of the class Zygomycetes. These fungi have an affinity for blood vessels, causing thrombosis and infarction. The cranio-facial form of the disease usually presents as nasal or paranasal sinus infections, most often during episodes of poorly controlled diabetes mellitus. Gangrene of the turbinates, perforation of the hard palate, gangrene of the cheek, or orbital cellulitis, proptosis, and ophthalmoplegia may occur. Infection may penetrate to the internal carotid artery or by direct extension to the brain, causing infarction. In the pulmonary form of disease, the fungus causes thrombosis of pulmonary blood vessels and infarcts of the lung; pulmonary mucormycosis most often occurs in intensely immunosuppressed patients. In the GI form, mucosal ulcers or thrombosis and gangrene of stomach or bowel may occur.

Diagnosis is confirmed by microscopic demonstration of distinctive broad, nonseptate hyphae in biopsies and by culture of biopsy tissue. Wet preparations and smears may be examined. Cultures alone are not diagnostic because fungi of the order Mucorales are frequently found in the environment.

2. **Infectious agents**—Some species of *Rhizopus,* especially *R. arrhizus (R. oryzae)* have caused most of the culture-positive cranio-facial cases of mucormycosis. Probably *Mucor, Rhizomucor, Rhizopus* and *Cunninghamella* spp. are the chief causes of mucormycosis in other sites. *Apophysomyces elegans, Saksenaea vasiformis* and *Absidia* spp. have been reported from a few human cases of mucormycosis.

3. **Occurrence**—Worldwide. Incidence may be increasing because of longer survival of patients with diabetes mellitus and certain blood dyscrasias, especially acute leukemia.

4. **Reservoir**—Members of the order Mucorales are common sapro-phytes in the environment.

5. **Mode of transmission**—By inhalation or ingestion of spores of the fungal agents by susceptible individuals. Direct inoculation by intrave-nous drug abuse and at sites of intravenous catheters and cutaneous burns are seen occasionally.

6. **Incubation period**—Unknown. Fungus spreads rapidly in suscep-tible tissues.

7. **Period of communicability**—Not directly transmitted from per-son to person or between animals and people.

8. **Susceptibility and resistance**—The rarity of infection in healthy individuals despite the abundance of the Mucorales in the environment indicates natural resistance. Corticosteroid use, metabolic acidosis, defer-oxamine and immunosuppressive therapy predispose to infection. Mal-nutrition predisposes to the GI form.

9. **Methods of control**—

    A. Preventive measures: Optimal clinical control of diabetes mellitus to avoid acidosis.

    B. Control of patient, contacts and the immediate environment:

        1) Report to local health authority: Official report not ordi-narily justifiable, Class 5 (see Preface).
        2) Isolation: None.
        3) Concurrent disinfection: Ordinary cleanliness. Terminal cleaning.
        4) Quarantine: None.
        5) Immunization of contacts: None.
        6) Investigation of contacts and source of infection: Ordi-narily not profitable.
        7) Specific treatment: In the cranial form, clinical control of diabetes; amphotericin B (Fungizone®) and resection of necrotic tissue have been helpful.

    C. Epidemic measures: Not applicable, a sporadic disease.

    D. Disaster implications: None.

    E. International measures: None.

ENTOMOPHTHORAMYCOSIS DUE TO *BASIDIOBOLUS* sp. ICD-9 117.7

ENTOMOPHTHORAMYCOSIS DUE TO *CONIDIOBOLUS* spp. ICD-9 117.7

These two infections have been recognized principally in tropical and subtropical Asia and Africa, are not characterized by thromboses or infarction, do not usually occur in association with serious pre-existing disease, do not usually cause disseminated disease and seldom cause death.

Entomophthoramycosis is a granulomatous inflammation caused by *Basidiobolus ranarum (haptosporus)*, a ubiquitous fungus occurring in decaying vegetation, soil and the GI tract of amphibians and reptiles. The disease presents as a firm subcutaneous mass, fixed to the skin, principally in children and adolescents, more commonly in males. The infection may heal spontaneously. Recommended therapy is oral potassium iodide.

Entomophthoramycosis due to *Conidiobolus* spp. (rhinoentomophthoramycosis) usually originates in the paranasal skin or nasal mucosa and presents as nasal obstruction or swelling of the nose or adjacent structures. The lesion may spread to involve contiguous areas, such as lip, cheek, palate or pharynx. The disease is uncommon and occurs principally in adult males. Recommended therapy is oral potassium iodide or amphotericin B (Fungizone®) IV. The infectious agent, *Conidiobolus coronatus*, occurs in soil and decaying vegetation.

For both forms of Entomophthoramycosis, incubation periods and modes of transmission are unknown. Person-to-person transmission does not occur.

DEFINITIONS
(Technical meaning of terms used in the text)

1. **Carrier**—A person or animal that harbors a specific infectious agent in the absence of discernible clinical disease and serves as a potential source of infection. The carrier state may exist in an individual with an infection that is inapparent throughout its course (commonly known as **healthy** or **asymptomatic carrier**), or during the incubation period, convalescence, and postconvalescence of an individual with a clinically recognizable disease (commonly known as **incubatory carrier** or **convalescent carrier**). Under either circumstance the carrier state may be of short or long duration (**temporary** or **transient carrier**, or **chronic carrier**).

2. **Case fatality rate**—Usually expressed as a percentage of the number of persons diagnosed as having a specified disease who die as a result of that illness. This term is most frequently applied to a specific outbreak of acute disease in which all patients have been followed for an adequate period of time to include all attributable deaths. The **case fatality rate** must be clearly differentiated from **mortality rate** (q.v.). Synonyms: fatality rate, fatality percentage.

3. **Chemoprophylaxis**—The administration of a chemical, including antibiotics, to prevent the development of an infection or the progression of an infection to active manifest disease. **Chemotherapy**, on the other hand, refers to use of a chemical to cure a clinically recognizable disease or to limit its further progress.

4. **Cleaning**—The removal by scrubbing and washing, as with hot water, soap or suitable detergent or by vacuum cleaning, of infectious agents and of organic matter from surfaces on which and in which infectious agents may find favorable conditions for surviving or multiplying.

5. **Communicable disease**—An illness due to a specific infectious agent or its toxic products which arises through transmission of that agent or its products from an infected person, animal, or inanimate reservoir to a susceptible host, either directly or indirectly through an intermediate plant or animal host, vector, or the inanimate environment (see also Transmission of Infectious Agents).

6. **Communicable period**—The time or times during which an infectious agent may be transferred directly or indirectly from an infected person to another person, from an infected animal to man, or from an infected person to an animal, including arthropods.

In diseases such as diphtheria and streptococcal infection in which mucous membranes are involved from the initial entry of the infectious agent, the period of communicability is from the date of first exposure to a source of infection until the infecting microorganism is no longer disseminated from the involved mucous membranes, i.e., from the period before the prodromata until termination of a carrier state, if the latter develops. Some diseases are more communicable during the incubation period than during actual illness.

In diseases such as tuberculosis, leprosy, syphilis, gonorrhea, and some of the salmonelloses, the communicable state may exist over a long and sometimes intermittent period when unhealed lesions permit the discharge of infectious agents from the surface of the skin or through any of the body orifices.

In diseases transmitted by arthropods, such as malaria and yellow fever, the periods of communicability (or more properly **infectivity**) are those during which the infectious agent occurs in the blood or other tissues of the infected person in sufficient numbers to permit infection of the vector. A period of communicability (**transmissibility**) is also to be noted for the arthropod vector, namely, when the agent is present in the tissues of the arthropod in such form and locus (**infective state**) as to be transmissible.

7. **Contact**—A person or animal that has been in an association with an infected person or animal or a contaminated environment that might provide an opportunity to acquire the infective agent.

8. **Contamination**—The presence of an infectious agent on a body surface; also on or in clothes, bedding, toys, surgical instruments or dressings, or other inanimate articles or substances including water and food. **Pollution** is distinct from contamination and implies the presence of offensive, but not necessarily infectious, matter in the environment. Contamination on a body surface does not imply a carrier state.

9. **Disinfection**—Killing of infectious agents outside the body by direct exposure to chemical or physical agents.

Concurrent disinfection is the application of disinfective measures as soon as possible after the discharge of infectious material from the body of an infected person, or after the soiling of articles with such infectious discharges; all personal contact with such discharges or articles minimized prior to such disinfection.

Terminal disinfection is the application of disinfective measures after the patient has been removed by death or to a hospital, or has ceased to be a source of infection, or after hospital isolation or other practices have been discontinued. Terminal disinfection is rarely practiced; terminal cleaning generally suffices (see Cleaning), along with airing and sunning of rooms, furniture and bedding. Disinfection is necessary only for diseases spread by indirect contact; steam sterilization or incineration of bedding and other items is recommended after a disease such as Lassa fever or other highly infectious diseases.

10. **Disinfestation**—Any physical or chemical process serving to destroy or remove undesired small animal forms, particularly arthropods or rodents, present upon the person, the clothing, or in the environment of an individual, or on domestic animals (see Insecticide and Rodenticide). Disinfestation includes delousing for infestation with *Pediculus humanus*, the body louse. Synonyms include the terms **disinsection** and **disinsectization** when only insects are involved.

11. **Endemic**—The constant presence of a disease or infectious agent within a given geographic area; may also refer to the usual prevalence of a given disease within such area. **Hyperendemic** expresses a persistent intense transmission and **holoendemic** a high level of infection beginning early in life and affecting most of the population, e.g., malaria in some places. (See Zoonosis.)

12. **Epidemic**—The occurrence in a community or region of cases of an illness (or an outbreak) clearly in excess of expectancy. The number of cases indicating presence of an epidemic will vary according to the infectious agent, size and type of population exposed, previous experience or lack of exposure to the disease, and time and place of occurrence; epidemicity is thus relative to usual frequency of the disease in the same area, among the specified population, at the same season of the year. A single case of a communicable disease long absent from a population or the first invasion by a disease not previously recognized in that area requires immediate reporting and epidemiologic investigation; two cases of such a disease associated in time and place are sufficient evidence of transmission to be considered an epidemic. (See Report of a Disease and see Zoonosis.)

13. **Fumigation**—Any process by which the killing of animal forms, especially arthropods and rodents, is accomplished by the use of gaseous agents (see Insecticide and Rodenticide).

14. **Health education**—Health education is the process by which individuals and groups of people learn to behave in a manner conducive to the promotion, maintenance or restoration of health. Education for health begins with people as they are, with whatever interests they may have in improving their living conditions. Its aim is to develop in them a sense of responsibility for health conditions, as individuals and as members of families and communities. In communicable disease control, health education commonly includes

an appraisal of what is known by a population about a disease, an assessment of habits and attitudes of the people as they relate to spread and frequency of the disease, and the presentation of specific means to remedy observed deficiencies. Synonyms: Patient education, education for health, education of the public.

15. **Herd immunity**—The immunity of a group or community. The resistance of a group to invasion and spread of an infectious agent, based on the resistance to infection of a high proportion of individual members of the group.

16. **Host**—A person or other living animal, including birds and arthropods, that affords subsistence or lodgment to an infectious agent under natural (as opposed to experimental) conditions. Some protozoa and helminths pass successive stages in alternate hosts of different species. Hosts in which the parasite attains maturity or passes its sexual stage are **primary** or **definitive hosts**; those in which the parasite is in a larval or asexual state are **secondary** or **intermediate hosts**. A **transport host** is a carrier in which the organism remains alive but does not undergo development.

17. **Immune individual**—A person or animal that has specific protective antibodies or cellular immunity as a result of previous infection or immunization, or is so conditioned by such previous specific experience as to respond adequately to prevent infection and/or clinical illness following exposure to a specific infectious agent. Immunity is relative: An ordinarily effective protection may be overwhelmed by an excessive dose of the infectious agent or by exposure through an unusual portal of entry; it may also be impaired by immunosuppressive drug therapy, concurrent disease, or the aging process. (See Resistance.)

18. **Immunity**—That resistance usually associated with the presence of antibodies or cells having a specific action on the microorganism concerned with a particular infectious disease or on its toxin. **Passive humoral immunity** is attained either naturally by transplacental transfer from the mother, or artificially by inoculation of specific protective antibodies (from immunized animals, or convalescent hyperimmune serum or immune serum globulin [human]); it is of short duration (days to months). **Active humoral immunity**, which usually lasts for years, is attained either naturally by infection with or without clinical manifestations, or artificially by inoculation of the agent itself in killed, modified or variant form, or of fractions or products of the agent. Effective immunity depends on **cellular immunity** which is conferred by T-lymphocyte sensitization, and **humoral immunity** which is based on B-lymphocyte response.

19. **Inapparent infection**—The presence of infection in a host without recognizable clinical signs or symptoms. Inapparent infections are identifiable only by laboratory means or by the development of positive reactivity to specific skin tests. Synonyms: Asymptomatic, subclinical, occult infection.

20. **Incidence rate**—A quotient (rate), with the number of new cases of a specified disease diagnosed or reported during a defined period of time as the numerator, and the number of persons in a stated population in which the cases occurred as the denominator. This is usually expressed as cases per 1,000 or 100,000 per annum. This rate may be expressed as age- or sex-specific or as specific for any other population characteristic or subdivision (see Morbidity rate and Prevalence rate).

    Attack rate, or case rate, is an incidence rate often used for particular groups, observed for limited periods and under special circumstances, as in an epidemic, usually expressed as percent (cases per 100). The **secondary attack rate** in communicable disease practice expresses the number of cases among familial or institutional contacts occurring within the accepted incubation period following exposure to a primary case, in relation to the total of exposed contacts; it may be restricted to susceptible contacts when determinable. **Infection rate** expresses the incidence of all infections, manifest and inapparent.

21. **Incubation period**—The time interval between initial contact with an infectious agent and the appearance of the first sign or symptom of the disease in question, or, in a vector, of the first time transmission is possible (**extrinsic incubation period**).

22. **Infected individual**—A person or animal that harbors an infectious agent and who has either manifest disease (see Patient or sick person) or inapparent infection (see Carrier). An **infectious person** or animal is one from whom the infectious agent can be naturally acquired.

23. **Infection**—The entry and development or multiplication of an infectious agent in the body of man or animals. Infection is not synonymous with infectious disease; the result may be inapparent (see Inapparent infection) or manifest (see Infectious disease). The presence of living infectious agents on exterior surfaces of the body, or upon articles of apparel or soiled articles, is not infection, but represents contamination of such surfaces and articles (see Contamination).

24. **Infectious agent**—An organism (virus, rickettsia, bacteria, fungus, protozoa or helminth) that is capable of producing infection or infectious disease.

25. **Infectious disease**—A clinically manifest disease of man or animal resulting from an infection (see Infection).

26. **Infestation**—For persons or animals, the lodgment, development and reproduction of arthropods on the surface of the body or in the clothing. Infested articles or premises are those which harbor or give shelter to animal forms, especially arthropods and rodents.

27. **Insecticide**—Any chemical substance used for the destruction of insects, whether applied as powder, liquid, atomized liquid, aerosol, or as a "paint" spray; residual action is usual. The term **larvicide** is generally used to designate insecticides applied specifically for destruction of immature stages of arthropods; **adulticide** or **imagocide**, to designate those applied to destroy mature or adult forms. The term insecticide is often used broadly to encompass substances for the destruction of all arthropods, but **acaracide** is more properly used for agents against ticks and mites. More specific terms, such as **lousicide** and **miticide** are sometimes used.

28. **Isolation**—As applied to patients, isolation represents separation, for the period of communicability, of infected persons or animals from others in such places and under such conditions as to prevent or limit the direct or indirect transmission of the infectious agent from those infected to those who are susceptible or who may spread the agent to others. In contrast, quarantine (q.v.) applies to restrictions on the healthy contacts of an infectious case. Recommendations which are made for isolation of cases (section 9B2 of each disease) are the methods recommended by CDC (CDC *Guideline for Isolation Precautions in Hospitals*, see Preface) as category-specific isolation precautions. (A recent CDC recommendation expanding blood and body fluid precautions for use with all patients ["universal precautions"] is found under "Blood/Body Fluid Precautions," below.) The recommendations are divided into 7 categories. Two basic requirements are common for all 7 categories:
    1) *Hands must be washed after contact with the patient or potentially contaminated articles and before taking care of another patient;*
    2) *Articles contaminated with infectious material should be appropriately discarded or bagged and labeled before being sent for decontamination and reprocessing.*

The seven categories are:

    a) **Strict isolation:** This category is designed to prevent transmission of highly contagious or virulent infections that may be spread by both air and contact. The specifications, in addition to those above, include a private room and the use of masks, gowns and gloves for all persons entering the room. Special ventilation requirements with the room at negative pressure to surrounding areas is desirable.

b) **Contact isolation:** For less highly transmissible or serious infections, for diseases or conditions which are spread primarily by close or direct contact. In addition to the basic requirements, a private room is indicated but patients infected with the same pathogen may share a room. Masks are indicated for those who come close to the patient, gowns are indicated if soiling is likely, and gloves are indicated for touching infectious material.

c) **Respiratory isolation:** To prevent transmission of infectious diseases over short distances through the air, a private room is indicated but patients infected with the same organism may share a room. In addition to the basic requirements, masks are indicated for those who come in close contact with the patient; gowns and gloves are not indicated.

d) **Tuberculosis isolation (AFB isolation):** For patients with pulmonary tuberculosis who have a positive sputum smear or chest x-rays which strongly suggest active tuberculosis. Specifications include use of a private room with special ventilation and the door closed. In addition to the basic requirements, masks are used only if the patient is coughing and does not reliably and consistently cover the mouth. Gowns are used to prevent gross contamination of clothing. Gloves are not indicated.

e) **Enteric precautions:** For infections transmitted by direct or indirect contact with feces. In addition to the basic requirements, specifications include use of a private room if patient hygiene is poor. Masks are not indicated; gowns should be used if soiling is likely and gloves are to be used for touching contaminated materials.

f) **Drainage/secretion precautions:** To prevent infections transmitted by direct or indirect contact with purulent material or drainage from an infected body site. A private room and masking are not indicated; in addition to the basic requirements, gowns should be used if soiling is likely and gloves used for touching contaminated materials.

g) **Blood/body fluid precautions:** To prevent infections that are transmitted by direct or indirect contact with infected blood or body fluids. In addition to the basic requirements, a private room is indicated if patient hygiene is poor; masks are not indicated but gowns should be used if soiling of clothing with blood or body fluids is likely. Gloves should be used for touching blood or body fluids.

A recent CDC recommendation states that blood and body fluid precautions be used consistently for all patients (in-hospital settings as well as out-patient settings) regardless of their bloodborne infection status. This extention of the blood and body fluid precautions to all patients is known as "Universal blood and body fluid precautions" or "Universal precautions." In this, blood and certain body fluids (any visibly bloody body secretion, semen, vaginal secretions, tissue, CSF, and synovial, pleural, peritoneal, pericardial, and amniotic fluids) of all patients are considered potentially infectious for HIV, HBV, and other bloodborne pathogens.

Universal precautions are intended to prevent parenteral, mucous membrane, and nonintact skin exposures of health care workers to bloodborne pathogens. Protective barriers include gloves, gowns, masks and protective eyewear or face shields. Waste management is controlled by local and state authority.

29. **Molluscicide**—A chemical substance used for the destruction of snails and other molluscs.

30. **Morbidity rate**—An incidence rate (q.v.) used to include all persons in the population under consideration who become clinically ill during the period of time stated. The population may be limited to a specific sex, age group or those with certain other characteristics.

31. **Mortality rate**—A rate calculated in the same way as an **incidence rate** (q.v.), using as a numerator the number of deaths occurring in the population during the stated period of time, usually a year. A **total** or **crude** mortality rate utilizes deaths from all causes, usually expressed as deaths per 1,000, while a **disease-specific** mortality rate includes only deaths due to one disease and is usually reported on the basis of 100,000 persons. The population base may be defined by sex, age or other characteristics. The mortality rate must not be confused with case fatality rate (q.v.).

32. **Nosocomial infection**—An infection occurring in a patient in a hospital or other health care facility and in whom it was not present or incubating at the time of admission, or the residual of an infection acquired during a previous admission. Includes infections acquired in the hospital but appearing after discharge, and also such infections among the staff of the facility.

33. **Pathogenicity**—The capability of an infectious agent to cause disease in a susceptible host.

34. **Patient or sick person**—A person who is ill.

35. **Personal hygiene**—Those protective measures, primarily within the responsibility of the individual, which promote health and limit the spread of infectious diseases, chiefly those transmitted by direct contact. Such measures encompass (1) washing hands in soap and water immediately after evacuating bowels or bladder and always before handling food or eating; (2) keeping hands and unclean articles, or articles that have been used for toilet purposes by others, away from the mouth, nose, eyes, ears, genitalia, and wounds; (3) avoiding the use of common or unclean eating utensils, drinking cups, towels, handkerchiefs, combs, hairbrushes and pipes; (4) avoiding exposure of other persons to spray from the nose and mouth as in coughing, sneezing, laughing or talking; (5) washing hands thoroughly after handling a patient or his belongings; and (6) keeping the body clean by sufficiently frequent soap and water baths.

36. **Prevalence rate**—A quotient (rate) obtained by using as the numerator the number of persons sick or portraying a certain condition in a stated population at a particular time (**point prevalence**), or during a stated period of time (**period prevalence**), regardless of when that illness or condition began, and as the denominator the number of persons in the population in which they occurred.

37. **Quarantine**—Restriction of the activities of well persons or animals who have been exposed to a case of communicable disease during its period of communicability (i.e., contacts) to prevent disease transmission during the incubation period if infection should occur.
    a) **Absolute** or **complete quarantine**: The limitation of freedom of movement of those exposed to a communicable disease for a period of time not longer than the longest usual incubation period of that disease, in such manner as to prevent effective contact with those not so exposed (see Isolation).
    b) **Modified quarantine**: A selective, partial limitation of freedom of movement of contacts, commonly on the basis of known or presumed differences in susceptibility and related to the danger of disease transmission. It may be designed to meet particular situations. Examples are exclusion of children from school, exemption of immune persons from provisions applicable to susceptible persons, or restriction of military populations to the post or to quarters. It includes: **Personal surveillance**, the practice of close medical or other supervision of contacts in order to permit prompt recognition of infection or illness but without restricting their movements; and **Segregation**, the separation of some part of a group of persons or domestic animals from the others for special consideration, control or observation—removal of susceptible children to

homes of immune persons, or establishment of a sanitary boundary to protect uninfected from infected portions of a population.

38. **Repellent**—A chemical applied to the skin or clothing or other places to discourage (1) arthropods from alighting on and attacking an individual, or (2) other agents, such as helminth larvae, from penetrating the skin.

39. **Report of a disease**—An official report notifying an appropriate authority of the occurrence of a specified communicable or other disease in man or in animals. Diseases in man are reported to the local health authority; those in animals to the livestock, sanitary, veterinary or agriculture authority. Some few diseases in animals, also transmissible to man, are reportable to both authorities. Each health jurisdiction declares a list of reportable diseases appropriate to its particular needs (see Preface). Reports should also list suspected cases of diseases of particular public health importance, ordinarily those requiring epidemiologic investigation or initiation of special control measures.

When a person is infected in one health jurisdiction and the case is reported from another, the health authority receiving the report should notify the other jurisdiction, especially when the disease requires examination of contacts for infection, or if food or water or other common vehicles of infection may be involved.

In addition to routine report of cases of specified diseases, special notification is required of all epidemics or outbreaks of disease, including diseases not listed as reportable (see Epidemic).

40. **Reservoir (of infectious agents)**—Any person, animal, arthropod, plant, soil or substance (or combination of these) in which an infectious agent normally lives and multiplies, on which it depends primarily for survival, and where it reproduces itself in such manner that it can be transmitted to a susceptible host.

41. **Resistance**—The sum total of body mechanisms which interpose barriers to the progress of invasion or multiplication of infectious agents or to damage by their toxic products. **Inherent resistance**—an ability to resist disease independent of antibodies or of specifically developed tissue response; it commonly resides in anatomic or physiologic characteristics of the host and may be genetic or acquired, permanent or temporary. Synonym: Non-specific immunity. (See Immunity.)

42. **Rodenticide**—A chemical substance used for the destruction of rodents, generally through ingestion. (See Fumigation.)

43. **Source of infection**—The person, animal, object or substance from which an infectious agent passes to a host. Source of infection should

be clearly distinguished from **source of contamination**, such as overflow of a septic tank contaminating a water supply, or an infected cook contaminating a salad. (See Reservoir.)

44. **Surveillance of disease**—As distinct from surveillance of persons (see Quarantine, b), surveillance of disease is the continuing scrutiny of all aspects of occurrence and spread of a disease that are pertinent to effective control. Included are the systematic collection and evaluation of:

    a) morbidity and mortality reports,
    b) special reports of field investigations of epidemics and of individual cases,
    c) isolation and identification of infectious agents by laboratories,
    d) data concerning the availability, use and untoward effect of vaccines and toxoids, immune globulins, insecticides, and other substances used in control,
    e) information regarding immunity levels in segments of the population, and
    f) other relevant epidemiologic data. A report summarizing the above data should be prepared and distributed to all cooperating persons and others with a need to know the results of the surveillance activities.

    The procedure applies to all jurisdictional levels of public health from local to international. **Serologic surveillance** identifies patterns of current and past infection using serologic tests.

45. **Susceptible**—A person or animal presumably not possessing sufficient resistance against a particular pathogenic agent to prevent contracting infection or disease if or when exposed to the agent.

46. **Suspect**—A person whose medical history and symptoms suggest that he or she may have or be developing some communicable disease.

47. **Transmission of infectious agents**—Any mechanism by which an infectious agent is spread from a source or reservoir to a person. These mechanisms are:

    a) **Direct transmission:** Direct and essentially immediate transfer of infectious agents to a receptive portal of entry through which human or animal infection may take place. This may be by direct contact as by touching, biting, kissing or sexual intercourse, or by the direct projection (droplet spread) of droplet spray onto the conjunctiva or onto the mucous membranes of the eye, nose or mouth during sneezing, coughing, spitting, singing or talking (usually limited to a distance of about 1 meter or less).

b) **Indirect transmission:**
1) Vehicle-Borne—Contaminated inanimate materials or object (fomites) such as toys, handkerchiefs, soiled clothes, bedding, cooking or eating utensils, surgical instruments or dressings (indirect contact); water, food, milk, biological products including blood, serum, plasma, tissues or organs; or any substance serving as an intermediate means by which an infectious agent is transported and introduced into a susceptible host through a suitable portal of entry. The agent may or may not have multiplied or developed in or on the vehicle before being transmitted.
2) Vector-Borne—(a) Mechanical: Includes simple mechanical carriage by a crawling or flying insect through soiling of its feet or proboscis, or by passage of organisms through its gastrointestinal tract. This does not require multiplication or development of the organism. (b) Biological: Propagation (multiplication), cyclic development, or a combination of these (cyclopropagative) is required before the arthropod can transmit the infective form of the agent to man. An incubation period (extrinsic) is required following infection before the arthropod becomes **infective**. The infectious agent may be passed vertically to succeeding generations (**transovarian transmission**); **transstadial transmission** indicates its passage from one stage of life cycle to another, as nymph to adult. Transmission may be by injection of salivary gland fluid during biting, or by regurgitation or deposition on the skin of feces or other material capable of penetrating through the bite wound or through an area of trauma from scratching or rubbing. This transmission is by an infected non-vertebrate host and not simple mechanical carriage by a vector as a vehicle. However, an arthropod in either role is termed a **vector**.
c) **Airborne:** The dissemination of microbial aerosols to a suitable portal of entry, usually the respiratory tract. Microbial aerosols are suspensions of particles in the air consisting partially or wholly of microorganisms. They may remain suspended in the air for long periods of time, some retaining and others losing infectivity or virulence. Particles in the 1- to 5-μm range are easily drawn into the alveoli of the lungs and may be retained there. Not considered as airborne are droplets and other large particles which promptly settle out (see Direct transmission, above).
1) Droplet nuclei—Usually the small residues which result from evaporation of fluid from droplets emitted by an infected host (see above). They also may be created

purposely by a variety of atomizing devices, or accidentally as in microbiology laboratories or in abattoirs, rendering plants or autopsy rooms. They usually remain suspended in the air for long periods of time.

2) Dust—The small particles of widely varying size which may arise from soil (as, for example, fungus spores separated from dry soil by wind or mechanical agitation), clothes, bedding, or contaminated floors.

48. **Universal precautions**—See under Isolation, Blood/body fluid precautions.

49. **Virulence**—The degree of pathogenicity of an infectious agent, indicated by case fatality rates and/or its ability to invade and damage tissues of the host.

50. **Zoonosis**—An infection or infectious disease transmissible under natural conditions from vertebrate animals to man. May be enzootic or epizootic (see Endemic and Epidemic).

INDEX

Note: Bold indicates main reference.